Praise for Advanced Breast Cancer

"I want you to know how much your book means to me. I am currently in treatment for breast cancer for the fourth time since 1987, second time for bone metastasis. I live in a small town and felt I was the only person in the world who couldn't get rid of cancer. Your book reassured me I had a lot of company, and has given me many role models for dealing with the disease. I thank you and those you profiled in your book for sharing their hopes and fears. When I mentioned your book to my oncologist, he asked me if I was frightened after reading about what I was facing. I had to reply that, to the contrary, it had given me courage to continue my fight."

— Judith Neilson, *metastatic breast cancer patient*

· · · · ·

"Your book truly is a gift to all women and those who love them. With tenderness and respect you wove the stories of these spirited survivors into an outstanding guide for fully living to life's end. The extensive resource list was a delightful surprise. What a joy to have the organizational web sites listed. As one of the early-diagnosed breast cancer survivors without a personal knowledge of chemotherapy, I found the glossary especially helpful."

— Rosemary Locke, *breast cancer patient and activist*

· · · · ·

"I found your wonderful book at UCLA Cancer Hospital. I am eternally thankful to UCLA for telling me about it. I had scoured book stores for sources of information on metastatic breast cancer. I believe yours is one of a few, if not the only, book out there that deals completely with metastatic breast cancer. I will be shouting its praises to anyone who will listen. I have read it twice."

— Judy Conklin, *metastatic breast cancer patient*

"I was afraid to even open the covers of this book—it seemed like it was going to be too difficult a journey. Silly me! You were right there with me, holding my hand, gently taking me down the path. I started it last night and look forward to reading the whole thing."

— Harriet Kay, *breast cancer patient*

. . . . .

"I started to read it and cannot put it down! As a woman who was diagnosed with a primary breast cancer last year, I have found the book reassuring, and feel that you have chased away some of the scary monsters in the breast cancer closet. As a friend of someone with metastatic disease, I have found something that I know will give her great comfort. I will be purchasing another copy of your book so that I may keep a copy for myself and add it to my private lending library."

— Norma Steele, *breast cancer patient*

. . . . .

"There is little information and support available for the advanced breast cancer patient. Each year I receive the Resource List from NABCO. I turned to the page on metastatic breast cancer/recurrence. Usually the only things listed deal with pain management and hospice. I have no pain and thankfully am not near hospice.

"I was pleased to find additional listings this year, including your book. Immediately I purchased it. I started reading and quickly realized what a treasure your book is, just what I was waiting for. I also told my husband and two daughters (27 and 29) that I'd like them to read it. I requested that the center where I am treated add this book to the patient library, which they said they will.

"You answered a need that was lacking for most of us on the breast cancer journey. And you did it perfectly. Bless you for that. I had been putting off getting involved with the computer. While reading I knew I couldn't delay any longer. So you are directly responsible for my joining the breast cancer email list. I thank you for that. It is a gift."

— Ruth Wolf, *metastatic breast cancer patient*

"Such a book was desperately needed, and I will be pleased to promote it through the many women I know who are living with a diagnosis of metastatic breast cancer, and others who are interested. It may prepare many of us for a road that we hope we will never have to face."

— Liz Whamond, *President, Canadian Breast Cancer Network*

· · · · ·

"This book, for me, has been a unique experience. It is a printed, living tribute to those whose words and thoughts are shared. It is a tribute, too, to loved ones who were kind enough to share experiences, a legacy to be proud of, shared, remembered, and learned from. Musa, I feel as though I know you, as I know those whose lives you shared. Thank you for the profound, gut-wrenching, eloquent lessons you teach through your writing."

— Carole East, *friend of a woman with metastatic breast cancer*

· · · · ·

"I just finished reading your latest book, and—wow!—what a good one it was. I wish I could get more women to read it. I did ask our cancer center to add it to their library. I think it is a fantastic book and a must-read for all so that everyone can understand the realities posed by metastatic breast cancer. As I have said before, the women with metastatic disease do face life issues differently than those of us who are disease-free."

— Lois Anderson, *breast cancer patient and activist*

· · · · ·

"While there are dozens, if not hundreds, of self-help books on breast cancer, relatively few discuss the realities of metastatic disease. This is the superbly-handled subject of Musa Mayer's sensitive and beautifully written [*Advanced Breast Cancer*]."

— *NABCO News*

ADVANCED BREAST CANCER

A Guide to Living with Metastatic Disease

ADVANCED BREAST CANCER

A Guide to Living with Metastatic Disease

Second Edition

Musa Mayer

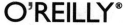

Beijing • Cambridge • Farnham • Köln • Paris • Sebastopol • Taipei • Tokyo

Advanced Breast Cancer: A Guide to Living with Metastatic Disease, Second Edition
by Musa Mayer

Copyright © 1997, 1998 Musa Mayer. All rights reserved.
Printed in the United States of America.

Published by O'Reilly & Associates, Inc., 101 Morris Street, Sebastopol, CA 95472.

Editor: Linda Lamb

Production Editor: Claire Cloutier LeBlanc

Printing History:

> September 1997: First Edition, under the title *Holding Tight, Letting Go*

> September 1998: Second Edition

Library of Congress Cataloging-in-Publication Data:

Mayer, Musa.
    [Holding tight, letting go]
    Advanced breast cancer: a guide to living with metastatic disease / Musa Mayer.
      —2nd ed.
      p. cm.—(Patient-centered guides)
    First ed. published under the title: Holding tight, letting go.
    Includes bibliographical references and index.
    ISBN 1-56592-522-X (pbk.)
    1. Breast—Cancer—Popular works. 2. Metastasis—Popular works.
I. Title. II. Series.
RC280.B8M353   1998
362.1'9699449—DC21
                            98-38919
                               CIP

To
Caren Buffum, Mary D'Angelo, and Jenilu Schoolman.
Women of grace, courage, and spirit.
Three among many.

Table of Contents

Pat and Chris Leach
Sharon and Lloyd Multhauf
Barb Pender
Barb Ragland
Ellen Scheiner
Jenilu Schoolman
Bob Stafford
Kathy Stone
Sue Tokuyama
Chris Tribur (Candace)
Gerry Wirth (Cindy)
Sandra Yandell

Preface

With Arms Held Out

A difficult subject

NOT LONG AGO, I visited a New York City boutique that sells prostheses, lingerie and bathing suits to meet the special needs of breast cancer patients with mastectomies. Because I had purchased from them before, I knew the two women who ran the store, and they remembered the memoir I'd written about my own experience with primary breast cancer. "What are you working on now?" one of the women asked politely. When I told them what this book was to be about, she grimaced and exclaimed, "Now, that's a depressing subject!" The other woman, who had been listening, turned her back toward me. Both these women have had mastectomies themselves, and make it their business to help hundreds of breast cancer patients look and feel their best.

That small moment was only one example of a reality I'd been aware of for years: Breast cancer strikes such terror into the hearts of American women that if they look at it at all, it is to turn instinctively toward those who are deemed cured, and focus more on the cosmetic realities of the disease than upon the threat to life itself.

Breast cancer entered my life in April 1989, when I was diagnosed with an infiltrating ductal carcinoma in my right breast, Stage IIA. I chose to have a modified radical mastectomy with simultaneous implantation of a tissue expander, later replaced with an implant. Although the cancer had not spread to my axillary lymph nodes, because of the three centimeter size and moderately aggressive pathology of the tumor, I decided to undergo six months of chemotherapy treatment with Cytoxan, methotrexate and 5-FU, or CMF. My treatment and recovery were considered uneventful, and I have experienced no recurrence of my cancer—but still, what had happened moved me to write and publish my story, focusing in particular on the emotional aspects of recovery. Beginning with the support group I joined during my treatment, and broadening to include the larger breast cancer community, my involvement with other women and men dealing with this disease has been redeeming and life-changing.

The elephant in the room

There's an elephant in the room.
It is large and squatting, so it is hard to get around it.
Yet we squeeze by with "How are you?" and "I'm fine"...
And a thousand other forms of trivial chatter.

—Terry Kettering[1]

The nine of us newly diagnosed breast cancer patients first met in a conference room at The Rusk Institute in New York City for a weekly group led by a social worker from the Cancer Rehabilitation Service of New York University Medical Center. When the Service lost its funding, we decided to continue gathering in a private home, without a leader. We were a close group and wanted to stay in touch.

Within a year, two of our members, Pat and Miriam, discovered their cancer had returned. Pat was diagnosed with metastases in the bones of her pelvis; Miriam's first metastases were to the internal mammary lymph nodes behind her sternum. Both joined what was then an experimental trial of the drug Taxol at Memorial Sloan-Kettering Cancer Center. Miriam, whose response to the Taxol was not very favorable, received other conventional chemotherapy. Pat, who had responded well to the Taxol, elected to undergo high-dose chemotherapy with stem cell rescue. In this procedure, sometimes called a bone marrow transplant, chemotherapy is administered in such high doses that the person would die if her own stem cells, harvested and frozen beforehand, were not reintroduced to rebuild the immune system.

In our group meetings, we found that Pat and Miriam's new status as metastatic breast cancer patients had an inhibiting effect both on them, and on the group as a whole. A perceptive group therapist might have remedied this, but we were a self-led group and it was hard to speak frankly about something we all feared so much. While Pat and Miriam discussed the details of their treatments with the group—though perhaps not as freely as with one another—they seemed reluctant to speak to the larger issues of their changed perspective, of the gulf that now apparently separated "them" from "us," or of their fears of the treatments they faced, of becoming disabled or dependent, of death and dying. By the same token, the rest of the group was inhibited in expressing concerns that might seem trivial by comparison. Even when Pat and Miriam weren't there, we didn't really discuss our fears for them, or for ourselves. It was the elephant in the room, too large and upsetting a topic for us to tackle unaided.

Gradually, as Pat and Miriam became more ill, because of their treatments and eventually because of the disease itself, they attended the group less and less. Each of them, we heard, was able to find some support from other women they met during hospitalizations, or in their doctors' offices, or from groups they briefly attended for metastatic cancer patients. Each of them withdrew into their families as time went on. A few of us in the original group kept in contact with Pat and Miriam and reported back to the others on the progress of their treatments and the latest test results.

It was Miriam's death, in December of 1992, as well as the celebration of my fiftieth birthday a month later on the same weekend as her memorial service, that inspired me to renew my efforts to complete the book I'd written about my own treatment and recovery and get it into print.

A year later, *Examining Myself: One Woman's Story of Breast Cancer Treatment and Recovery*[2] had found a publisher and was released. By then, Pat had successfully taken her insurance company to court to force them to pay for a second high-dose chemotherapy with stem cell transplant, after the first had failed. Several of us in the group had circulated petitions and marched in Washington for the National Breast Cancer Coalition's first drive to lobby the President and Congress for increased breast cancer research funding.

Sharing the experience of metastatic breast cancer

The following summer of 1994, I discovered the Internet and the newly created Breast Cancer Listserv, a remarkable group of hundreds of people all over the world whose lives had been touched by breast cancer: patients, family members and friends, researchers, nurses, doctors. Every day I received all the e-mail messages that other people who subscribed to the List had posted (sent) to the computer in Newfoundland that distributed the e-mail messages around the world.

Most of the participants on the List seemed to be, like me, information seekers whose anxieties were allayed somewhat by finding out the facts. I felt right at home. I knew a lot about breast cancer already, but now, with the benefit of all these diverse experiences and perspectives, I learned how much more there was to learn. What had been personal—specific to me and my support group—I now saw manifested on a much larger scale. What had been abstract became real, in the words of hundreds of women and men describing their lives. Sometimes what I found out was reassuring. More often, though, the imponderables of breast cancer treatment and the diversity of medical opinions seemed only to emphasize how important it was for patients to gain insight into their own minds and hearts as a basis for decision-making.

Except for those who were online to promote their books, and the few radiologists, surgeons, oncologists and researchers who generously gave of their time, it soon became clear that the population of the List was also split between people with primary and metastatic breast cancer. Most prominent were the many newly diagnosed patients, coping with the shock of diagnosis, the confusing onslaught of treatment choices, the effects of surgery, radiation and chemotherapy, and the often lengthy emotional recovery. Gradually, as time passed, these women (and men, for many of the people who posted were the computer-literate and supportive husbands of women with primary breast cancer—and a few were men with breast cancer) came to terms with what had happened and left the List.

When I first joined, those with metastatic breast cancer didn't post many messages about what they were going through to the List at large. There were occasional oblique references to treatment choices, and to the fact that they corresponded privately with one another. Sometimes, when people left the List, we knew they had become very ill and were in the final stages of the disease. From an obituary notice or a husband writing a last message from his wife's e-mail address, we might find out later that a woman had died. But often, no one had an address or phone number, and we were unable to find out what had happened. As we began to acknowledge the real intimacy of our bonds with one another, this became increasingly distressing.

I began to see that there was the same division of interests, the same ambivalence, on the List as in my own support group. Most of the time, women with metastatic disease (and their husbands or partners) were loath to discuss their problems and fears openly, even when invited to do so, for fear of demoralizing the newly diagnosed. Their messages would often be prefaced by disclaimers like, "I don't want to bring everybody down," or "I hope this isn't too depressing." It took a number of reassurances for a new level of dialogue to begin.

Not everyone was pleased about this turn of events. There were those who found that reading about advanced disease was too upsetting, who contemplated leaving, and who did, in fact, leave because of this unwelcome exposure. It was painfully clear that reminders of vulnerability did nothing to help them. There was talk back and forth about how to resolve this problem. No one, it appeared, wanted to split the group in two and lose a single newfound friend. For a while, we tried warning people by placing the code word "METS" (for metastases) in the subject line of the e-mail messages concerning the subject. But that didn't last long.

In the years since this threatening subject has been broached, women and men dealing with metastatic breast cancer have begun to discuss their problems and feelings very freely on the List. Their posts are often moving and eloquent. Those of us fortunate enough not to have had recurrences stand by with compassion, curiosity, admiration and, yes, fear.

Not long afterward, the Breast Cancer List made another evolutionary leap in articulating lives at the edge. A new unspeakable topic was broached, coded in the subject line of the messages as "D&D," for death and dying. Like the short lived "METS" designation of the previous year, this early formality has yielded further disclosures—more of the wrenching, revealing, human chartmaking for this unknown land. Caren Buffum, a teacher from Philadelphia who'd been living with metastatic disease for five years, was among the first to respond:

> I just want to add my voice to those who recognize the importance of being able to talk about this, not just at this time, but ongoing. Walking this line between fighting and acceptance is such a balancing act for me— sometimes I need to share how exhausted or discouraged I am—and sometimes I need to be able to hold out my arms to someone else who feels that way. I may want to hide my head in the sand, and sometimes I need to do just that—but I need to be able to take it out again and know that if I get scared, there are others ready with their arms held out.

How this book came to be

It was from this ongoing, free-ranging discussion group that the germ of the idea for this book was born, in part for selfish reasons, to assuage my own sense of helplessness and survivor's guilt in the face of continuing losses. Reading about these lives, I'd felt inspired and strengthened. I could sense how important what these women and men had to say was. I knew that out there, in the larger world beyond the List, were many thousands of women and men who felt isolated with the disease, and that their voices were not represented in the literature. I wanted to offer the moving stories I was privileged to read to those who needed to hear them, beyond the confines reached by an Internet mailing list.

I had also witnessed firsthand how invaluable metastatic breast cancer patients and their families found it to read about what others had experienced. At least some of the pain and fear they felt was eased by this companionship. Both physical and emotional barriers of isolation imposed by advancing disease and difficult treatments were breached when connection with others was only a few keystrokes away. Over and over, I'd seen despair and terror, when expressed and confronted, yield to acceptance and love.

Most of these women and their families believed, at the time they first found out the cancer had come back, that they were on a fast track to the grave. Now they were eager to share the news that many metastatic breast cancer patients can live for years following a recurrence, that the quality of their lives usually remains good until the disease is very advanced, and that skilled intervention can prolong life, often very significantly.

But who was I to take on a book like this? I was a writer, after all, not a health care professional or a cancer expert. Nor could I speak with the authority of direct personal experience, not being a metastatic breast cancer patient myself.

It was the trust given to me by the people I've interviewed, many of whom have become friends, that assured me that I could do it. They knew that I was a breast cancer survivor who had loved and lost many friends from this disease, friends whose lives I wished to honor through letting their words live on. They knew of my deepest beliefs: that mindful exploration of the self is crucial if we are to be fully alive, that living fully is the best and only antidote to mortality, and that those on the edge of life can tell us more about this than anyone.

And so they've let me into their lives, honoring me with their friendship. Mary D'Angelo, Ellen Scheiner and Penny Lebow had already been "real life" friends when I began this book. Although she never knew about this project, Jenilu Schoolman and I corresponded often in the year before she died. Months before I began work on this book, members of the Breast Cancer List started meeting in person, and forming close friendships. Glenn and Barb Clabo visited twice, following a long personal correspondence. Lisann Charland, JB Boggs, Sandra Yandell and Caren Buffum attended some of the writing workshops I offer to cancer patients. And in October 1996, at the first large gathering of the List, I had the great and poignant joy of meeting many of those I had interviewed for this book for the first time in person. Hugging and talking with Lucie and Cy Shuster, Bob Stafford, Kathy and Chuck Stone, PJ and Mike Hagler, Sharon and Lloyd Multhauf, Chris Tribur, Joleene Kolenberg, and Barb Pender was an extraordinary experience. Seeing them let me feel their confidence in me, which I hope has helped me to write about their lives with greater authority. It is a measure of their pride in this project that all have asked me to use their real names.

No writer comes to a subject without personal investment and bias. My own heedless strategy has often been to rush headlong in the direction of whatever I fear, to find out anything and everything about it. This was no exception. Still, I wondered if my own fears of recurrence might distort my perceptions, or lead me to sentimentalize some of the more difficult realities of metastatic disease. How could it not be alarming to know all the various ways this relentless disease can strike, or how toxic and debilitating some of the treatments can be? How could it not be sad to lose people I'd come to care about? All this is certainly true. But I also know that having a life-threatening illness prepares the crucial and neglected arena for some of our deepest, most difficult engagements. With psychiatrist Arthur Kleinman, I have come to believe that, "Nothing so concentrates experience and clarifies the central conditions of living as serious illness."[3] For me, it has been inspiring, even comforting, to know that ordinary people are able to find the resources within themselves when they need to, for the journey all of us must make.

What to expect from this book

This book is based on the firm belief that knowing more about metastatic breast cancer, and reading what other people have experienced with the disease, will be of help, both practically and emotionally. It subscribes to the idea that with good support and a sense of kinship with others, you will likely surprise yourself with your resilience in facing what lies ahead. Some of this book won't be easy to read. Some parts will be scary, or depressing. But some parts will be enlightening and uplifting, too.

If you are dealing with metastatic breast cancer, it's likely that you've been feeling more alone since being diagnosed with advanced disease. Understandably, you are frightened and confused. What lies ahead, you ask yourself. How will I cope? How will my family manage? Though each person, each case, is different, it does help to know that others have gone ahead and will freely and honestly share what they've learned.

If you have the kind of temperament that tends to magnify the unknown, creating unrealistic terrors, it will be reassuring to know more about the realities of metastatic disease, even when they are not encouraging. Those realities usually seem doable, taken day by day, in contrast to whatever unnamed and amorphous dread you may have been carrying. It's an odd paradox, perhaps, but hearing about the experiences of those who are living what you fear most can often be strangely comforting. These women and men have learned to *live* with the disease, sometimes for many, many years. During part of this time, they may be immersed in symptoms and cancer treatments, but at other times, they are able to carry on with their lives quite normally.

If you know that you do better by taking information in slowly, and shielding yourself from some of the harsher realities, many sections of this book may still be meaningful. Having placed your trust in your treatment team, you may not want to know a lot of medical details or how the disease may progress or be treated. Hearing how other people cope with side effects may help, however, or you may want to read how husbands really feel about their wives' illness. The sections on sources of hope and spirituality may speak to you. Something another person shares that helps them remain optimistic may be of real help. Just because you don't want to read all the "gory details" doesn't mean you have to isolate yourself from what other people who've been there before you have to say. The key is in knowing yourself, and what you need. As so many have observed, cancer can be a great teacher in this regard.

If you are the husband or partner of a woman with metastatic breast cancer, you are in distress as well. This is happening to you, too. Often, the emotional needs of husbands and other family members are swept aside in the pressing struggle to deal with the disease. Throughout these pages, husbands and partners talk candidly about the stresses illness has placed on their marriages and families, and the ways they and their wives or partners have found to support one another at every stage of the disease.

Through the stories in this book, you'll come to see that women and men are still able to live their lives with metastatic breast cancer, however grim the prognosis may at first appear, and that while a cure may be remote, a recurrence does not mean the immediate death that people imagine. You'll learn that there is always hope for something, whether an extended remission, a long awaited graduation or wedding or grandchild, a newly cherished friendship, or even the beauty of a single day, or hour. Hearing from these extraordinary but ordinary people offers the hope that you, too, can cope with this disease. These stories can help you find the strength and tenacity within yourself to meet the challenge of such a crisis. These people are not superwomen or supermen. If they can do it, so can you.

In these pages, you will find three important kinds of tools: practical information, common ground, and new sources of inspiration and hope.

Practical information. From the complex tangle of information on metastatic breast cancer and its many treatments, this book will endeavor to help sort out what is known from what is not yet known. There is nothing simple about this disease. Though certain generalizations can be made, breast cancer is not a single disease, and its course is unpredictable.

Every case is highly individual—because of the pathology of the tumor, the mechanism of its spread and your own unique biology. All of these are subject to change over time. Not even the most skilled oncologist can accurately predict exactly which treatment will work at a particular time and what the course of disease is likely to be. Ongoing research enables doctors to make educated guesses about the most effective treatments, based on statistical probabilities of success. But no treatment works in every case. Because new research is constantly evolving, current state of the art treatments as of this writing may well be outdated by the time you read this. Instead, this book will focus on how to find out what you need to know about your particular disease and the best treatments available to you at the time you need them.

Once there were few treatment options for women with metastatic breast cancer. Now there are many hormonal and chemotherapy regimens, some of which are accepted as a standard of care, and others which are controversial, highly toxic, and still unproven, since they are undergoing clinical trials. Treatment choices are often extremely difficult, and require a degree of self-knowledge as well as unbiased medical consultation and information.

Because treatment information tends to be both time and case sensitive, this book will focus, instead, on developing a process for gathering good, sound information: through seeking other medical opinions, searching for and reading research studies, asking your oncologist to share his or her reasoning with you, investigating clinical trials, asking for information through the telephone and Internet, and talking with other people who are struggling with the same issues.

By contrast, since many of the side effects and other problems associated with treatment for metastatic breast cancer are similar from patient to patient, you are likely to find useful and reassuring information by reading what others have experienced and how they have coped.

Because there have been some exciting and hopeful developments in breast cancer treatment in the year since this book's first publication, this revised edition includes several sections containing updated information about changes in conventional treatment, as well as new drugs and promising clinical and laboratory research. In particular, the ongoing development of targeted and relatively non-toxic treatments shows new promise for transforming a lethal disease into a manageable, chronic condition.

Appendix B, *Resources*, is keyed to the subject matter discussed in each chapter, and will suggest other sources of reading and information.

Common ground. As diverse as treatment decisions may be, the psychological and spiritual issues people face as they contend with life-threatening illness are universal. Because you are human, you can empathize with others, relate their struggles, disappointments and triumphs to those in your own life, and draw conclusions about your own situation. Maybe you have been feeling out of control, frightened and isolated. Reading about other people going through this will help you to understand that your feelings are normal, given the circumstances, and that no one needs to feel alone with this disease. As you learn more and develop strategies for handling the changes in your day-to-day life, feelings of anxiety and loss of control may lessen. Reading about the ways other people have managed to cope may give you ideas on what you can do for yourself and those you love. Certainly, hearing the stories in this book will make you feel less alone.

Sources of knowledge and hope. This book is all about life, about learning how to *live* with disease. It is based on the possibility of transformation in the most painful of circumstances. But it is not about staying "positive" and keeping "negative" thoughts and feelings away. This aspect of life, coping with serious illness, is pretty messy and confusing, for anyone. Denying this turns out not to be a very effective strategy, and has the effect of making people who are ill feel even more isolated. Real help comes from hearing real stories, and from learning you are not alone. So there won't be any simple formulas and how-to lists in this book. Nothing you can clip on the refrigerator with a magnet.

Out of the pain and depths of illness, new and hard-won bonds of love can sometimes be forged. Moments of beauty and clarity of mind can be savored. Meaning and renewal of faith can be pursued. In this book, you'll see over and over again how ordinary people in difficult circumstances are able to call upon resources in themselves they never knew they possessed. They have learned to reach out to others to give and receive support and help. They have moved from paralyzing anxiety and despair to a state of acceptance and intense aliveness in the moment. They have found ways to strengthen their faith and spirituality, to prepare and support their families and friends. They have done it, and so can you. No one has to take this journey alone.

Ordinary heroes

Most of us would agree that the people who live in the pages of this book are heroes, yet not a single one would claim that label. There is nothing more human, more real, than confronting the loss of health and independence, of able-bodied, pain-free life, and ultimately of everything and everyone held dear—whether this comes prematurely or at the end of a long life. These heroes find nothing so remarkable in their ability to do this. On a day-to-day level, they are only doing their best.

In an interview, and with characteristic modesty, foreign correspondent Terry Anderson, held hostage in Iran for so many months, spoke of his captivity in a way that is familiar to many of those who have to cope with life-threatening illness. "I don't think of myself as a hero. A hero is someone who makes difficult choices. I had no choices—I was chained to the wall. I did what I had to do, to get by."

In her bafflement and frustration at how others responded to her nearly twelve years of dealing with breast cancer, Caren Buffum wrote:

> I understand what a person thinks they mean when they say "I couldn't go through what you are going through," but what does that really mean? Would they commit suicide if they had to deal with cancer? Who thinks they can go through this? From my side of things, I don't feel at all noble or brave or whatever quality I am being assigned. I consider myself to be coping well, and yet, I have not met too many cancer patients who are not in some way coping admirably, all things considered.

About the people in this book

A caveat, before we proceed. Throughout the chapters that follow, readers should note that the experiences of the people whose voices come alive on these pages may not be typical of the larger population of all women and men dealing with metastatic breast cancer. While it's my hope that the forms their disease has taken, and their emotional responses to illness, are representative—at least of women and their partners who are willing and motivated to read and discuss their advanced breast cancer—this small group of people is not randomly chosen.

Throughout the book, I refer almost exclusively to those with metastatic breast cancer as "she." Breast cancer does occur in men, however, though men represent less than one percent of cases, about 1,400 each year in the United States. Clearly metastatic breast cancer is largely a women's disease. Although I have included the experiences of a man with metastatic breast cancer—a man who is committed to getting the word out that men are also at risk—for simplicity's sake, I have elected to use female pronouns when speaking in general terms.

In general, breast cancer is also a disease associated with aging. Although it appears to be the case that pre-menopausal women with breast cancer sometimes have more rapidly growing, aggressive, hormonally negative cancers, it is still true that three quarters of women diagnosed with breast cancer are over 50 years of age, and that the overall incidence is significantly higher in older women. It goes without saying that metastatic breast cancer is likely to have an entirely different meaning in the twilight years of a long life than it does for a 40-year-old woman with a young family still to raise.

These women and men I've written about here, as a group, differ significantly by virtue of being younger, more well-educated and affluent than the population at large. By and large, their life circumstances are probably representative of the demographics of American Internet users, where minorities and lower-income people are not well represented. Certainly, the people I interviewed are more articulate and self-disclosing, more willing to grapple with the difficult issues head-on. Most of them have enjoyed stable, long-term relationships and have supportive families. They have had only minor problems with access to good medical care, and health insurance coverage. Care should be taken not to generalize, therefore, from these experiences to those of all people in similar medical circumstances. Not only is the disease itself variable, but the responses to illness are as unique and individual as the portraits on these pages.

Most women with metastatic breast cancer would probably not choose to be in contact with others who have the disease, whether in support groups or elsewhere—although by doing so they might well feel supported and decrease their sense of isolation. Nor is it likely that they would wish to be interviewed for a book such as this—although telling their stories might give them a needed opportunity to externalize their thoughts and feelings, and provide a structure to contain fearful events. And it's unclear whether they would be motivated to read about the experience of others—although they, too, might find echoes there, and common ground, if they did. They might even come to a place where the solace of these echoes might outweigh the anxiety of hearing what can happen in the course of the disease.

Telling the truth about life

In October of 1996, I met many of the people interviewed in this book for the first time. We gathered in a Chicago hotel for the first of what we hope will become an annual event. Though they had never met face to face, or even talked on the telephone before, people came from as far away as Germany and Hawaii, so important was the Breast Cancer List in their lives. Some used canes to walk, some sported wigs, scarves, or proudly shaven bald heads, or showed other signs of the ravages of treatment or disease. But faces shone. Eyes gleamed. People couldn't stop talking and hugging one another. We all agreed that everyone looked different than we'd expected, but that hardly mattered. Never had physical form seemed more clearly the container for spirit. Long before we met in Chicago, we'd passed the stage of superficial chit-chat, and shared our deepest pains and joys. The weekend soon became an extraordinary outpouring of love and laughter.

Sunday morning, Bob Stafford, who was a pastor in a small town in Indiana before metastatic breast cancer forced him to retire, held a service in which he spoke movingly of the love he'd found on the List, and of those who had died. Drawing close to the end of his life, and in daily pain, his thoughts had turned to finding grace, to walking with God. The next day, when we had all returned home, Bob wrote to the List, confessing to feeling a little let down, now that the festivities were over. One of the many people who wrote back with encouragement was Barb Pender, a woman of strong religious faith, also struggling with metastatic disease.

> Like I said Sunday morning, I know what the Lord looks like—I walked down Michigan Avenue with Him, shopped at Marshall Fields with Him, talked with Him till 2:30 in the morning, broke bread with Him, sat in the Hard Rock Cafe with Him, laughed with Him, cried with Him—and my dear brother Bob, you must only look in the mirror to see Him yourself, for you are wonderful!

These people have learned to live with what the two women in the New York mastectomy salon were unwilling to face. For people who face life-threatening illness, and their families, this is much more than just a "depressing subject." It is the reality they must live with every day. It is my hope that this book and the stories you find here will offer new information and some relief from isolation, and that you will gather strength from the remarkable tenacity and spirit that animates the words of these women and men who have generously shared their lives so that others could feel less alone.

Bob Stafford said it well:

> I think when you get into this position, all phoniness is gone. There is no one to impress or delude. You can become transparent because it doesn't matter what people think about you. I see it in people who are very sick that I come in contact with. They will tell you the truth about life and themselves.

Acknowledgments

SINCE I BEGAN INTERVIEWING for this book in March 1996, scores of metastatic breast cancer patients and their husbands and partners have joined the Breast Cancer Discussion List on the Internet. In their messages to one another, they continue to build a legacy of support and information for all who seek help. They are a continuing inspiration, as eloquent as any of the people I found to interview before they joined. For the insight that they always give me into their courage, persistence and humor, I am grateful to them all. I wrote this book for them and those they love.

Stories are the heart of this book. For the thirty-two people I interviewed over the last year-and-a-half, no words can express how significant this sharing between us has been for me, on every level. By offering a window into their hearts and souls, they have given me—and all who read this book—an immeasurable gift. I will always be grateful to them. Although they are named in the book, of course, I want to thank them all here as well, for each has left an indelible mark on me. They are: Kim Banks, Lucie Bergmann-Shuster, JB Boggs, Caren Buffum, Lisann and Leo Charland, Glenn and Barb Clabo, Bob Crisp, Mary D'Angelo, Bonnie Gelbwasser, Nancy Gilpatrick, Terry Houlahan, PJ Hagler, Pam Hiebert, Scott Kitterman, Joleene Kolenburg, Pat and Chris Leach, Sharon and Lloyd Multhauf, Barb Pender, Barb Ragland, Sylvan Rainwater, Ellen Scheiner, Jenilu Schoolman, Bob Stafford, Kathy Stone, Sue Tokuyama, Chris Tribur, Gerry Wirth, and Sandra Yandell. Although I didn't interview them at length, with their gracious permission, I also quoted from the words of Joan Bengston, Karen Caviglia, Monica Driver, Laurie Feldman, Jacque Fisher, Carole Greene, Shari Kahane, Penny Lebow, and Bill Sherman.

There are many other people who helped with this book, by sharing what they knew, asking the right questions and pointing me toward resources I hadn't thought of. Roz Kleban, of Memorial Sloan-Kettering Cancer Center, shared her perceptions about leading support groups for metastatic breast cancer patients. Dr. Sam Waxman, of Mt. Sinai Medical Center in New York City, offered an oncologist's perspective on treatment options and the difficult decisions metastatic patients face. Dr. Fred Schwartz, Medical Director of the Visiting Nurse Service of New York Hospice Care, shared his wisdom and compassion on palliative treatment and end-of-life care. Barbara Quirarte, a hospice volunteer from Oregon, offered her perspective.

Over the course of writing the book, there were a number of people I met on the Internet whose help proved invaluable. Lauren Langford, Nancy Oster, Ginette Eldridge, Jessica Fiorelli and Harriet Kay helped me to find information I needed, put me in touch with other resources, and helped me to discover the questions I needed to ask. Marianne Brosseau lent depth and breadth to my information seeking, and challenged me to revise my notions of patient advocacy. Karen Gray gave me the benefit of her keen and skeptical mind, as did Loren Buhle. Sue Hunter offered not only unflagging friendship and humor, but paid the kind of skilled, careful attention to the text that only an anxious author can truly appreciate.

I owe an immense debt to O'Reilly & Associates for their foresight in developing the Patient-Centered Guides. For a publisher to take a risk with a book on a difficult to market, "untouchable" subject like metastatic breast cancer is as commendable as it is unusual. This would never have occurred, I suspect, if Linda Lamb, my editor, had not seen for herself the powerful healing made possible by the Breast Cancer Discussion List and shared in my dream of bringing this to the world beyond the Internet. Linda's friendship, support and editorial acumen throughout this difficult and often painful project, her capacity to see clearly what I was trying to say, has been what has made this book possible. Her assistant, Carol Wenmoth, has been attentive, thorough, thoughtful and always right there when I needed her.

A number of breast cancer survivors and health care professionals were kind enough to read and comment on the manuscript draft to help improve it. Among them are Kathleen Allen, Barbara Brenner, Susan Claymon, Kathleen Ford, Deborah Kahane, Mary Jane Massie, Sue Matorin, Fred Schwartz, David Spiegel, Samuel Waxman, and Jackie Weber.

This book represents a new direction in my writing, and involved a great deal of agonizing, long hours and self-doubt. It also took me into what is clearly scary and dangerous territory for any breast cancer survivor. Without my husband Tom's unfailing interest and quiet encouragement, I could never have found the strength to challenge myself. As always, I am deeply grateful to him.

CHAPTER 1

Voices of a Forgotten Population

ALTHOUGH BREAST CANCER HAS BECOME A TOPIC widely covered in the media, the message is almost always cheerful, emphasizing early detection and the high likelihood of cure. The reality of metastatic breast cancer is almost never publicly talked about, and considered "too downbeat" by mass media to attract an audience. In this chapter the social context of the disease will be examined, and the ways in which the "politics" of breast cancer isolates people dealing with metastatic and high-risk breast cancer.

Psychological and social factors both play a part in the denial and fear surrounding metastatic disease. Even in the breast cancer community of advocacy and support, there is often a sense of division between those diagnosed with primary disease and those whose disease has recurred. These larger issues—fear, discomfort, isolation, discrimination—create a climate of silence that prevents the real stories of people living with metastatic disease from being told. As the stories in this book unfold, patients and their spouses and partners break this silence, speaking in depth about their lives, their families, their feelings, their hopes and their fears.

A cheerful message of survivorship

Boo! It's October, it's Halloween, it's Breast Cancer Awareness Month. And I'm the bogey-woman who needs to be kept in the closet.

Karen Caviglia, a breast cancer activist, wrote these words in 1995 for a Massachusetts newsletter a few months before her death.

Two years ago, sitting in the Memorial Oncology Clinic receiving CMF treatment for breast cancer during October, I was still spinning with the news of my metastasis. It didn't seem that I could get away from breast cancer anywhere—it was a media frenzy. Specifically I remember an enthusiastic TV reporter commenting that Olivia Newton-John had "beat" breast cancer. Since it had only been two years for her and I had gone five and a half years apparently disease-free, I was muttering uncharitably under my breath, "We'll just see what happens. It may not be over yet."

If you've been feeling angry and left out by the cheerful emphasis on breast cancer survivorship in the media, you are not alone. These days, television specials, magazine articles and books on breast cancer seem to focus exclusively on the importance of early detection and on the process of treatment and recovery in primary breast cancer—that is, the experience of women diagnosed with early stage breast cancer for the first time. The focus is almost always upbeat, the outcome positive.

From watching TV and reading the newspapers, you'd think breast cancer was rarely a fatal disease any more. Throngs of happy survivors sporting pink visors participate in runs and walks around the country each October to benefit various support and research organizations. Not a month goes by without news of some heartening medical "breakthrough" in treatment or diagnosis that on examination usually turns out to be far less promising or novel than it is touted to be.

Thirty years ago, before Betty Ford, Happy Rockefeller and a few other early pioneers of self-disclosure helped to make public revelation of the disease a commonplace occurrence, having breast cancer was perceived as a shameful secret. The name of the disease was spoken only in whispers. The equation in the public's mind was still cancer equals death. The disfiguring radical mastectomy was the surgical norm, cobalt radiation treatments left burns and scars, and receiving chemotherapy usually meant the disease was terminal.

Times have changed. More than half of diagnosed women are now considered candidates for breast-conserving surgery, and adjuvant chemotherapy, given following mastectomy or lumpectomy with radiation, has become the standard of care in many cases of primary breast cancer. Radiation is now far less damaging, and there are new, effective drugs to counter the nausea and low blood counts caused by chemotherapy. Scores of women in public positions have admitted having the disease, from Sandra Day O'Connor to Gloria Steinem. Women and men all over the country have banded together in support groups and advocacy organizations. In recent years, the American Cancer Society has developed extensive educational programs on mammography and early detection, and is doing everything it can to promote the notion that breast cancer need not be fatal if discovered early. This message is important and laudable. To reduce the stigma and fear associated with the disease, these public service campaigns have helped the pendulum to swing from the former grim inevitability to a new glib perception of cheerful survivorship.

This is not false; it is merely simplistic. Clearly, it is reassuring to women terrified of breast cancer to know that so many do recover. The hope is that this new optimism encourages women to be less afraid to examine their breasts, and to seek screening for early detection, when the treatment is most likely to be curative. And newly diagnosed women clearly take great comfort in the longevity and vigor of long term survivors.

But the nasty secret that inspired those whispers in the past hasn't changed one bit: women are still dying of this disease, and in huge numbers. Breast cancer remains the most common cancer in women, and the leading cause of death for women between the ages of 40 and 55. In 1998, the National Alliance of Breast Cancer Organizations (NABCO) estimates that 43,500 American women will die of the disease.

Yet it is the disease-free survivors we hear from the vast majority of the time. What of the tens of thousands of women whose breast cancer comes back each year, who face a much more grim prognosis? Where are their voices? Who speaks for them? Who speaks for you? Karen Caviglia struggled to break this silence in a letter she wrote to the Breast Cancer List:

> As we approach Survivor's Day—I myself have invitations to four celebrations—I'm prepared to deal with an onslaught of the Pollyannas. Once upon a time I too thought that my breast cancer was a blessing in disguise—but then it metastasized. Talk about struggling to accept. Well now I'm very positive day to day—it's easy when I'm not in pain—and I'm determined to live as long and as well as I can, but my doctors say I'm incurable so I accept that sooner or later, and certainly sooner than I want, it's gonna get me. And please don't talk to me about getting hit by a bus or that mortality is 100 percent.

Rosalind Kleban, a social worker at Memorial Sloan-Kettering Cancer Center in New York City who leads a support group for metastatic breast cancer patients, became acutely aware of the impact of Breast Cancer Awareness Month on the women she works with:

> During October, when we are inundated and flooded with stories, one of the women in my group said that she had a question, and you could see that she was not comfortable raising it. She was somewhat embarrassed, didn't know if it was foolish to ask. Her question was: "Are we survivors?" When she said that, all the other women in the room turned away or put their heads down. It was a question that touched them, embarrassed them, something that they had struggled with, too. I asked her what she meant by that. She said, "Well, all you hear about are survivors. I don't know if I am a survivor. I'm alive. But I don't feel like they do. Somehow, they are victorious. I am not victorious."

It is a story Kleban has heard repeatedly from her patients with metastatic disease, a sense of stigma that she herself has come to feel passionately about.

> They are the forgotten population, shunted aside because they have blown it. They have failed. These other people have won the battle. They're the people we applaud, whom we put on television to talk about breast cancer. Women with metastatic breast cancer connote a failure of the system, of medical knowledge and science, which, clearly, the system doesn't feel good about. The view is that once you have metastatic disease, it's a death sentence, and that it's really over.

Even at one of the most prestigious cancer treatment and research centers in the United States, these ambivalent feelings about metastatic disease are evident, Kleban admits.

> In trying to help support the primary people, we do keep it quiet. We say, "You're going to be fine." I myself will say that, in order to promote hope. On Wednesday in our metastatic group, one of the women was saying, "Well, it happens even here." In the chemotherapy unit, on the desk where patients check in, there is a flyer that talks about the adjuvant group (for primary breast cancer patients) that meets every Thursday at one o'clock. There's no mention of the metastatic group. I'm afraid of scaring the others. The metastatic group is listed in our brochure, however. To be very honest, I am more comfortable with that. It's folded. You have to look to find it.

The universal symbol of breast cancer awareness in recent years has been the pink ribbon, appropriated from the ubiquitous AIDS red ribbon. Breast cancer activists frequently object to this symbol. "This is not a pastel-colored disease, and little strips of cloth will not end the epidemic,"[1] wrote Barbara Brenner, Executive Director of Breast Cancer Action of San Francisco. Of all the pink ribbon pins made over the last several years, only one manages to convey the dual reality that breast cancer patients really face, and it is that of the Ottawa-based Breast Cancer Action group, that uses an upside-down pink ribbon, in the shape of a teardrop, the pink lined with black.

In the clamor for competing needs, every public message takes on a political cast. Advocacy groups, when they emphasize the mortality figures in an attempt to impress officials with the urgency of this public health problem, know full well they strike a delicate balance between alarmism and complacency. Officials from the cancer establishment tell us that breast cancer is hardly the epidemic activists claim it to be, and that the alarming increase in breast cancer incidence over the past thirty years (from one in fourteen in 1960 to one in eight today) is mostly the result of better screening that picks up the disease years earlier. They speak of the innovations in treatment that save lives, of promising new drugs and ever-more aggressive treatments. Breast cancer activists, skeptical of profiteering by the cancer "industry," remind us that the death rate from breast cancer has remained constant over the years, that the promise of microbiology and genetic research has yet to be realized, and that treatments still consist of "slash, burn and poison," to use the oft-repeated characterization of surgery, radiation treatment and chemotherapy.

Denial, fear and popular perceptions

But the problem extends far beyond any individual disease, and stiffens the invisible resistance that works against the abilities of advocacy groups to rally supporters—especially those representing people who may die of their illnesses. American society does not deal well with life-threatening diseases of any kind, preferring to gloss over the realities, just as it idealizes those who are struggling with them, and the nature of those struggles.

In the first paragraph of her essay *Illness as Metaphor*, writer and breast cancer survivor Susan Sontag speaks of serious illness as the "night side of life" and "that other country," a foreign terrain to be explored by each of us, eventually.[2] This strikingly self-evident fact is largely ignored. Most people live their lives as if no such event will come to pass, and are utterly shocked when it does. Thus, a disease considered incurable seems particularly to inspire silence and denial. Consequently, without a supportive group or community of some kind, people dealing with metastatic cancer of any kind are likely to find little in their daily lives to provide any reflection of their altered reality—and this despite the fact that cancer strikes one in three, and is certainly a commonplace occurrence.

As a culture, Americans live in a perpetual state of denial of personal mortality. This is true despite—or perhaps because of, for this surely deadens people to real pathos—the violence of our popular entertainment and the barrage of catastrophes that perpetually assault us through our media news. This is not likely to change. Social scientists say that cultural avoidance of the personal impact and meaning of serious illness derives from individual psychological tendencies. The emerging research suggests that unwarranted optimism and even denial may be an innate protective mechanism.

"Normal people believe to an unrealistic degree that the future holds a bounty of good things and few bad things," claims psychologist Shelley Taylor in her book, *Positive Illusions*. "Depressed people are actually realists, having lost the positive biases that normally shelter people from the harsher side of reality."[3]

"Patterns emerge from the scientific evidence that would seem to indicate that, just as individuals and families deceive themselves, so do larger groups of people, so do whole societies," psychologist Daniel Goleman writes. "If there is a lesson to be drawn from the new research, it is the urgent need for compelling antidotes to self-deception. The more we understand how natural a part self-deceit plays in mental life, the more we can admit the almost gravitational pull toward putting out of mind unpleasant facts."

On a large scale, denial can even become the enemy of a democracy, which depends on the free flow of information. "Censorship," Goleman continues, "seems the social equivalent of a defense mechanism. Now that cognitive psychology is showing how easily our civilization can be put at risk by burying our awareness of painful truths, we may come to cherish truth and insight, more than ever before, as the purest of goods."[4]

Philip Slater, in his influential social commentary *The Pursuit of Loneliness*, examined our tendency, as Americans, to hide away from view that which is difficult, and he gave it a memorable name: "The Toilet Assumption—the notion that unwanted matter, unwanted difficulties, unwanted complexities and obstacles will disappear if they're removed from our field of vision."[5]

Beyond the cliché-ridden language of popular culture, there's precious little written about the real experience of life-threatening illness. Arthur Frank, a medical sociologist who suffered a heart attack at 39, then was diagnosed with testicular cancer a year later, offered one explanation of why we find it so difficult to articulate this aspect of our lives, even to those we expect to understand it most—our doctors. Illness is the total experience of living with the disease, he reminds us. Yet it is only the physical facts of disease, and not the illness, that medicine deals with.

> Physicians are generally polite about answering questions, but to ask a question one must already imagine the terms of an answer. My questions end up being phrased in disease terms, but what I really want to know is how to live with illness. The help I want is not a matter of answering questions but of witnessing attempts to live in certain ways. I do not want my questions answered; I want my experiences shared. But the stress and multiple demands on physicians and nurses too often push such sharing outside the boundaries of "professional" activity.[6]

The ensuing silence, this lack of "illness talk," affects both public and private life. On the rare occasions when advanced breast cancer does find its way into the media, it is to show an optimistic and valiant veteran of high dose-chemotherapy, convinced that the treatment has saved her life. Or a soft-focused lens will be turned on some sad elegy about a noble, uncomplaining (deceased) cancer "victim," often a celebrity.

Those who, while mortally ill, project courage, selflessness and transcendence, keeping their inner struggles private, usually provide the prettied-up images we see. Inevitably, both the courageous and the saintly models turn into expectations in the minds of ordinary people—just one more chance for you to feel you don't quite measure up. In your own day-to-day life with metastatic breast cancer, it's not quite so simple; all kinds of complicated and messy feelings intrude.

In real lives, along with precious moments of peace and transcendence, there is also pain and anger and a terrible sadness. In real lives, terror and self-doubt keep daily company with courage. In real lives, family support is given by human beings, by husbands who are tired and frightened too, by children who withdraw into themselves, whose schoolwork suffers. In real lives, despite the love and support, there is still, at times, a wrenching loneliness, and the fear of becoming dependent and burdensome on those you love.

In real lives, the boredom and dehumanization of hours and days spent in hospitals and laboratories and doctors' offices swallows time and energies. In real lives, waiting becomes the constant, a training in patience and perseverance that comes in just two flavors: tedium and anxiety. The tedium involves the endless waiting for appointments, for insurance payments, for your records to find their way into the right hands, for all the health care bureaucracy to grind in its slow and inefficient way. The anxiety occurs as you wait for a painful procedure to begin or to end, and to see what the scans and tumor markers will show this time, to find out whether this or that combination of drugs has worked to slow or stop disease progression, and if it has, for how long.

Even with the best, most compassionate medical care, there are bound to be times you feel out of control, at the mercy of tests and divergent medical opinions, times when you despise the weariness and sickness of constant treatment, and are overcome with the fear of what lies ahead, as you struggle to keep some measure of hope, and live with your disease as best you can. In the real lives of people with metastatic breast cancer, all these feelings are commonplace, yet rarely shared with others.

Most older Americans recall a post-war era bright with medical miracles. Whole generations grew up expecting the steady advancement of medical progress in every field. If men could walk on the moon, fulfilling Kennedy's promise, surely victory in Nixon's "war on cancer," declared thirty years ago, did not seem beyond reach. But for metastatic breast cancer patients today, those ideals now seem painfully naïve.

Our culture still looks back with nostalgia to these simpler, more optimistic times. Mass media, in response to these widely felt longings, strives to reduce complex information into easily digestible, feel-good soundbites and to churn out dramatic breakthrough stories. Thus, a newly renamed tumor marker test becomes, in the hands of network news, an "innovation of great promise." The discovery of the P53 oncogene, implicated in the wild cellular growth of some tumors, holds out "exciting new hope" for women with familial breast cancer. On closer investigation, these claims turn out to be premature. The real story is always far more ambiguous.

The real story about metastatic breast cancer

Lost in the hype about questionable new treatments, and in the focus on screening and primary care, are the lives and experiences of those living with metastatic breast cancer, which are far more diverse and vital than is generally supposed. A 1995 study sponsored by the National Alliance of Breast Cancer Organizations (NABCO) surveyed 200 women with metastatic breast cancer and their caregivers. Most of those surveyed "believe the public sees these women as being near death—with little or no time to live." But this simply isn't the case. Fully 20 percent of newly diagnosed metastatic breast cancer patients live five years or more.

"Prevailing public perception," according to the study, has it "that advanced or metastatic breast cancer is an immediate death sentence—often perpetuated through inaccurate media portrayals." But the survey overwhelmingly refutes this image, with "74 percent of respondents reporting that women with breast cancer are, in fact, not limited in normal daily routine." Amy S. Langer, Executive Director of NABCO, concludes that "many patients with metastatic breast cancer are able to manage their illness as a chronic disease, and maintain an active and satisfying work, family and personal life for several years."[7]

Yet their lives are often dominated by the fact of their illness. Like many of the women interviewed for this book, PJ Hagler dismissed cancer from her mind after she recovered from her initial ocurrence of breast cancer, diagnosed back in 1984. She no longer consulted an oncologist. But six years later, extensive lung metastases were found, and six years after that, tumors in her liver. Recently, undergoing a difficult course of treatments, PJ felt frustrated and sad that some of her friends and family members seemed unable to understand the reality she was forced to live with.

> *They think it's not healthy for me to put so much focus on cancer. How do you do that? They don't seem to have an answer for that. For some reason Taxol and other chemos and being bald, sick, tired, and in unreal pain seems to keep my mind focused on cancer from the moment I wake until I take the last of my pills and go to bed at night. I have lived with cancer for twelve years and good Lord willing I would like to live another twelve years, at least. But every day I do live, I live with cancer.*

Jenilu Schoolman, diagnosed with a liver recurrence three years after her mastectomy, was initially told she had only months to live. Defying all predictions, she underwent treatment and entered an extended remission that lasted nearly eight years. This was new territory for her.

> *Frankly, remission is an awkward place because I am not busy dying. In fact, beyond the normal wear and tear of aging, I now look and feel as well as I did before I became ill. But I have not been able to go ahead with my life simply as though nothing had happened.*

These two women at different stages of their disease—one struggling with the constant reminder of treatment side-effects, the other with the ambiguities of remission—had something in common: their lives had been permanently changed, and they both keenly felt the absence of stories documenting experiences like their own. When she looked, Jenilu found virtually nothing had been written for people in this "uncharted land," as she called her life in remission—so she set out to write her own story, "Within Measured Boundaries." Such a record might help others discover an echo of their own lives, she reasoned, or offer an uncomprehending family member or friend a sense of what it is like to live with metastatic disease.

Where are the resources?

In 1989, when my own breast cancer was diagnosed, the burgeoning of resources for breast cancer patients was just beginning in the United States. Eight years later, when I wrote the first edition of this book, the then-current guide from the National Alliance of Breast Cancer Organizations[8] listed fully twenty-two pages of resources for patients, including books, pamphlets, videotapes, businesses, magazines, service organizations, as well as some 350 support and advocacy groups around the country. The half page that was headed "Metastatic Breast Cancer/Recurrence," however, listed three resources for pain control, two sources of hospice information, one reference to advance directives and living wills, and a pamphlet from the National Cancer Institute, written for all cancer patients, entitled "When Cancer Recurs: Meeting the Challenge Again."[9]

Should this come as a surprise? Societal reactions only reflect personal, individual responses, writ large. Before you became ill, like most people, you probably were uneasy with the realities of life-threatening illness. You may have found yourself tongue-tied and lapsed into awkward silence at the bedside of someone you loved. Maybe you felt compelled to keep up a facade of false cheer during strained hospital visits. Or maybe you even avoided seeing your very ill friends, sending cards and flowers from a distance, especially at the end of their lives. There is so much to say at these times—and yet it is still so difficult to speak about what is painful and frightening, so hard to acknowledge the feelings.

Caren Buffum, having exhausted treatments for her liver metastases, recognized this:

> Most people who have not had to deal with these issues either want to believe the best for me (so they don't want to hear from my "I think the end is near" side) or they see me as dead already so they have these unbearable looks of pity on their faces.

So did Glenn Clabo, whose wife Barb's disease had already spread at the time of her initial diagnosis with Stage IV breast cancer:

> I find myself wondering why our closest friends are rejecting us and our needs at a time when we need them the most. How can people, so called longtime friends, pull away from those that they have claimed to love and cherish?

Once sensitized, evidence of discomfort and denial about metastatic breast cancer seems to be everywhere. Lucie Bergmann-Shuster, whose breast cancer metastasized after twelve years, describes running an errand near her home in San Jose, California.

> The post office had a little flyer sitting on the counter for the breast cancer awareness stamp. The flyer has three personal accounts of women and supports each with a very positive note. "With education, awareness and the support of family and friends, breast cancer is no longer the death sentence it once was," the pamphlet says. "They get treatment, and they go on with their lives.... The survival rate is improving daily.... Breast cancer...it's a fact of life...not an end to life." Nowhere in this flyer does it mention the tens of thousands of women who die of the disease. While the pamphlet tells no lies, it certainly distorts the truth. To me it is soft pedaling this monster that is still claiming far too many lives.

Division in the breast cancer ranks

Now that these resources are more widely available, women with breast cancer often join support groups or advocacy organizations following their diagnosis, appreciating the support, information and camaraderie this offers. But having metastatic disease may make you begin to feel estranged from other breast cancer survivors who have not had a recurrence. What is happening to you is, of course, particularly frightening for them. You may find yourself instinctively pulling back, and censoring what you say, for fear of upsetting them. Their concern for themselves and the fear your situation creates in them may interfere with their ability to give you the support you need, at least until you and they can talk openly about it.

What makes this particularly poignant is that these are likely to be the same women who understood so well how you felt when your healthy friends could not, when you were first diagnosed. However understandable these reactions are, it still hurts to feel this distance. Some support groups disintegrate under this stress. Others manage to survive, however, and benefit from the experience of confronting the reality of the disease, a reality that will become a part of any group of breast cancer patients who continue to know one another over a span of years.

Social worker Roz Kleban tells this story:

> One young woman joined a post-treatment group I was leading. She recurred after three or four sessions, seven months after her adjuvant treatment had ended. She came to the group dressed to the nines for this meeting. "I know all of you are afraid of recurrences," she said. "And I just want you to know that it's much, much, much, worse than you can ever imagine. I'm your worst nightmare."
>
> The response to her from another young woman in the group was magnificent: "You are not my worst nightmare. A recurrence is, indeed, my worst nightmare, and I'm sorry it happened to you. My fear is that when I recur, I am just going to fall apart emotionally and be so desperate, and make it worse on myself, my husband, my children. But looking at you somehow encourages me, because as horrible as you're telling me you feel—and I do appreciate that—look at you, you're dressed, you're

put together. It's clear to me that you're coping: you got up in the morning, put your clothes on, you're going to work tomorrow. You're letting me know it's possible to do it."

Still, dread begets dread, and interferes with rational thought. We play games with numbers in our heads. If American women as a whole read the one-in-eight or one-in-nine lifetime incidence figures and are filled with apprehension, it is even more true that the more than a million American women who already have been diagnosed with breast cancer dread recurrence more, fearing and obsessing about the statistics they are given. Prepared for pessimism by losses already incurred, they know intimately what it is like to lose against favorable odds. And the odds, as it turns out, aren't all that favorable anyway.

In the women's magazines, it is common to see figures of 80 to 90 percent survival rates, and even higher. According to the American Cancer Society, "The overall five-year survival rate for breast cancer is approximately 83%. The rate can be as high as 96% if the cancer is detected early, before it has spread to other parts of the body." Sounds positive, doesn't it? That is, until you realize it is not disease-free survival they are talking about, and until you examine how the numbers change over time. The ACS report continues: "In spite of this advance, some breast cancers, even localized ones, will recur after five years. The overall 10-year breast cancer survival rate is 65%, and after 15 years, the rate is 56%."[10]

These figures make it clear that breast cancer can, and does, recur many years after the original diagnosis. There is never a time when those diagnosed with the disease can rule out the possibility of recurrence. Once metastasized, breast cancer is no longer considered a curable disease, but a chronic condition that will sooner or later result in death for all but two or three percent of the women with this diagnosis. Of course, as humorists and sages often point out, life itself is an incurable condition.

What this means to you

If you feel isolated, judged or discriminated against as a person with metastatic disease, being aware of these larger issues may just help you to identify what's going on. If your friends or family members ask how you are, but don't seem to want to know the answer, if they change the subject or say, "But you're fine now, aren't you?" rather than listening to you, you can know that it is their fear talking. It doesn't excuse such behavior, but it makes it easier not to take it personally.

What can you do about it? Speak frankly, take action as needed and seek out others who understand your feelings. Telling your story and hearing the stories of others, whether in a support group or elsewhere, can provide surprising help and real comfort—but it's not an easy thing to do. Many women discover a sense of healing and purpose in advocacy efforts, working with others to advance legislation relating to breast cancer, secure increased funding for research and raise public awareness. Speaking publicly, or even privately, about any illness that is rarely cured, where length of survival is extraordinarily variable, where medicine too frequently defaults on its promise of life-saving treatments, means confronting others with what they'd rather not think about. It means being mindful of walking the thin edge between preserving hope and facing reality, between optimism and truth-telling, between challenge and acceptance. This balancing act is what all metastatic breast cancer patients and their families, caregivers and physicians face every day.

From this dynamic relationship came this book's original title: *Holding Tight, Letting Go*. Holding tight to those you love, to integrity, courage, to what matters most to you, to the promise of remission and even cure, to life itself. Letting go of your illusions of control, of immortality, of health and youth and beauty—and of the guaranteed future. Letting go of regrets and expectations, into the present moment in which you live, into your final moments and the mystery beyond.

CHAPTER 2

Dread, Uncertainty and White-Water Rafting

LIVING WITH UNCERTAINTY is the hallmark of breast cancer. Fear of recurrence is a given for all breast cancer patients, and rightly so. According to the most recent long-term incidence and survival statistics available from the National Cancer Institute, more than half of women diagnosed with breast cancer in 1974 eventually experienced a recurrence.[1] While treatment advances and earlier detection since then have improved these rates, the risk is still very high. Most recurrences will happen in the first two or three years following primary diagnosis, but some occur as late as twenty years or even more following initial diagnosis with breast cancer.

This chapter explores what it's like for high-risk patients to live with the knowledge that their cancer is likely to recur. The signs and symptoms of recurrence and the sense of vigilance that women feel are discussed, in the context of the basic unpredictability of the disease. Friends and family often deny this reality, which can provoke a sense of distance and isolation for patients. The gulf that separates the woman in remission from the "normal" world seems unbridgeable at times. Psychiatrist David Spiegel's research with metastatic breast cancer patients is reviewed here, with his findings that women can learn to live, and live well, with the disease—often prolonging their lives beyond expectations.

Like the women and men interviewed in this book, perhaps you will find within the uncertainties of breast cancer some room for hope. Perhaps you will come to feel that despite the dread, there is still a real and meaningful life to be lived, even in the shadow of metastatic disease.

The future is always uncertain

"Living with a serious illness takes effort and devours time," writes medical sociologist Kathy Charmaz. "It also means overcoming stigmatizing judgments, intrusive questions, and feelings of diminished worth."[2] In *Good Days, Bad Days*, an exploration of the subjective aspects of chronic illnesses, Charmaz conceptualizes the differing, often progressive stages of illness as *interruption* of life, *intrusion* upon daily activities, and, finally, total *immersion* in disease symptoms or treatments. This simple but useful three-part formulation can help make sense of the differing challenges you may face during the course of metastatic breast cancer, as well as many other chronic illnesses.

Unless you are among the 10 percent of breast cancer patients diagnosed at Stage IV, meaning that your breast cancer had already spread when it was first discovered, chances are that you've already experienced some version of the trajectory familiar to breast cancer patients: finding a lump, biopsy, diagnosis, mastectomy or lumpectomy, radiation, chemotherapy, reconstructive surgery, emotional healing. The interruption of primary breast cancer can be characterized by these three elements: "Temporary crisis. Life-saving treatments. Full recovery."[3]

But with breast cancer the future is always uncertain, for if you have a disease that may return two, five, ten or even twenty years later—as it did for two of the women interviewed in this book—you can never know when or if you are cured. For many breast cancer patients, the notion of full recovery is always tempered by the ever-present threat of recurrence, which intrudes in pervasive but subtle ways upon the rest of life.

Every woman who has had breast cancer fears recurrence. Perhaps dread is a better word, particularly for high-risk patients. Depending on the kind of person you are, your coping skills, the information you've been given, the stage of disease at initial diagnosis, the treatments received, and the risk factors quoted to you, your anxiety about the disease coming back will be more or less manageable and present in your life. Often your fears will be heightened around the time of quarterly or biannual checkups with your doctors. Particularly in the first two or three years after diagnosis, any unusual or persistent ache or pain or swelling is cause for concern. That these thoughts and feelings may be the norm in an abnormal circumstance is often overlooked.

Some of the people in your life may be oblivious, even impatient, about what seems to them to be a negative preoccupation with disease, even after a high-risk diagnosis. Yet among the women and men interviewed for this book, this level of anxiety is commonplace, pervasive—and some would even say protective, as it does tend to increase awareness of symptoms that may indicate a problem requiring swift intervention.

Nowhere is this more poignant than in recently treated women who are at high risk for recurrence. Sue Tokuyama, 34-year-old mother of two young children, works as a database marketing director and has recently been transferred by her company to Arizona, from New York City. Diagnosed with a Stage IIIB carcinoma with thirteen of twenty-six lymph nodes involved in October 1994, she underwent high-dose chemotherapy with stem cell reinfusion (also referred to as bone marrow transplant, or BMT) in an attempt to forestall the further spread of her disease.

Three years after her treatment, with no sign of disease, Sue still lives in a state of constant anticipation. Dread and hope combine daily to create heightened awareness of her mortality. When she was first diagnosed, Sue began a journal.

> I wanted to create "artifacts" of myself, so that if I should die soon, my children, then 18 months and 3 years old, would have as much of me as I could possibly capture in words, pictures, art, videotape. Until recently, I was the person behind the videotapes, the voice-over. I've now, with little subtlety, staged a good deal of the taping, to capture me—by myself and with the kids. I wanted them to hear me say that I love them, to hear the sound of my laughter.

Whatever happens in the future, whether or not she has a recurrence, being ill has altered her life in profound ways, Sue feels.

> Breast cancer has given me fear—fear of death, fear of pain, fear of loss. Aches and pains have greater significance. The specter of death repels even those who love us best. When we most need to feel part of life, we are reminded of our separateness. But there definitely are days when I feel that breast cancer has broadened the emotional range of my experience. In other words, the lows are very low, and the highs are exhilarating. In a real sense fate has upped the ante—and I am far less casual about how I play every hand. I am a lot less willing to write off a "bad day." That day will never come again.

Physician and psychotherapist Ellen Scheiner, then 63, had been retired for several years from her medical practice as an internist in Manhattan due to increasing problems with scoliosis and a right arm paralyzed by a birth injury, when she found an enlarged lymph node under one arm late in 1993. A biopsy and subsequent mastectomy revealed that invasive lobular carcinoma was present in all fourteen axillary nodes removed from beneath her arm.

> *My surgeon was too upset to call me and made my internist, whom I had known since residency, tell me the news, by telephone. I'm certain that any other patient would have been invited to the doctor's office to receive such devastating news. I was alone at home.*

Three years after undergoing a rigorous experimental chemotherapy protocol, Ellen is still regaining her strength but is thus far disease free. A student of Buddhism, she feels that meditation has helped her to cope with her fears of recurrence and the loss of physical control she experienced during her treatment.

> *The truth is that no one is certain of anything. Being a cancer patient shoves that truth in your face. Sometimes you are in the boat and can steer, sometimes you are in the water, almost drowning, and sometimes simply floating. In any case, it drives you along. You don't manage the process; you don't do it, it does you. Your need to feel in control is almost superfluous. What helps to get through is the life force that is the river in which you are a passenger.*

Bonnie Gelbwasser, 53, lives in Massachusetts with her husband Herman and is assistant director of a news service at an independent technological university. Like Sue Tokuyama, Bonnie had been diagnosed at Stage IIIB and treated with high-dose chemotherapy with stem cell reinfusion. Bonnie had inflammatory breast cancer, however, an uncommon and aggressive form of the disease which rapidly spreads into the lymphatic channels in the breast. She had felt a little uneasy all along about letting herself, as a high-risk patient, be interviewed for a book on metastatic breast cancer. It was almost as if she were tempting fate. Now she was having her first real scare since her diagnosis in 1993.

> *Life takes funny turns sometimes. One of my ribs is fractured. I'm going in for a CT scan tomorrow. If the scan indicates changes to bone,*

they'll do a biopsy. If the biopsy is positive, it means the cancer has returned. My honest feeling is that I will not survive very long. I am fighting like crazy to keep focused on the possibility that the good 50 percent odds will come out in my favor. But Wednesday is a long way off and I am very, very frightened. So much for strength and courage. The marshmallow in me is very much in evidence—quite a turn about from the gutsy, in-your-face kind of person I presented to you.

On biopsy, the bone sample turned out to be benign, but Bonnie was sobered by the experience.

The reality, which I did not grasp until last week, is that those of us with inflammatory breast cancer do not have a long "shelf life." The other side to this is that my doctors and their support staff are going to do everything they can to push back my "expiration date." Life goes on.

For the high-risk patient, these fears are never really resolved, only set aside, temporarily. Four months later, after a pleasant summer on Cape Cod, Bonnie wrote:

Sunday was the second anniversary of my ABMT and I had the great pleasure of celebrating this one with my kids: a daughter who just got her diamond, another daughter visiting from Arizona with her significant other, and my son and his new girlfriend. The talk was not of cancer and bone marrow but of wedding dresses and the scenery in Sedona! How far we've come. Life could not be better.

Though she cannot know what the future will bring, Bonnie is learning to let go of her fear and allow herself to live again—for now.

Your life is never the same

"I had a woman come to see me once," Memorial Sloan-Kettering social worker Rosalind Kleban recalls, "She went all over the City, shopping for new protocols, whatever was the newest treatment. On Monday she went to a psychic healer, on Tuesday, she went to somebody who did Therapeutic Touch. I listened to her and I said, 'Why are you doing all of this?' She said, 'I have to live. I have a young child. I have to live.' I pointed out to her that that was a wonderful goal, but the fact of the matter was that she wasn't living. There was not a day that was not a cancer day."

In women at risk of recurrence, persistent thoughts of cancer often represent a sort of preparation for the worst. But, as Kleban points out, there is no real preparation for such a shock. One of her patients refuses to have the implanted catheter (a device that makes it easier for chemo to be administered and blood drawn) removed, although she is two years post-treatment.

> She will not take her port out. "Why should I take it out if I know the cancer is coming back?" A lot of women have that sort of attitude. It emanates from a sort of unconscious "evil eye" syndrome. They don't want to be too confident. When they were first diagnosed, they were caught unawares. You were having one terrific life, thinking it would go on forever, and you were caught, so to speak, with your pants down. And it's never going to happen again. So that when they come to you, and tell you it's in your lung, you can say, "Well, I knew it anyway." In my experience here, that never helps. Because when they do tell you it's in your lungs, it's the same thing: there is no preparation. None whatsoever.

Now divorced, former coordinator of a math and science summer camp program, Barb Pender, of Oceanside, California, spent most of her adult life raising her three children. In 1992, when she was 42 years old, two aggressive tumors were found in one breast and suspicious calcifications in the other. Bilateral mastectomy was followed by an experimental protocol of four treatments of high-dose Cytoxan and Adriamycin. Less than a year later, however, Barb experienced her first recurrence, in the form of nodular densities in her lungs, discovered during a routine chest x-ray as she prepared for a revision of the reconstructive "tram flap" surgery in which her own abdominal muscles had been used to form new breasts.

> Once you are diagnosed with cancer, your life is never the same. We can no longer have a headache from stress—It's going to the brain. We can no longer have a backache from sleeping on the wrong side—It's in the bones.

> Unfortunately, there are no guarantees when dealing with breast cancer, but I had 17 lymph nodes positively involved and it would have been naive of me to think I wouldn't see it again somewhere.

More surprising, perhaps, is that even after the two high-dose chemotherapy treatments with stem cell reinfusion which followed, some of the people in Barb's life could not, or would not, comprehend the severity of the disease she was dealing with:

> About a year ago, I was worried that a lump I felt under my good arm was a recurrence. My sister quickly snapped, "Gosh, Barbara, can't you have an ass or an elbow hurt like a normal person?" I had to think for a minute and replied, "No, I'm not a normal person. Normal people don't lose parts of their bodies and replace them with other parts of their bodies. Normal people don't have daily doses of chemicals that would kill off an elephant."

If you've had friends or family members react like this, perhaps you can take some comfort in the fact that this is not an unusual response. Many cancer patients feel hard-pressed in trying to communicate their reality to others who may be less than eager to hear about it. Psychologist Camille Wortman, who has studied social responses to breast cancer patients, writes:

> In [one] study of the perceived support available to breast cancer patients, 72 percent of the respondents reported that they were treated differently after people knew they had cancer. Of these, 75 percent indicated that they were misunderstood by others and over 50 percent reported that they were "avoided" or "feared."[4]

This is not to say that family and friends can't learn to move past these fears and become extraordinarily empathetic and supportive, as later sections of this book will make abundantly clear, but only that initially you may encounter fear and emotional distancing from people you were close to before, at the very time your own needs may be the greatest. A study of medical self-help groups found that "people with serious illness, especially cancer, are often faced with isolation from friends and family because of fear of contagion, fear of expression of intense emotions, or because the others don't wish to be reminded of their own vulnerability."[5]

Dr. Harold Benjamin, founder of the Wellness Community, a program that provides emotional and psychological support to cancer patients, put it more bluntly:

> In a way, cancer patients are abandoned, if we understand that word to mean that they are treated differently than they were before the diagnosis. Some family and friends find the cancer patient's situation so upsetting that they make sure they don't see him or her very often. Others

*maintain contact, but the relationship becomes strained and the conversa-
tions limited to the "right things" they think they are supposed to say.[6]*

A patient at the Wellness Community said:

> *When they ask you how you are, and you answer "OK," that's the
> end of that conversation. They really don't want to know. To people who
> love you, actually knowing how you feel would be more devastating than
> they could bear.[7]*

Adding to feelings of isolation is the constant self-questioning that often
attends a high-risk diagnosis or a period of remission or stabilization from
metastatic disease. Is this new symptom normal aging or something to be
concerned about? Am I being alarmist, or should I make an appointment
right away? Should I share my concerns with my family?

For Pat Leach, 53, a retired psychiatric nurse living with her husband in
Connecticut, there had been subtle premonitions that all was not well long
before her recurrence was found five years after her treatment for primary
breast cancer.

> *After my initial diagnosis in 1984, after treatment and talks with my
> oncologist, I felt extremely hopeful that I had beaten the disease. My
> oncologist told me I fell into the 85 to 95 percent cure rate range because
> of size of tumor and my negative nodes. I continued to feel terrific for
> three or four years, then slowly, it seemed, the thoughts of recurrence
> crept in—I was more emotional, my mood was labile, I cried a lot. When
> I think back on it, it was almost as if my body and mind were trying to
> tell me something. Got a call from my oncologist—"Your tumor marker is
> elevated, I think we should do a bone scan." I knew, deep down. I only
> had to wait a couple days for the scan and my oncologist called the next
> day—metastases in left hip.*

Many women are successful at putting breast cancer back in some far
removed corner of their minds, however, particularly after some years have
elapsed. Some may even have been told, or convince themselves, that they
are cured.

Mary D'Angelo, 48, a high school English teacher from Queens, New York,
recalled being convinced her cancer was gone after her treatment for primary disease was completed, despite a large tumor and several lymph nodes
that showed spread of the cancer.

When the chemo was over, I remember saying to my doctor, "Well, you won't be seeing much of me!" He said, "We'll be seeing you at least every three months for the rest of your life."

Going back for check-ups seemed pointless to her, but she did as he asked. A strong-willed woman who had survived growing up in a family disrupted by a profoundly disabled child, Mary was determined not to dwell on what had happened to her. Until the day, four years later, when she was told she had tumors in her liver, Mary simply refused to consider the possibility that her cancer would return.

Is vigilance better than denial? It is useless to speculate, for evidence suggests that these coping styles are firmly a part of personality makeup long before disease strikes. Under the stress of illness, it's most likely that you will tend to fall back on what has worked in the past, on the habitual ways of comforting yourself that feel most natural. For anxious cancer survivors, avoiding thoughts of recurrence seems inconceivable, and comfort comes by way of information seeking and contact with one another. For someone who copes by conscious avoidance and distraction, however, weekly attendance in a support group may well be depressing, and personally researching cancer might seem inconceivable. Better by far would be an excursion to do something enjoyable.

Since living with breast cancer is usually a long-term proposition, you may find yourself doing better as you learn to live more and more fully in the present. Neither avoiding thoughts of illness, nor obsessing about it when it doesn't demand your attention, you can learn to achieve a balance between these extremes much of the time. When you need to, of course you will give your attention to the disease and its consequences. There are doctors to see, tests and treatments to undergo. Then, when you are free to, you can focus on the people and activities that are precious in your life.

Signs and symptoms

There are clearly certain physical symptoms that do warrant investigation. Dr. Susan Love notes that while patients fear any new change in their bodies after a diagnosis of breast cancer, "if you know that the symptoms of breast cancer metastasis are usually bone pain, shortness of breath, lack of appetite and weight loss, and neurological symptoms like pain or weakness or headaches, there are at least limits to your fear." [8]

Other symptoms to look out for are persistent abdominal pain and a cough that won't go away. Any change in your mastectomy scar, a lump or a rash where the incision is should be reported to your oncologist. If you've had a lumpectomy, examine the treated breast just as you do your other breast, for lumps and thickenings and changes in the skin or scar.[9]

If you find yourself concerned about every new ache and pain, you may sometimes envy your more oblivious friends who seem able to avoid the constant fear of recurrence. But being oblivious can be problematic too, when it extends to denying or overlooking symptoms. Sometimes neither patient nor physician is vigilant enough.

Free of cancer for six years, but plagued with long-term pain in her hip and chest, Lisann Charland felt betrayed when her doctor missed the early signs of recurrence. A computer systems analyst who lives in Mountain View, California with her husband Leo, Lisann admits that

> *I did not know that breast cancer could spread to other parts of the body. I did not even know the word "metastasize" until that time. I felt angry at all the visits and tests I had done, and yet he could not find anything wrong with me sooner. I felt like I had been hit by a truck and my world was falling apart before me.*

Four years after that, when she got the telephone call that confirmed a recurrence to her liver, Lisann decided to contain her fears until she could meet with her doctor, so as not to unduly worry her husband.

> *I got out of bed and paced the house, looking for any types of books that would tell me what the liver functions were. I went in and out of the garage opening boxes and could not find anything. My husband was fast asleep while all this was going on. I had a sleepless night. I cried and felt so helpless as the night dragged into morning. Where did I go wrong? Why was this happening to me again? What had I done to deserve this?*

Barbara Ragland, now retired on medical disability from her job at the University of Nevada, was 63 years old when her breast cancer, first diagnosed in 1974, returned in the form of two small bumps at the site of her original radical mastectomy.

> *The surgeon performed the biopsies in his office under a local anesthetic so we were talking all the time. When he had excised the one and transected the other, I asked him if they looked like cancer. He said,*

"That's what we have the pathologist for." I said, "I know. However, we've known each other for almost twenty years, and I want to know what you think." He said it looked like cancer. My first reaction was disbelief. I knew if I made it to the five-year mark after the first cancer, my chances were good; and then when I had made the ten-year mark, I thought it was gone forever.

Bob Crisp, a professor of computer systems engineering at the University of Arkansas, researched his wife Ginger's illness thoroughly when she was first diagnosed in 1993.

We always knew the risk was there. I probably understood it better than Ginger as I did all the reading. I knew her cancer was aggressive so I guessed that if a recurrence would happen, it would probably show within two years. At the end of one year, I started to breathe a bit easier. I was not necessarily expecting it nor was I thinking we were in the clear. Ginger had resumed all of her activities and life had returned to normal. The docs gave us little information about recurrence, odds, what to expect....Most of what we knew was what we—mostly me—read.

It is not uncommon, among the typically avid information seekers on the Breast Cancer List on the Internet, for patients or their spouses to become quite expert on particular aspects of the disease and its treatments. This depth of knowledge can work both for and against you, as we'll discuss in a later chapter. At times, having access to the latest information can relieve anxiety and confirm treatment choices. Combined with assertive behavior, such information can and does break down the increasingly formidable barriers to getting the best medical care and adequate insurance coverage.

At other times, however, knowing too much can actually decrease your confidence in a particular treatment or physician, when it becomes apparent just how much is still uncertain and unknown about the disease. It can lead to the sort of hypervigilance that Ellen Scheiner, as an internist specializing in the treatment of cancer patients, experienced as she evaluated her condition and the treatment she was receiving while undergoing intensive chemotherapy:

During the last hospitalization my gums were bleeding and I did not dare to ask my platelet count. I fantasized bleeding into my brain—one of the disadvantages of knowing too much.

Even for lay people, reading or hearing that metastatic breast cancer is still rarely considered curable can eat away at any remaining hopes, despite the wide variability of the illness and the fact that metastatic breast cancer is best managed as a chronic, treatable disease. Social worker Rosalind Kleban observes this problem in the women she counsels all the time.

> Most of the women I work with are research oriented and go immediately to the literature. Although they are extremely bright and intellectual, and under any other circumstances could understand the real meaning of variability in statistics, given the emotional state they are in, they just can't. They see everything as grim and black.

Others, depending on their emotional makeup, may see information like this as a challenge, and become determined to live long enough for the new treatments they are convinced will come. Still others pursue with renewed vigor a process of fashioning new kinds of hope and meaning from the time remaining to them.

Some physicians are very clear about risks with their patients. Kim Banks was only 34 years of age at her first recurrence. A freelance writer, Kim lives with her husband, Richard, in Colorado.

> My husband and I had just celebrated our one year anniversary when I was diagnosed with breast cancer, and we hoped to start a family. When I had made it to the two year mark with no signs of recurrence, I had started to allow myself to think about having a child again. My first doctor was very adamant about my waiting on children. He also emphasized that the diagnostic tests on the original tumor showed an aggressive cancer and then there were the four positive nodes that showed it had started to spread through my lymph system.

After her treatment was completed, Kim's hope for motherhood began to flower again, though her doctors had warned her she might experience a recurrence.

> I felt I had followed what my doctor told me and that the cancer was behind me. Before the recurrence I was the epitome of the eternal optimist, so even though I feared recurrence, I was still shocked that it had happened to me. My doctors and their staff were never overly pessimistic, which helped me to keep an optimistic attitude and go about life without constantly worrying about a recurrence.

Sometimes no one has a clear idea of what is going on, at least initially. "I had not been well for a long time," says Lucie Bergmann-Shuster, 51, who lives with her husband, Cy, in Northern California. Twelve years after her initial diagnosis, Lucie had been experiencing vague but persistent abdominal discomfort and tiredness for many months. Finally, she became concerned about her family history after reading a paper on the Internet about the risks of ovarian cancer for pre-menopausal breast cancer patients ten years after diagnosis. She asked her doctor to arrange for a transvaginal ultrasound and pushed for the definitive surgery which revealed metastatic spread to her ovaries and surrounding tissues and nodes. "Seems to me that getting the bad news was more of a relief after nearly a year of anguish," Lucie said later.

"Breast cancer in all its manifestations is an unpredictable disease"

"We can't accurately predict the course of any individual's illness," writes Dr. Susan Love, whose book is considered by many to be the breast cancer bible. "This is true of initial disease, and metastatic disease is even more unpredictable."[10]

Maddening as this may be, the variability and unpredictability of metastatic breast cancer is also a source of hope. Uncertainty—the perceived enemy of the primary breast cancer patient—can become a friend of sorts when you have metastatic breast cancer. Story after story of women far outliving expectations, of new treatments proving effective, of unexplained remissions, have led the group of survivors I interviewed to look at statistics and predictions with skepticism, and dismiss the "deadlines" they may receive from pessimistic and occasionally insensitive physicians.

"That is the philosophy in my group: this is it, how can we live with this?" social worker Roz Kleban says. "This group is not a preparation for death, not that we can't talk about that. But the big chore here is, 'How can we live with this?' All the reading in the world is not going to give you certainty. The chore is, 'How do we live with uncertainty.' That's the goal here."

Trust in the process

While there are certain typical patterns or courses of disease for metastatic breast cancer, you can take heart at the diverse forms of progression, stabilization and even reversals the disease can take. Though it's not clear why this should be true, many of the women interviewed for this book have far outlived even the most optimistic predictions of their physicians. It's possible that this has something to do with the way they've chosen to cope with their illness.

A now famous study, conducted by Stanford University psychiatrist Dr. David Spiegel, published in the British medical journal *Lancet* in 1989, offers the tantalizing possibility that some of the life choices you make may actually influence the course of disease.

An earlier study Spiegel had done in the late 1970's involved eighty-six women with metastatic breast cancer, randomly assigned to participate or not in weekly therapy groups over the course of a year. The intent was not, at that time, to look at the prolongation of life, but to try to improve quality of life by providing emotional support, connection with other patients and a safe haven for facing what must be faced. In fact, at the end of the year, the fifty patients receiving the group therapy had less pain and anxiety, and were clearly coping better than the thirty-six patients who did not. This was not surprising. "The aim," as Spiegel explains of his ongoing work with patient groups, "is to help people tolerate their anxiety, fear, sadness and grief long enough that they can make the most out of whatever remains of their lives."[11]

People who are very ill desperately want control of their lives, Spiegel says. By assuming control of some aspect of their lives, cancer patients can move from a passive stance to an active perspective. A number of research studies, beginning with that of psychologist Steven Greer and his British research team in 1979, have suggested that cancer patients who adopt an active role in their treatment and in their lives—exhibiting what researchers called "fighting spirit"—may actually live longer and weather their treatment better.[12] These findings are still quite tentative, however, and there is no evidence that changing one's attitude leads to curing the disease, or that personality or attitude play any role in causing the disease.

For Spiegel, control has three dimensions. Mental control involves delving into and facing your deepest feelings, so that you can move from "feeling like a victim of intrusive fears to becoming someone who can master and direct your own thoughts, feelings and activities." In physical terms, control may mean learning self-hypnosis and relaxation techniques to help cope with pain and the side effects of treatment. And in the social arena, control means deepening and improving the relationships that matter most, while letting go of those that are unrewarding or merely obligatory.

Earlier in this chapter, Ellen Scheiner used the metaphor of going down a river to describe what very aggressive chemotherapy felt like to her. Following a rafting trip he and his wife took on the Salmon River, David Spiegel also found wisdom in this metaphor, using it to describe his patients' experience of life-threatening illness as a whole. This passage, from the Introduction to *Living Without Limits*, offers this potent metaphor for negotiating cancer:

> The exhilaration of negotiating our way around the rocks made us acutely interested in the skills of our guides in steering the rafts. They pointed out that the most common mistakes novices make is to waste energy pulling against the current of the river. The force of the water leaves little doubt about which direction you will take. It is similarly gratuitous to row downstream; the river will take care of that. The way a good guide steers is by moving the boat **perpendicular** to the flow of the stream. This means that you accept the direction, but the quality of your trip is influenced enormously by which portion of the onrushing flow you ride. Moving a mere five feet to the left can allow you to avoid a disastrous collision with a rock. Indeed, we learned that there are portions of most streams along the banks that actually flow lightly in the opposite direction so that you can move upstream a bit simply by getting near the edge.

Cancer patients and indeed everyone facing mortality and illness could, Spiegel reasoned, benefit from this existential perspective:

> The ultimate direction has been determined and opposing it is exhausting and futile. However, the nature of the trip and how safe and pleasant it is can be enormously influenced by maneuvering within this fundamental direction. It is even possible to slow the trip down. Some illnesses are curable, some are chronic afflictions that one lives with for

> many years, and some may lead to death fairly rapidly. Many medical
> treatments can make a difference in the odds, but sooner or later the out-
> come for all of us will be death. Where we have enormous control is in
> how we live whatever life we **have**.

A 1984 psycho-oncology conference in New York prompted Spiegel to consider some of the harm New Age claims of "mind over matter" might be
causing to patients. His concern was that people embracing these theories
were being made to feel like failures as their cancer progressed. Simplistic
mind/body approaches attributing cancer to stress, recent personal losses,
depression and passivity, lack of a will to live, or even to an unconscious
need for illness bothered Spiegel deeply. Thinking to debunk these theories,
he embarked upon a re-examination of his study of metastatic breast cancer
patients from over a decade earlier. He was convinced that survival statistics
would demonstrate that psychosocial interventions, such as his therapy
groups, while improving quality of life, made no difference in length of survival.

As the analyzed data began coming in, the results astonished him. "The two
survival curves overlapped initially," Spiegel reported, "but diverged mark-
edly at twenty months. By four years after the point at which the women
were enrolled in the initial study, it turned out that all of the patients in the
control group had died, but fully one third of the patients who had received
group therapy was still alive." When all the results were in, the divergence
between the two study populations was striking: the women randomly
assigned to the group lived nearly twice as long as the controls.[13]

Since 1989, several small scale studies using group therapy and support with
lymphoma and melanoma patients have confirmed these findings. More controlled studies are in process, but there is every reason to believe that, while
the direction and flow of the river are incontrovertible, David Spiegel is
right, and there is still quite a bit of room for maneuvering. Unlike research
on the safety and toxicity of chemotherapy drugs, you don't have to wait for
all the study results to be in to safely take advantage of this promising information. This treatment is truly non-toxic. It turns out that the very activities
that improve quality of life may also enhance quantity of life. No effort is
wasted.

We have no way of knowing what it was that prolonged the lives of those
fifty women in Spiegel's study. It may have been their contact with one

another, the support of others who understood and sympathized from their own experience. It may have been the cathartic act of expressing difficult feelings of loss and grief, or the steadying impact of facing what is most feared in a supportive setting. It may have been that their openness in the group led to improvements in other relationships, with family and friends. It may have been that the group helped the women clarify priorities and determine how best to use the time they had. It may have been the empowerment of seeking and exchanging information that gave a sense of greater control. It may have been the encouragement they received from other group members to assert themselves and insist on the best medical treatment and compassionate care. It may have been that through working through painful, often repressed or denied feelings in the group, a fuller and deeper sense of connection with meaning and spirit became possible. It may have been any or all of these things, in some indefinable combination that was different for each person.

One thing seems clear, however: that all these goals are worthwhile for anyone facing metastatic breast cancer to consider. As a result of his findings and observations, Spiegel feels strongly that support groups should go hand in hand with conventional surgery, radiation and chemotherapy. "It is my personal belief," he maintains, "that group support should be routinely recommended as part of cancer care."[14]

Still, you may find support groups disturbing. It's painful to get attached to others you may lose, and at first you may find that your own fears can be heightened by what you learn there. Most people soon discover, however, that the benefits of a well-led support group far outweigh these drawbacks. But if a group is not for you, there is no reason to believe that there is anything intrinsically magical about this particular form of support. It's probable that many of the benefits of groups can be sought in other forms—individual counseling, for example, with a skilled therapist experienced in working with cancer patients.

Sharon Multhauf, 54, a retired school teacher who lives with her husband Lloyd and two teenage children in Northern California, used some of the same imagery to express what life has been like for her before and after metastatic breast cancer.

> *On the trail, I looked at the map and decided where I would go.*
> *On the river, I had to go where I was taken.*

On the trail, I stopped and rested when I got tired.
On the river, I couldn't stop, the flow was so constant.

On the trail, I knew that I could turn around and go back down the mountain if the way was too rough.
On the river, there was only one direction.

Hiking is within my scope—I can imagine, I can plan, and I can walk.
But in a rudderless boat with no oars on an unknown river, what can I do?

No one gets out of this life (boat) alive, so I'm going to work on my navigation skills and settle in for the ride.

But it's a wild ride this river takes you on—no mistaking that—and you have precious little control over whether you are one of the fortunate ones who stand on the bank, watching, or whether you find yourself in the water, paddling furiously. Avoiding the sight of the rockier and more turbulent parts makes the run no easier. Learning to navigate skillfully may, however. But before you can learn to navigate, it will help to learn a bit more about what you are dealing with. The facts and details of the disease are indeed painful to read, as the next chapter will make clear. This illness can be relentless.

In a good support group, fear and pain, once shared and experienced, yield to a sense of connection and purpose. The process, like the river, carries people along.

Trust in the process.

CHAPTER 3

Seventeen Stories of Metastatic Breast Cancer

WHILE THERE ARE CERTAIN COMMON PATTERNS of disease, metastatic breast cancer can manifest itself in many ways and in many parts of the body, affecting almost any organ or tissue. This chapter offers a brief road map and a primer for some of the more common metastatic sites and what they mean.

This probably won't be an easy chapter for you to read. It may seem dense with unfamiliar medical information, and the details of the many possible sites for recurrence may make the disease seem more aggressive than it is. A discussion about metastatic process will be followed by a list of the various ways in which metastatic breast cancer usually makes itself known. To personalize this, and make it less daunting for you, this will be done through telling the stories of some of the people whose lives are featured in this book. A section on prognostic factors follows, the ways in which your doctors may be able to look at how your disease may progress and respond to treatment. The remaining sections will cover Stage IV disease at primary diagnosis, local recurrence, regional recurrence, distant recurrence or metastasis, and the various metastatic sites: bones, lung, liver and other less common sites.

What is metastatic breast cancer?

When breast cancer cells spread from the primary tumor in the breast through the lymphatic system or the circulatory system to other parts of the body, establish themselves there, and begin to multiply, they are said to have metastasized. Most cancer deaths are due to the effects of metastases resistant to treatment. Metastases must find favorable conditions to grow. According to Drs. Lee Ellis and Isaiah Fidler, "To grow beyond the size of 1-2 mm., primary tumors and metastases must develop an adequate blood supply through the process known as angiogenesis."[1]

"The process of metastasis isn't random," explains Dr. Loren Buhle, creator of the Oncolink Cancer Information Service at the University of Pennsylvania. "Instead, it is a cascade of linked sequential steps that must be traversed by the tumor cells if a metastasis is to develop. Each step involves multiple tumor-host interactions. To be successful, a metastatic tumor cell must leave the primary tumor and invade local host tissue. It must then enter the circulation, survive in the circulation, arrest at the distant vascular bed, extravasate (or spread) into the organ interstitium (space between the organs) and/or parenchyma (the organ itself) and multiply to initiate a metastatic colony. Interruption of the metastatic cascade at any of these steps can prevent the production of clinically symptomatic metastasis."[2]

Micrometastases, presumed "seeds" from the primary tumor that later grow into tumors at distant sites, are still too small to find on any scan or blood test. Often, it will be years before these new tumor sites grow large enough to be detectable. The rate of growth, or "doubling time," of a cancer is not necessarily constant, either. Sometimes, metastatic tumors will lie dormant or quiescent, until, for reasons as mystifying as the reasons they became dormant in the first place, the tumors begin to grow again. At other times, the disease progresses rapidly and relentlessly.

While the pathophysiology of metastasis is beyond the scope of this book, some general observations may be helpful. According to Dr. Alan Aaron, the two theoretical models that have been most frequently cited in discussing advanced breast cancer are the "anatomic-mechanical" theory proposed by J. Ewing in 1928, and the "seed and soil hypothesis" proposed by Paget in 1889. "The mechanistic approach states that metastasis develops in the first organ a tumor cell encounters."[3] As Dr. Aaron observes, this theory, while it clearly plays a role, has been shown to be oversimplified, and has given way to a second theory, known as "chemotaxis," based on the Paget hypothesis, meaning that cancer cells are chemically attracted to certain specific sites within the body.

Some scientists now believe that this happens because of certain molecular patterns on the surface of cells, as pathologist Dr. Erkki Ruoslahti explains:

> Physical trapping of cancer cells in the blood vessels at the site of
> metastasis is not the whole story, however. If it were, cancers would not
> spread so diversely through the body. Indeed, some types of cancer show a
> striking preference for organs other than those that receive their venous

blood—witness the tendency of metastatic prostate cancer to move into the bones. Once again, the explanation seems to rest with the molecular address system on cell surfaces. A specific affinity between the adhesion molecules on cancer cells and those on the inner linings of blood vessels in the preferred tissues could explain the predilection of the cells to migrate selectively. Different concentrations of growth-promoting factors and hormones in various tissues may also play a part.[4]

Having spoken of the variability of metastatic disease, let's take a look at the few generalizations about the spread of breast cancer that we can make.

When you are diagnosed with primary breast cancer, particularly if the tumor is in the upper, outer quadrant of the breast—the part of your breast nearest to your arm—it is likely to spread, if it spreads at all, first to the axillary lymph nodes under your arm, which are the nearest nodes that drain the lymphatics in this part of the breast. This is, of course, why these lymph nodes are biopsied at the time of surgery, so that determining the extent of disease can suggest optimal treatment. The cancer may be contained there, or micrometastases may escape and begin to establish themselves elsewhere.

This isn't always the route of spread, by any means. If your tumor was located more centrally in the breast, under the nipple, or in the inner quadrants, you may experience an undetected spread to the internal mammary nodes located between the ribs and beneath the sternum. Doctors used to believe that cancer always spread through the lymphatic ducts, beginning in the breast and radiating outwards. Now we know that isn't always true, for nearly 30 percent of women with no cancer evident in their lymph nodes following axillary dissection eventually go on to develop metastatic disease. Clearly, the cancer can spread microscopically through the bloodstream and perhaps even pass through the lymphatic system without detection. Your cancer may already have been systemic—that is, affecting your whole body—by the time you were first diagnosed. This is the rationale behind giving strong chemotherapy to women with large, or rapidly dividing tumors, particularly those younger women whose tumors are not estrogen or progesterone receptor positive, or who have several or many lymph nodes affected. Since chemotherapy is most likely to be effective the first time around, as adjuvant treatment following primary diagnosis and surgery, oncologists will try to identify those women at highest risk for recurrence, using the best tests and prognostic indicators available, so that these high-risk patients may receive the best available prophylactic, or preventative, treatments.

In the last chapter, we heard from Sue Tokuyama, Bonnie Gelbwasser, and Ellen Scheiner, all of whom had multiple lymph nodes positive for the spread of cancer when they were first diagnosed. These nodes are strongly suggestive of metastatic spread, which is the reason all three women elected to have unusually aggressive chemotherapy regimens. While the long-term survival rate is certainly lower for these women than for women with fewer or no positive nodes, there are many cases of very long-term remission and even apparent cures—though doctors usually don't like to use this word, because breast cancers can recur after many years.

At the time of this writing, physicians and patients are hopeful that high-risk women with Stage IIB and Stage III diagnoses and ten or more positive axillary lymph nodes will have extended disease-free survival from high-dose chemotherapy with stem cell or bone marrow rescue, but the results of these studies are not yet in. Two large scale studies, undertaken by the Cancer and Leukemia Group B (CALGB), the Eastern Cooperative Oncology Group (ECOG) and the Southwest Oncology Group (SWOG), are comparing this treatment with conventional chemotherapies and, as of this writing, are still enrolling patients. Preliminary results appear to indicate some success.[5]

Many stories, common threads

The stories you are about to read represent some of the diverse ways in which recurrent breast cancer can present itself. As you will see, these stories differ greatly in the details of illness onset, and are as unique as are the people afflicted. The timing of the disease, the organ systems affected, the physical manifestations, and even the means of discovery, all vary greatly.

Yet there are common threads. The ways that people effectively come to terms with life-threatening illness suggest shared themes and concerns. More universal—and more crucial in your life than any of the specific details of the disease onset—is the emotional impact of such a diagnosis, and the struggle, confusion and ultimate decisions that go into seeking out the best doctors and making good treatment choices. This material will be covered in the next chapters.

Reading about the disease in all its manifestations is emotionally trying. As you read, please keep in mind that every one of these people recovered from the brutal shock of her diagnosis, reported here and in the next chapter, and went on to find effective ways of coping with the progression of the disease and its emotional impact.

Primary diagnosis: Stage IV

In about 10 percent of primary breast cancer cases, the cancer is found to have already metastasized to distant sites when the diagnosis is first made. Doctors refer to this as Stage IV breast cancer. Patients diagnosed this late in the disease process often experience a rapid progression of the disease that is difficult to gain control over. Still, they can sometimes be treated to partial or complete remission, particularly if the disease is still very limited and hormonally responsive.

Kathy Stone, 53, a former fiscal administrator for the University of California before her disability retirement, lives with her husband Chuck, a retired fire marshal, in a community near San Francisco. Together, they've raised two sons and two daughters, all grown and out in the world, and have four grandchildren, two of them teenagers.

In July 1994, several carcinomas were found in Kathy's left breast, along with a patch of inflammatory cancer. All 28 axillary nodes were affected, and there was cancer in the supraclavicular lymph nodes under her collar bone, so the cancer was said to have metastasized already. In August of 1995, after a year of treatment, widespread new metastases were found in her femur, hip, pelvis, sacrum, spine, ribs and cranium, as well as a soft tissue tumor in the lymph nodes in her neck.

IBC

Eight months later, this is what Kathy wrote one of the newcomers on the Breast Cancer Discussion List:

> I, too, was diagnosed as Stage IV from the onset, and it scared the shit out of me, but I have started living each day and stopped getting ready to die. I have decided that whatever takes me and whenever it is will still be a mystery to me. None of us is guaranteed the next moment.

At the time of her diagnoses in October of 1995, Barb Clabo, 47, a computer operator, and her husband, Glenn, a business manager for the Naval Sea Systems Command, lived in Northern Virginia, with their 19-year-old son, Chad, and their daughter, Jamie, 20, in college nearby.

Barb's oncologist told her that all of the 12 lymph nodes sampled showed spread of her cancer. One particular word stuck in her mind from this conversation. "He told me my prognosis was 80 percent failure," she recalls. "What the hell did he mean by failure? Failure equals death? The doctor ordered an MRI of my brain, and a CT scan of my chest, explaining that there was an excellent chance of mets (metastases), and they had to search to see where." The tests showed cancerous lesions in her liver and spine.

Nancy Gilpatrick, 43, a social worker on leave from her private practice, who was living with her boyfriend in Utah, was diagnosed with breast cancer in November of 1995. Stunned as she was by the diagnosis, it never occurred to her that the hip pain she'd been experiencing for two months could be a bony metastasis of her breast cancer. Sudden, increased pain turned out to be a fracture of the pubic bone. In March of 1996, Nancy reported, "I had another bone scan and CT of the abdomen. There was new disease and the original tumors looked like they had grown. This was only a few months from the original tests. I was dealing with an incredibly aggressive cancer." One month later, a fracture to her left hip forced her to use a walker and wheelchair. She was told she would have to wait until the effects of her high-dose chemotherapy subsided enough for her to heal from surgery required to repair her pelvis and hips. "I have not had one doctor's visit since the diagnosis that was positive," she exclaimed in pained frustration.

Pam Hiebert, 49, an electronic publishing technician, lives with her life partner, Sylvan, in Oregon. In 1993, Pam was diagnosed with a hormone sensitive breast cancer that had already spread to her left femur and one rib. Her disease was stabilized with tamoxifen for three years. On a first name basis with her oncologist, Pam re-read her chart of the first days after her initial diagnosis. "Ralph ended his summary of my condition and prognosis by writing, 'This patient is going to be very difficult to keep alive.' I beat his odds!"

But spring of 1996 brought stiff necks, headaches, and a rise in tumor markers. Awaiting new tests, Pam wrote in her journal:

> Tomorrow is just the mechanics of a procedure. I have the same amount of hours in this day as I would ever have. Use your day well and let others do their job. They can't pass a verdict on you. You are of free will. You live the life meant for you. Live the moment. Love the moment.

And later, the same day, further self-inquiry in the form of a poem:

> What if they find something and it's bad?
> What if I don't have a lot of time left?
> What if they want to push ahead to high-dose?
> Who will I be?

What if they find nothing new?
and they just shrug?
What if I just let go...returned to work...
To think about the summer?
What if I rush to fill my tamoxifen Rx again?
Who will I be?

What am I now that I won't be tomorrow?
Except more knowledgeable.

The scans brought certain knowledge of the end of remission and evidence of further spread to her bones, and a change to a new hormone, Arimidex.

Looking at prognosis

For most women with metastatic disease, however, a period of months to years, sometimes many years, elapses between primary diagnosis and the discovery of advanced disease. Recurrence, when and if it happens, may be local, regional or distant, and may be singular, involving a single site in one part of the body, or widespread, involving many lesions in several parts of the body. The extent of the disease and where it is located give some measure of how serious the prognosis may be, and how rapidly the cancer may progress. In a study of over a thousand women whose cancer had recurred, researchers found that, "Involved axillary lymph nodes at the time of initial diagnosis and/or lack of ERs (estrogen receptors) may indicate a highly malignant tumor or a weak host defense, either of which might be related to short survival after relapse."[6]

Another very important prognostic factor is time to recurrence. If many years have elapsed between the initial diagnosis and recurrence, this can mean that the cancer cells are relatively slow to reproduce themselves, and have a long doubling time. Often, though not always, this indicates slow disease progression.

Still another crucial factor is whether or not the tumor needs the hormones estrogen or progesterone in order to grow. While this is not an absolute measure, a tumor can be said to be estrogen and progesterone receptor positive or negative (ER or PR + or -), depending on the findings in the initial pathology. Having an ER+ and/or PR+ tumor is thought to be a positive prognostic sign. This is because hormonal treatments can slow, stop or even regress the growth of these tumors, sometimes for long periods, before chemotherapy drugs, which are more toxic to normal body cells, have to be used.

The tumor's response to the various treatments used in metastatic breast cancer is one of the most significant factors in prolonging life. Some women's cancers are very sensitive to chemotherapy treatments, some are sensitive only to some, and still others are resistant to almost every drug. Eventually, almost all tumors mutate to become resistant to the drugs used to treat them, and will no longer respond. The oncologist's job is to determine which drugs, used in which sequence, will produce the longest partial and complete responses (remissions), combined with the best quality of life.

When I asked my oncologist, Dr. Samuel Waxman, who divides his time between research and clinical practice, to characterize how he looks at the treatment of metastatic breast cancer, he spoke of what he does as a complex and subtle process.

> *I try to convert the disease to a chronic condition. I've certainly had patients with advanced breast cancer for many years, in different areas, and they can live with it for a long time. We don't know why. I am sure it's not just my treatment. I am sure there are things going on that we don't know how to measure in a given patient. I don't think it's witchcraft. It's the biology of the tumor and the biology of the host. That, and the fact of the instability within the cancer cell population and its ability to become more de-differentiated and less responsive and more resistant to the treatments we use. Even a given population of cancer cells in the same patient is totally heterogeneous. That's why the problem is so complicated.*

Treating this complex disease is the focus of much ongoing research, and forms a body of knowledge that is constantly changing. The standard and experimental treatments and what is known about them will be discussed in some detail in the sections on treatment.

Local recurrence

A local recurrence can happen when tumor cells remain in the original site and, over time, grow to become a measurable tumor. While requiring further treatment, a local recurrence doesn't by itself mean the disease has become systemic and life-threatening. A percentage of women who elect to have breast conserving surgery (lumpectomy or similar limited surgery which removes the tumor and enough surrounding tissue to provide clear margins) will have some part of the tumor grow back from cancer cells that were left behind, despite radiation therapy to the remaining breast tissue. Residual cancer cells, over time, can grow a new tumor without spreading through the circulatory or lymphatic system. One extensive study, published in the *Journal of Clinical Oncology*, found that 10 to 20 percent of patients will have locally recurrent disease one to nine years after lumpectomy and radiation.[8]

Doctors generally treat local recurrence as a failure of the initial treatment, and do not consider it a true spread of the cancer. Usually treated with a "salvage mastectomy," this kind of limited recurrence is thought to have little impact on overall mortality when it is found growing in residual breast tissue contiguous to the primary tumor. Researchers have not yet determined, however, whether an invasive local recurrence in the remaining breast tissue can easily spread to other parts of the body. Though evidence is inconclusive, it is reasonable to assume that spread may be possible.

While a second primary breast cancer in the same breast may be referred to as a local recurrence, it is really a new cancer and is treated in much the same way as a new breast cancer in the other breast might be. Breast conserving surgery is not an option, however, because the breast cannot be irradiated a second time, and the risk of local recurrence is unacceptably high without radiation treatment.

After mastectomy, which always leaves some small amount of breast tissue, a local recurrence is also possible in the remaining skin and fat, and can be treated with excision and radiation if the diagnosis is clear.

The problem in this instance, though, is that sometimes a new tumor in the mastectomy scar does not arise from residual breast tissue, but from spread of cancer through the circulatory or lymphatic system. This can be a disturbing sign, because in the majority of cases it is a harbinger of systemic, metastatic disease. Unfortunately, it is not always possible to tell the difference between these two very different circumstances. "It is impossible to tell whether local recurrence results from cells that persist locally or from those that have passed through the general circulation to return to implant at a favorable site," according to Dr. Edward Scanlon.[10]

One day, Barbara Ragland looked in the mirror and saw something strange at the site of the scar from the Halstead radical mastectomy she'd had nineteen years before.

> *There was a raised bump and a short distance from that was a depression—like a hole where the skin was pulled in. It didn't dawn on me that it could be recurrence. When the internist first saw the tumors (which were obvious by just looking at my chest), she really showed concern. I thought she was just being very cautious when she ordered tests and sent me to the surgeon. I didn't think it would turn out to be cancer. I'd had annual checkups from my surgeon for nearly 20 years and the radiologist had checked me annually for 10 years. When the pathology report came back, the surgeon's nurse called me at my office. She said, "I have bad news—it's cancer." I asked which tumor was cancerous and she told me both were.*

Regional recurrence

Sites of regional recurrence include the muscles of the chest wall, the internal mammary lymph nodes under the breast bone and between the ribs, and those up above the collar bone, known as supraclavicular nodes, and the nodes in the neck. The remaining skin and scar tissue can be affected as well.

A regional recurrence is considered more serious than a local recurrence, for it usually indicates that the cancer has spread past the confines of the breast and axillary lymph nodes. Here is how the Physician's Data Query of the NCI expresses these relative degrees of risk and severity: "Patients with chest wall recurrences of less than three centimeters, axillary and internal mammary node recurrence (not supraclavicular, which has a poorer survival), and a greater than 2-year disease-free interval prior to resection have the best chance for prolonged survival."[11]

Kim Banks was diagnosed at 32 with an aggressive two-centimeter infiltrating ductal carcinoma. Two axillary lymph nodes showed spread of the disease, so she underwent chemotherapy. She decided on a latissimus dorsi breast flap reconstruction, in which a muscle from her back was brought to the front of her body to shape a new breast.

Though her tumor tested positive for estrogen and progesterone receptors, Kim was among the minority of women who have serious side effects with the estrogen antagonist, tamoxifen. She gave up taking tamoxifen as a possible preventive agent against recurrence because it increased her migraine headaches. Two years later, the cancer was back in between her pectoral muscles in the shape of a flat coil about four inches in length. Before a course of chemotherapy could be completed, metastases to her spine were detected.

Distant recurrence or metastasis

A distant metastasis, most often to bone, bone marrow, lungs or liver, and to soft tissue and other organs somewhat less frequently, is the most alarming kind of recurrence, for it indicates that there may be more widespread dissemination of the cancer.

The liver and lungs are common metastatic sites for many cancers, probably because the role they play in purifying and nourishing the body means that these organs are highly vascular. They act as filters for the entire blood supply, which passes through them. Breast cancer also appears to be attracted to bone and bone marrow tissue when it metastasizes, a characteristic referred to as "osteotropism." The bones of the spine, ribs, pelvis and skull, and the long bones of the legs and arms are most commonly affected. Metastases to the brain and eye are not unusual, particularly as secondary sites.

Bone metastases

Nearly 25 percent of breast cancers metastasize first to the bone, and most others eventually show some bone involvement.[12] "The bony skeleton is a site of symptomatic disease in three quarters of patients who develop secondary breast cancer," according to a 1994 review article in the *British Medical Journal*.[13] In the previously cited article in the *Journal of the American Medical Association*, Dr. Alan D. Aaron quoted the figure as 84 percent: "Clearly, certain cancers exhibit osteotropism and predictably metastasize to bone."[14] Both breast and prostate cancers show this attraction to bone in equal proportion.

Bone metastases may be of two types: osteolytic or osteoblastic. Osteolytic lesions actually form holes in the bone as the cancer replaces healthy bone, and give the bones a typically moth-eaten look on x-ray, and making them susceptible to fracture, particularly the weight bearing bones of the legs, hip and pelvis. Osteoblastic lesions, while they lead to an increase in bone density, can also lead to fractures. Both kinds can cause pain.

Sharon Multhauf found it hard to distinguish the pain she already had from her cancer pain. Over the years, arthritic symptoms had developed, with pain that would come and go, and change with the weather. Then, in 1987, Sharon was diagnosed with invasive lobular and ductal breast cancer at age 44, and treated with lumpectomy, radiation and six courses of chemotherapy. Because none of her lymph nodes had showed any evidence of spread, Sharon hoped that the cancer was gone. After more than seven disease-free years, she felt reasonably certain the cancer would not return.

> *Ever since I was in my 20's, I've had bouts of low-back pain, and there was always a logical explanation for them. Sometimes I pulled muscles, sometimes I slept in a bad bed while traveling, sometimes I worked several days in an awkward position or sat through long car trips, or any one of many other things.*

In 1994, a hardening in her radiated breast led to a biopsy and diagnosis of a local recurrence. As indicated earlier, local recurrence is usually thought to be from cancer cells left behind from the original surgery, and does not mean, in itself, that the cancer has spread through the blood and lymphatic system to regional or distant metastatic sites. What happened next gives a picture of how complex a diagnosis of bone metastases can be.

> *I had the biopsy and mastectomy in December, but didn't have a bone scan until after the surgery. It showed new activity in the sacrum, pelvis and hip joint. But since I had so much arthritis, they did an x-ray to see if they could tell the difference. Nothing showed up on the x-ray. I guess only certain bone lesions—the kind that eat holes in your bones—show up on x-rays, and mine were the other kind. So, the definitive test was the MRI. With that, they were able to distinguish among the three different things that were causing my pain. One was the arthritis, which occurred only at joints, and only on the surface of the bone. The second was two herniated lumbar disks which were pressing on a spinal nerve. But the third was metastatic areas in the sacrum, pelvis and hip. They showed up quite differently from the way the arthritis looked.*

Sharon looked away from the MRI computer screen while she was undergoing the scan.

I remembered the horrible feeling when I had my first bone scan and the monitor was positioned so that I could see it from the table. I had looked at the monitor and had seen all the bright spots on my skeleton and deduced the worst. That's what comes from not knowing how to read the signals. What was glowing in the 1987 bone scan was my arthritis— matched pairs up and down the skeleton at the joints.

A fellow breast cancer patient, fearful that her own pain might signal a return of her cancer, asked Sharon to describe the pain associated with bone metastases. Sharon wrote back:

The best I can say is that the pain from my bone mets seems to be dull, deep, persistent and localized, as opposed to the radiating pain I sometimes get from the compressed spinal nerves or the joint aches of arthritis. I also don't think everyone's experience is the same on this question. I do, however, remember that when my mother had bone mets from lung cancer, she used to wake up at night with pain. This never happened from her (or my) arthritis.

According to Dr. Aaron, "Patients with bone metastasis generally present to the clinician with pain. The pain is characteristically described as dull in character, constant in presentation, and gradually progressive in intensity. Night pain and pain not relieved by rest are especially worrisome. Spinal involvement may present with localized back pain or extremity paresthesia (tingling or pins-and-needles sensation) from nerve-root compression."[15]

Susan Love offers this commonsense advice: "If you have pain that lasts for more than a week or two and doesn't seem to be going away, and isn't like whatever pains have been familiar to you in your life, you should get it checked out."[14]

Bob Stafford's breast cancer was first diagnosed in 1988, when he was 37 years old. Like most people, he hadn't known that men could get breast cancer when he first showed his family doctor the pea-sized nodule on his chest. Indeed, the disease is rare in men (less than one percent of breast cancers occur in males) and it is almost unheard of in men his age. Now 45, he is retired from his work as a pastor and counselor in a rural community near South Bend, Indiana, where he lives with his wife, Sherry, and teenage son and daughter. Following a mastectomy and chemotherapy, Bob made a good recovery, until March of 1991.

My right hip started to hurt. I thought it might be a congenital hip problem because my mother has problems with her hips. I started using over-the-counter pain medicine before I finally went to the clinic to see a family doctor. He prescribed medicine for arthritis and it seemed to help for a while. But the pain continued to increase. One time I played golf with a couple of men from work. One of the men felt so sorry for me that he would carry my clubs as well as his own. Finally, the family doctor suggested the possibility the cancer could be back and scheduled a bone scan. Apparently, there were several hot spots including my left ribs which I had been complaining about also.

Before seeing him, his oncologist arranged for a biopsy of one of his ribs, and Bob and his wife began the long wait for the test results.

The worst thing about cancer is the waiting. We had to wait until the following Monday to get the results from the doctor even though we were told he knew the results. It was one of the longest weekends in our lives. When we finally got hold of him he said he wanted us to meet with the oncologist and we knew immediately what that meant.

When we finally made it to the oncologist's office, his opening remark was, "Well, I guess I didn't want to see you as much as you didn't want to see me." Then he shared the results. There was cancer in the bones. The bone scan had shown spots on the hips, ribs, spine, clavicle, sternum and skull.

Penny Lebow, 50, a member of Tigerlily, my own face-to-face support group in New York City, found her recurrence seven years after her initial diagnosis in 1987 with a large, six-centimeter invasive lobular carcinoma. Penny, a social worker now on disability, and her longtime life partner, Mark, now live in Maine, a move they had dreamed of making for years.

At my yearly oncology checkup at the end of December 1994, I discussed the fact that I was having pain attributed to arthritis in my left hip when I did certain exercises in my aerobics class, and wanted to follow up with the orthopedist, with whom I had an appointment the next day. She encouraged me to see him and was not concerned about it being cancer. The orthopedist recommended a bone scan, which showed increased "hot spot" activity in my left hip and pelvis.

A subsequent MRI also revealed a suspicious area. Finally, a bone biopsy confirmed that the cancer was indeed back, but it had been a long, difficult month of waiting and hoping for Penny and Mark.

Up until the second MRI results, my oncologist maintained that "you can knock me down with a feather if this is cancer." When I told her I planned to bring a feather to our treatment conference, she didn't laugh.

Lung metastases

"Sixty to 70 percent of patients who die of breast cancer eventually have it in their lungs," writes Dr. Susan Love. "The lungs are the only site of metastasis in about 21 percent of cases."[15]

Often the first sign or symptom of lung metastases is a dry cough or shortness of breath, subtle at first, then gradually increasing over a period of days or weeks. At other times, a nodule or nodules in the lungs may be asymptomatic, only showing up on a routine chest x-ray. Multiple nodules are suggestive of the spread of breast cancer, while a single nodule must often be biopsied to rule out the possibility of a primary lung cancer.

Sometimes the tumor manifests itself as fine widespread lesions, called lymphangitic spread because it seems to have spread to the lungs through the lymphatic system, and is not easily detectable on x-rays or scans. This may be accompanied by what is called a malignant pleural effusion, an accumulation of fluid in the pleural cavity surrounding the affected lung, causing decreasing exercise tolerance and shortness of breath.

Very occasionally, thoracotomy, surgical removal of part of a lung, is a feasible treatment for a single, discrete lesion. Most of the time, though, there are several tumors, and systemic treatment with chemotherapy and hormonal treatment is recommended.

Caren Buffum recalled the discovery of her lung metastases in December 1991, six years after her initial Stage I diagnosis.

I had a persistent cough, of a dry and ticklish kind, like I'd inhaled dust. Eventually I saw my GP about it and he ordered x-rays, saying it might be bronchitis (though in retrospect, he may have suspected mets). The x-rays revealed what appeared to be tumors in the lungs, so we went to CT scans, which confirmed the tumors there and also picked one up in the liver. I still have (four and a half years later) a sort of ticklish feeling that compels me to cough. Sometimes it also feels kind of like a burning sensation at the bottom of my windpipe. I've had some back pain which could be attributed to the lung mets, but since it hasn't been persistent, it could also be from chemo, aging, bad posture...

In December 1990, PJ Hagler was anxiously awaiting her husband Mike's return from a business trip. In recent days, she'd been short of breath and felt a searing pain in her back that kept her up at night. Though she'd told no one, she feared a return of the breast cancer she hoped she'd beaten six years before, in 1985, when she'd had her second mastectomy.

When she and Mike went for the doctor's appointment, after he returned from his trip, the doctor's tests were inconclusive; there was some fluid, perhaps a bit of pleurisy. PJ was put on antibiotics. An oncologist could find nothing definite, despite numerous scans and other tests. A broncoscopy showed very little more.

I grew to hate that word "inconclusive." It always meant another doctor, another test and another "We're not sure."

After three months of uncertainty, PJ consulted a thoracic specialist, who ordered a thoracentesis performed, to draw the accumulated fluid from the pleural sac surrounding the lungs. This test is still vivid in PJ's memory:

While you are leaning across a table very much awake, they insert a very large needle and draw the fluid off the lung to test it. I prayed that if pain was any indication of a good conclusive test, this would be the winner. Mike held tight to my hands as I leaned on this table and they continued to draw more and more fluid. I saw about one and a half liters of fluid put into a big jar. I was told I should be able to breathe a little better with the fluid off my lung. They did their tests on the fluid and that awful word came back—"inconclusive." By then I was walking with a cane most of the time if I walked much at all. I used oxygen at home and didn't go to work anymore.

A second thoracentesis a month later drained four liters of fluid that was highly suggestive of metastatic spread of cancer, but the site of recurrence was still unclear. In April, after four months of uncertainty and pain, PJ underwent open chest exploratory surgery.

Tiny, pinpoint tumors were found all over the pleura, or sac, around her right lung, which was shriveled and no longer functioning. A port had been implanted to administer the chemotherapy. Two days after her surgery, when PJ was again able to focus on what was happening around her, the thoracic surgeon, the oncologist and her husband Mike agreed that it was time to discuss the results with her.

Mike was going to try telling me alone but just couldn't do it. They told me the cancer was back. Mine was a very unusual cancer, the doctor said. It was quite bad but we were just starting the fight. I was asked to talk to Mike, and write down any questions. We were told that the oncologist would be back in an hour to start the chemo and give me the answers and fill in all the gaps in what would go on for the next few months. After the doctors left, Mike and I just sat in silence for awhile. I was in shock. Numbing shock. We cried, held on to each other and just shut the door and cried. When I could stop, my first question was had he been told before I woke up. He just nodded, and squeezed my hand.

My fears were realized. I had cancer again and they couldn't just cut it out of me this time. We held hands and prayed harder and with more emotion than we had ever prayed before. We wrote some questions that in hindsight were quite meaningless. But I didn't know what to ask. The oncologist came into the room and he and Mike just sat down by the bed. Dr. K. asked me for my questions. Not on the list but the first thing I asked was, "Am I going to die?" Mike started to cry again so I figured this meant yes. But Dr. K said he honestly didn't know if I would die from cancer or something else. He didn't know when I would die any more than he knew when he would die. He said we will do all we can do.

For Joleene Kolenberg, the diagnosis of lung metastases at age 66 was much more straightforward. She and her husband took early retirement from their work at a Christian college in Chicago, and bought 15 acres in the country near South Bend, Indiana. Jack had finished building their new home and they'd settled in to enjoy their daughters and three grandchildren, when Joleene was first diagnosed with breast cancer in November 1992. Five out of the seventeen lymph nodes sampled showed spread of the cancer, so the CAF (Cytoxan, Adriamycin and 5-FU) protocol, followed by tamoxifen, was used in addition to her mastectomy.

Life had begun to seem normal again, when in May of 1995, during a routine x-ray, several nodules were discovered in one of her lungs. Since he couldn't be sure the nodules were a spread of her breast cancer, and not granulomas, which are benign, her doctor advised a "watchful waiting" approach, following her closely with monthly x-rays. By December, when Joleene began to cough and experience shortness of breath, it was clear her cancer was back. The nodules had grown.

The first half of 1996 brought difficult treatments that left Joleene housebound and footsore from her chemotherapy. It gave her time to reflect.

> When I was first diagnosed with cancer, I really fussed and cried. I was 62, and I wanted to live until I was 72. I don't know why I picked that number. Now that I'm 66, I think maybe 72 is too soon. My youngest grandchild is 12 today and I'd like to see her graduated, (6 more years). I think if we love life, we can never really say when we will be ready to leave. I am not afraid of dying, and am ready to die, but as some have said, just not ready to leave yet.

Liver metastases

Oncologists often consider metastases to the viscera, or organs of the abdomen, especially the liver, among the most serious of prognostic signs. After bones and lung, the liver is the third most common metastatic site, presenting as the first recurrence in about 25 percent of cases and eventually present in about two-thirds of women with metastatic disease. Since much of the liver must be replaced by cancerous tumors before symptoms become unmistakable, the signs are often subtle at first, involving gastrointestinal distress, loss of appetite, weight loss and fever. Pain, caused by liver enlargement, may appear in the upper right quadrant of the abdomen. Routine blood tests that measure liver functions can often point to early metastatic signs, and liver scans, in which radioactive dye is injected before pictures are taken of the liver, can sometimes confirm these findings. A liver biopsy is often needed, however, to distinguish between metastatic tumors and other irregularities.

Mary D'Angelo was as determined as she was overoptimistic. She put off her initial diagnosis for more than a year after finding a lump, then later decided to ignore the possibility her cancer could come back.

> I didn't deal with having had cancer at first. I just went and did the chemo and thought, well, everyone is a fool, this is never going to happen to me again, but I will do everything they say.

*Then the counts (tumor markers) started going up and up, and they
sent me for scan after scan. That was kind of horrible. With a private
oncologist, they send you to labs and you have to make all the appointments yourself. Everyone was always so ill-trained, I felt; they couldn't
get the needles in...but I was never frightened, just annoyed and inconve-
nienced.*

*They finally got the scan back—the liver, or abdominal scan—and
said, "Oh, you're in big trouble." I remember asking my oncologist, "Well,
what does this mean?" He said, "If you don't get treatment, you could be
dead in about three months." So I was horrified, because he had spent six
months sending me for bone scans—three of them, I think—and they kept
coming back okay. Finally, he'd sent me for the abdominal scan and they
discovered the metastases in my liver.*

For Lisann Charland, the diagnosis of liver metastases in 1994 represented a
second recurrence after a lengthy remission. Four years before, and six years
after her initial diagnosis with breast cancer, bone metastases had first been
discovered and treated. In her case, the discovery of liver metastases happened quite inadvertently, and not from symptoms or routine screening
tests.

*Between August and October 1994, I met with the breast surgeon in
conjunction with the oncologist. I also requested that the silicone implant
be removed since I could not handle the "controversial" issues going on.
Upon agreement of the details of surgeries and approval by the insurance, the breast surgeon scheduled an MRI of the chest/pelvic area in
preparation for surgical removal of the silicone implant. The plan was to
do a tram flap after satisfactory healing of the surgery.*

Instead, events took an entirely different, more ominous turn. Lisann vividly
remembers every detail of those traumatic days.

*At 8:20 p.m., on October 24, 1994, the breast surgeon notified me
that a 6.5-centimeter mass on the liver had been detected by the MRI. She
recommended I put the surgery on hold, and go to the oncologist immediately. I saw the oncologist the next day to discuss the CT scan, possible
surgery, i.e., plan of action. The oncologist did not feel the mass was cancerous because it looked like a perfect circle on the scan. However,
because of my history and to be safe, he felt a biopsy was in order.*

> *On November 9, a CT guided liver biopsy was performed at El Camino Hospital, an experience I will always remember. The doctor did not feel it was cancer. But the results of the biopsy were metastatic adenocarcinoma, consistent with lobular carcinoma from my primary breast cancer.*

Other metastatic sites

Bob Crisp recalls that he hadn't been too concerned at the first signs of his wife's recurrence.

> *Ginger noticed a lump under her left armpit, opposite from the mastectomy side. Neither of us were particularly worried as it being on the opposite side didn't make sense. Ginger went to Little Rock by herself (rare, as I nearly always go with her for tests, etc.) but this seemed routine. Well, they did the needle test and it showed positive.*

An open biopsy was scheduled. Before surgery, Ginger discovered what looked like a rash on her right breast, confirmed by the surgeon as inflammatory breast cancer a few days later in the operating room.

> *When the surgeon came out to talk to me, I sensed from his demeanor that this was very serious. Also, when he told me that the only surgery was the excision of the node, then I knew we had something worse than we had expected. I was devastated and broke down. I went to the chapel room to be by myself for a while and cried.*

> *Ginger came out of surgery slowly. Kent (the surgeon) had told her about what he had found but she had been too groggy to comprehend. So I was with her when they brought her to her room. She told me that Kent had told her, but she hadn't comprehended what he said. This moment will be forever printed in my mind. It was very difficult to tell her what was found and that it was bad. I managed to do it without too much emotion. Shortly after, I left the room, went to the waiting room and lost it again. Very difficult. It was one of the worst days of my life.*

Scott Kitterman, 33, a systems analyst and Navy Reserve Officer, lived with his wife, Mary, 43, a retired aerospace engineer and fellow Reserve Officer, and their two-year-old daughter, Sylvia Joy, in a Maryland suburb of Washington, DC. Like a number of husbands interviewed for this book, Scott made it his business to research his wife's illness and the available treatments. Mary was diagnosed in March of 1995 with a Stage IIIA locally advanced infiltrating ductal carcinoma.

Actually, at first they said it was inflammatory breast cancer, then IBC
they said no, it's really locally advanced. Lately they've decided it really
was inflammatory. Mary has gotten to the point with this that she relies
on me to give her my best advice on what course to take. The situation is
so scary that she needs me to take some of the decision-making burden off
her shoulders.

They decided on aggressive treatment, believing that "hitting it hard" and early was their best shot at a long remission or cure. Mary had gone directly from mastectomy with immediate tram flap reconstruction and combination chemotherapy to high-dose chemotherapy with peripheral stem cell transplant.

Mary had completed 9 of 30 local radiation treatments when relapse
hit. She had a series of bad headaches, vertigo spells and light sensitivity
that were initially thought to be some kind of localized herpes zoster
(chicken pox/shingles virus) infection. These are common in the first year
post-BMT. Wrong. On March 15, 1996, we got the pathology report that
there were malignant cells in her cerebrospinal fluid. She had carcinoma-
tous meningitis. Further tests also revealed a walnut-sized lump related to
the lymphatic system under her sternum.

Lucie Bergmann-Shuster had been in remission for twelve years, and it didn't occur to her or her doctors that the vague symptoms she was feeling might signal a return of the breast cancer.

I had not been well for a long time. My zest, my joy, my exuberance,
my vitality had been failing me. Medically, my condition could be best
described as nonspecific ailments. My diagnosis of mets to the ovaries was
confirmed in December, but as early as March of that year I opted to
move my regular annual checkup into April as I was not feeling well and
thought a month early might be of benefit. I rationalized some of my "dis-
ease" away, attributing the sense of body/mind disconnectedness to the
grieving process in the aftermath of my mother's death in the first week of
January. Still, there were body signals which needed to be brought to the
attention of my physician.

A barrage of tests revealed nothing of concern, and with the help of an anti-depressant, Lucie felt a little better for a while. By chance, during an exchange about Internet health resources, she came across a paper about risk factors after a premenopausal breast cancer diagnosis.

> There was a 47 percent increased risk of getting ovarian cancer a decade later for women with familial lines of breast cancer. That information kept coursing through my mind for the next week and I decided to review my familial medical past and my present discomforts.

It was not until after many more tests and exploratory surgery that a definitive diagnosis was reached—there was cancer in the ovary, and in the surrounding tissues. Lucie's own instincts and information-seeking style had led her to the right diagnosis. But was this a primary ovarian cancer, or a metastasis of her breast cancer? At first, because the original slides from her primary breast cancer diagnosis were presumed lost, she was treated for ovarian cancer. But the slides were found, as it turned out, and the disease turned out to be a metastatic spread of her breast cancer.

What now?

A diagnosis of recurrence leaves the patient and her family in a state of shock and grief. That which has been most feared is now a reality, and the future is in question. That moment is always etched indelibly on the minds of all who experience it. Bob Crisp recalls it this way:

> Ginger's diagnosis occurred on the same day as the Oklahoma City bombing, which saturated the news. Ginger saw that and knew that life could end anytime, anywhere, very unexpected. So it gave her strength that her condition was not as bad, and that, unlike those poor persons, she was still alive and there was always hope. Funny how something tragic like that might affect her and give her perspective.

The next chapter follows these patients and their families in the days and weeks after getting the bad news—the shock, panic and grieving, the first, fumbling attempts at adjusting to the changed reality, the frenzied search for information and resources, as they move toward decision-making about treatment.

CHAPTER 4

The Shock of Recurrence

FINDING OUT THAT BREAST CANCER has recurred or spread beyond the breast is always a terrible blow. Almost all breast cancer patients know already that this means their prognosis, which may have been good, is no longer nearly as hopeful. Unless they've known others with metastatic breast cancer, they may even assume that a recurrence signifies imminent death. It takes time, accurate information and support to work through these early reactions.

This chapter will explore the nature of that reaction—from the feelings of unreality, numb shock and terrible grief, to a desperate sense of urgency that time may be short. I'll talk about the kinds of support and information that people find helpful during this stressful time, and the variety of ways in which they begin to adapt, cope and develop strategies for dealing with the reality of metastatic disease.

As you read these stories about how people have reacted and coped to the bad news, you will likely find echoes of your own responses. You will also discover how all of these people surprised themselves by their strength, flexibility and resilience in dealing with this crisis—and perhaps you will see the beginnings of these qualities in yourself.

Getting the bad news

> Getting the "bad news" was beyond any act of courage I had ever faced. It was so far beyond the ordinary that it held no boundaries and took its own mystical and supernatural turns. It was more like a time before words, a time composed of tones and gut feelings. It was so personal. These strange people in white coats pronouncing death, my death, in such a straightforward manner. I spent the major part of the first days wandering around, dazed, trying to absorb and put into framework a death sentence that was being foisted upon me.

This was how Pam Hiebert, diagnosed with Stage IV Breast Cancer, described her emotional response to getting the news about her bone metastasis from her surgeon.

> *Before this phone call I had discussed the cancer diagnosis in her office and it seemed so bizarre, for she kept repeating "We have ways of treating this." All I heard were the numbers, 35 percent chance of being alive in two years. Now I realize statistics are only a crude picture, like little stick figures made up to represent a class of people someone else can look at and line up. I remember at one point getting really angry at this surgeon for not having a solution and I blurted out, "I don't want to hear this. I'll just have to find some people who can tell me better things."*

> *The initial visit with Ralph, my oncologist, came the day after I had found out about the metastasis. I had become aggressive and would no longer answer the phone for results. I wanted action, now! and readily agreed to an earlier appointment with a male oncologist instead of a female colleague of his, whose immediate appointments were booked. I was in such a fit that my skin was itchy all over and I felt extremely nauseous. Sylvan left me lying on a black leather sofa in his waiting room, while she let the nurses know I had arrived. Lying there, staring at the ceiling, I couldn't focus; my mind would only whirl around in macabre pictures. I absolutely could not figure out what was happening to me. Then, Sylvan came back and began to rub my feet and talk to me, letting me know we would soon see a doctor.*

These feelings of unreality in response to the shock of a diagnosis of recurrence are not unusual. "People go through various stages in their attempt to adjust to a serious illness," writes psychologist Margaret Backman. Drawing on studies in the literature of coping and adaptation to illness, Dr. Backman describes the responses of one of her patients as typical of what many people experience at this time: "Following the diagnosis, there was a period of shock, of disbelief, an inability to face the reality of what was happening. She felt like an outsider, looking in at the scene. Emotions were cut off, isolated from what was happening around her. There was a sense of cognitive dissonance, a temporary dissociation of the self from the body and from feelings, expressed numbly as 'This can't be happening to me.' "[1]

Jenilu Schoolman reported similar feelings. She characterized the initial period after her diagnosis with metastases to her liver as a time of panic.

No word more clearly describes my initial reaction to the news. I felt like I had been run over. Like I was about to throw up. Faint. Run in circles. My mind raced and I couldn't calm down. What to do? What to do first? Whom to talk to? What to say? I could not cry or scream. Only move blindly from one racing thought to another.

The people closest to me seemed to panic right along with me. We talked about everything, fast, furiously, intensely. And we ran as though our tails were on fire. This, even though I was very weak from an open liver biopsy and the cancer itself. My life had a weird, dreamlike quality just then. It was a juxtaposition of opposites.

Rivers of tears

According to Dr. Backman, the initial stage of shock and disbelief tends to give way to a period of grief and sometimes despair within a day or two. Again describing a patient of hers, newly diagnosed with serious illness, she writes: "Feelings of anger alternating with hopelessness and deep depression affected her eating and sleeping. She was emotionally flooded with disturbing and persistent thoughts of what was to be: thoughts of self, family, friends, job, upcoming treatments, prognosis. The future appeared bleak, as if there were no way out."[2]

Jenilu wrote:

The deep tide of awareness that my death was real kept rising and falling. I wrote good-bye letters to people I wanted to say good-bye to and began to cry when I realized this was not some melodramatic play. I had assumed that I, like my mother, would survive breast cancer. I never dreamed that it would kill me. Through the adrenaline haze of panic, a deeper pain began to penetrate my psyche as what was happening entered my being. This was the end of my life. This was real.

After her first metastasis was found in the bone of her hip, Lisann Charland experienced many of these same strong emotions.

The "Why me, Lord?" questions came back over and over again in my mind. Where did I go wrong? What could I have done to prevent this? The guilt and helpless feelings left me crying rivers of tears. Poor Buddy cried along with me and felt helpless and angry at what was happening again to me. I wanted to run away to my family—I needed my mommy. I had not even told my mom and dad of the recurrence. After the crying sessions, I begged Buddy for a divorce. I felt doomed, and did not want to be a burden to him. He had been a wonderful husband throughout all the obstacles sent our way. He deserved better than that. He would not hear of my divorce request, and encouraged me to keep my spirits up. He was staying with me for better or for worse. We lived on coffee only for two days.

Four years later another sickening shock came when Lisann's coworkers were presenting her with flowers and a cake as she returned to work after a hospital stay for some tests.

As we began to eat the cake, my phone rang so I stepped out of the lunchroom to answer it since I was awaiting the results of the biopsy. My office is very close to the little lunchroom on the second floor. It was my oncologist and he had the liver biopsy results. He was very sad but had to tell me the results were positive and to return to the office for further treatment discussions. I felt the second shoe just dropped. I felt my world closing in on me. All my plans were shattered. I was going to die for sure this time since this disease had attacked one of my major organs. I closed my office door and tossed a pencil in the ceiling like a dart. I wanted to scream. I slammed my hand on the desk, and walked out of the office in tears. By then, everyone had recognized that it was bad news. I apologized to the group for not being in the mood to stay and enjoy their welcoming gift and began to clear my desk. I felt very sad and apologized many times for "ruining the party."

Pat Leach described the day she found out her cancer had metastasized to her hip after five years:

I was devastated. My husband cried and cried and that gave credence to the seriousness of it all and that I would die. My kids were shocked—they cried, we cried. But they were all hopeful. I felt very good physically so it was hard to believe this was happening. I ran the gamut of emotions and feelings every day—fear, despair, how would I cope with the pain, with dying. I spent a lot of time, still do, thinking about Chris and the kids and how they were going to cope with my suffering and death. And I thought a lot about what I would miss—Chris' arms around me, laughing and playing together, weddings, births—I felt and still feel that life without me would be horrible for my family.

Sometimes the bad news comes all at once, at other times in devastating steps. That is how it was for Glenn and Barb Clabo. Permanently etched in Glenn's memory is the scene when Barb found out, by telephone, that the cancer was in all twelve of her biopsied lymph nodes.

> Barb was sitting in the computer room when she got the news, and I was in the living room. When I walked in, she just plain broke down and cried deep sobbing tears for a long time. It was the same as when I had to tell her her Mom had died. I just held her and couldn't say a word. Anything said would be stupid and most likely not heard. I felt so damn helpless and totally useless. All those caveman instincts came out. I had to help her and make it better. I had to stop her from crying and make her happy. Pretty damn stupid, us men. She finally started to ask questions and I gave her some hope. I really was trying to give us both some hope by talking out loud, and she heard some things that made her feel better.

The next bit of bad news, that her cancer had already metastasized and was at Stage IV, was also delivered by the surgeon.

> On the way to see the surgeon we discussed whether Barb should ask if there were any test results. I went into protection mode and said no. Let's wait until we see the oncologist I thought we could have a few good days without knowing. The surgeon examined her and said everything was coming along fine.... He was looking through her medical record and writing something and mentioned a test result would drive her oncologist to treat her aggressively. Barb asked what the test result said. He said that there were indications of liver mets! Matter of fact, without much hesitation he just told my love that her cancer had spread to a major organ! Is this how it happens to everyone? I wanted to choke him but Barb just went into her questions about are they sure it isn't something else. Barb was the cool one this time. I was so filled with anger that I don't remember anything for a few hours.

Barb was still holding out hope that these lesions that had turned up on tests of her liver might not be what they feared:

> I asked, could it be something else? He said maybe, but since I had so many positive nodes that it was highly likely to be mets. Biopsy was the only way to be sure that it was mets but he didn't recommend it because it

*is a painful procedure and it wouldn't change the oncologist's treatment. I
kept my composure in the office but broke down in the car. Again more
panic and fear. Would I ever get any good news?*

*I kept asking the oncologist the same question over and over but in
many different ways. I felt, in my mind, that I had to make sure he
understood my question. I asked him if these lesions could have been
caused from gall bladder problems. He finally had to be very blunt with
me and tell me that I had mets to the liver.*

These few examples, with the others given in the last chapter, suggest the
devastating immediate emotional impact of a diagnosis of metastatic disease.
Although everyone responds a little differently, what these stories tell us is
that it is normal to experience a sense of numbness, unreality and disbelief
when you first hear the bad news. This is the psyche's way of protecting
itself. These feelings are often followed by deep grief, anger and even despair
for a time. It's important to get loving emotional support, if you can. Having
someone with you and holding you, perhaps sharing in these strong emotions, is what helps most.

While you are absorbing the bad news, it may be difficult to think clearly
and make sense of the information you need to decide about treatment. If
you allow yourself time to express the normal feelings of grief and anger, and
get the emotional support you need, you will feel calmer later on, when it is
time to talk to the doctor, research your treatment, and make decisions.

Three a.m. plans and the dubious future

"It has been assumed that recurrence is more distressing, disabling, and dis-
couraging than the shock of the first diagnosis of cancer," wrote Dr. William
Worden, a psychiatrist who teaches at Harvard Medical School and practices
at the University of Massachusetts Medical Center. Worden studied the experience of patients with several kinds of recurrent cancers, breast cancer being
one, and compared his 102 subjects with newly diagnosed patients from an
earlier study.[3]

*Surprisingly, there was a sizable group of recurrent patients (30 per-
cent) who found the experience less traumatic than their original diagnosis. These were patients who were less surprised by the recurrence, who*

had not let themselves believe that they were cured, and who, in some respect, were living under the proverbial Sword of Damocles.

Lucie Bergmann-Shuster had suspected recurrence for a long time, and experienced the confirmation of her fears, when it came, as a kind of relief. As she awaited the surgery that would give definitive word about whether the mass on her ovary found in the scans was a recurrence of her breast cancer, she was already beginning to prepare herself and her husband for what might lie ahead.

In the intervening week between Thanksgiving and the sail just before the surgery, I had plenty of time to take stock of my dubious future existence. The possibility of life curtailed was very real, although hardly shocking or jolting. I tend to adjust readily to situations, and my body had already told me all year long about what was soon to be confirmed. In these times, I do visualization and what if scenarios in my mind and from that I chart a course of action.

The memories of my mother's death nearly a year prior comforted me with the knowledge that dying was not such a terrible and frightening affair at all, especially with the aid of a hospice provider. My husband and I would talk about my end stages, and he offered to stay with me, possibly taking a leave of absence from work for the duration of the terminal portion. I proposed that somewhere along the way, we might have to hire outside help to handle the household chores and assist with shopping and perhaps even cooking.

It occurred to me that neither my husband nor hired help would be able to continue the upkeep of the garden of which 82 roses in the ground was but a portion of the total garden upkeep. Similarly, our house with its three bedrooms was a bit much for just two people and certainly excessive for the one survivor, my husband. The memories of our life together would haunt him in each room, each niche, and its many shadow plays of morning and afternoon light. So I proposed that we sell our home, and do the little cosmetic lifts needed to make it attractive in the real estate market and then move into a two bedroom condo. Part of the downsizing would be selling off the antiques and furnishing anew but sparsely in a minimalist style. That scenario was painful for me, but whatever loss I would perceive would lighten the future burden for him and that gave me release.

Diagnosed with Stage IV breast cancer that had already spread to her supra-clavicular lymph nodes, Kathy Stone was able almost from the start to acknowledge and accept what had happened to her:

> For the most part my feelings were almost always based on the acceptance that I had cancer. It was a fact...I couldn't **make** it go away. As I read and learned more, and found out just what breast cancer was and what it could mean, was capable of doing...my feelings bordered more on the sad, the mortality part of it, being scared, the unknowing. I can honestly say I haven't yet felt really "cheated" or had the "why me?" syndrome. I think that is because I've always felt that everyone has something really difficult in their life to take care of and no one is exempt. This is part of life, even if it may mean an earlier death than I had planned on...and even that isn't a given to any of us at any time.
>
> I never thought I felt angry about having cancer until the past couple of months...then a few things happened that showed me that maybe I was angry. Even now, I'm not sure if I'm angry that I **have** cancer, or more angry with how it is perceived by others.

As women and their families emerge from the haze of unreality and numb shock, and move through the initial grief and anger, they often begin to experience a sense of great urgency. Although it is rarely the case, death seems imminent. Not knowing if treatment will be effective in bringing about a complete or at least a partial remission, people feel a deep imperative to prepare and plan for what they fear lies ahead. Often, in retrospect, these plans seem irrational or precipitous, but at the time, they fulfill a real need for mastery, and reflect the presence of a heightened sense of mortality.

For Jenilu Schoolman, time was suddenly foreshortened, and she felt a tremendous pressure to complete whatever was undone.

> In the next few weeks, my behavior mirrored my thoughts as I dashed about making sure my will was in order, making funeral arrangements, trying to make sense of my rather messy financial affairs, trying.... I had so many decisions to make; most of them felt bizarre. What music did I want at my memorial service? Where did I want such a service? Who would do the service? What did I want done with my remains?
>
> While lying awake at night, all the horror of dying at a comparatively young age would overwhelm me. I would think of all sorts of prob-

lems the next few years would bring to those I love, and I knew I would not be there to help.

I became compulsive at anticipating my family's needs and tried to dream up solutions only to realize more fully that my death meant I would have no part in helping those I love. Worst of all, I knew my death would cause great pain and I would not be there to comfort.

I have a farm and I worried about its future. Could my business partners maintain the farm? If so, how? What could I do to ensure the security of those people and those things I love? What about simple problems like wood for the next winter? I heat with wood and generally cut it myself. Who would do that chore if I weren't here? Should I breed the goats or not? Did my partners need more or less to care for? Was there anything I could do to help ease the pain of loss for the people I love?

If this sounds odd and illogical, lots of things do at three in the morning. As I tried to prepare myself to die, I tried to prepare my family to go on living. I picked and froze enough raspberries and blueberries to last two years. I made and froze a year's worth of coffee cakes, thinking they'd be useful when people visited after I died, never dreaming I'd be alive to eat them myself.

Where do I start? What do I do first?

Most of us, when faced with a personal crisis, medical or otherwise, find our way through it as best we can. Social scientists, studying how people respond in these circumstances, have found that some situations make coping much more difficult, and that those who cope successfully tend to use certain common strategies.

Harvard psychiatrist William Worden's study of coping showed that stressors associated with high levels of emotional turmoil were:

Degree of sickness (including symptoms, disability and confinement).
Lack of emotional support.
Presence of concurrent concerns unrelated to illness.
Pessimism and fears about death.
Lack of spirituality.
Relative youth.

All of these stressors were significantly correlated, he found, with self-blame. "This self-blame is interesting," Worden commented, "in light of current popular literature that espouses the need to take responsibility for the condition of one's health, whether good or bad."

Worden also found that neither elapsed time since primary diagnosis nor prognosis for recovery had much to do with how hopeful patients felt. If anything, patients who went long periods of time before recurrence, who were most likely to have considered themselves cured, were among the most hopeful, contrary to his initial hypothesis.

In looking at how people coped, Worden found certain factors that helped a great deal, factors we will come across over and over in these pages: 1) knowledge of the medical system and how to negotiate it, 2) understanding of cancer treatments and side effects, and 3) familiarity with the extent and availability of a support system. "Support continues to be an important mediator of distress," Worden observed, "and the support systems for recurrent patients had already been tested at the time of their original diagnosis. By the time the cancer recurred, these patients knew with some degree of certainty what support would be available."[4]

The women and men I spoke with shared these same urgent needs for information and support. As the first force of the emotional impact of the diagnosis begins to lessen, most people newly diagnosed with recurrence feel an intense and urgent need to *do* something, to take some sort of concerted action. Uppermost in their minds, of course, are questions about treatment, prognosis and selecting the best medical team—issues that will be discussed at some length in the following chapters. At the same time, as they go through the often maddening hurry up and wait process of testing, consulting and seeking opinions on treatment, they are also reaching out to others for emotional support, and embarking on a search for meaning.

Reaching out for support can take many forms. Often it can mean seeking out new sources. Disappointed with the response of their friends, and sensing a need for more emotional support, as well as for information, Glenn Clabo subscribed to the Breast Cancer Discussion List on the Internet.

I received an onslaught of welcome messages and a very warm welcome feeling. I think that this day was the day that made me realize that we weren't alone and that I needed people's help. I learned that I could just state my feelings much better though written words than I could verbally.

If they are fortunate enough to have a close and resilient relationship, couples reach out for one another, experiencing an intimacy deepened by crisis. For Glenn, news of the spread of the cancer to Barb's lymph nodes provoked great rushes of tenderness and anguish that sought expression in words, the depth and passion of which surprised him.

How could I keep giving Barb hope knowing it wasn't going to be good news? I knew that it was very probable that the cancer was somewhere else. I wasn't ready for this. I was supposed to die first.

I started writing a poem. I never liked poems or attempted to write a poem before. What made me do this is still beyond me. I do know that I was embarrassed by it and didn't show it to her or anyone else for a long time. Even though I now know it isn't any good, I'm not embarrassed by it anymore. It says so much that I can't say. The world be damned.

A Monster Without Heart

Side by side though our lives
We before the other
Our souls have grown to be just one
Just one and not another

I fight this fight beside you now
I run through every wall
When you cry, you cry our tears
When you trip, I fall

I feel your fear, your hurt, my love
I want to take your pain
Listen for my scream, my love
I feel the pain the same

Get the hell away from her
I've loved her from the start
I'm not yet through holding her
You monster without heart

Get the hell away from her
You'll never win her heart
Our soul has grown to be just one
As one it will not part.

"Where do I start? What do I do first?" After crying out these words, Lisann Charland reached out for support.

> *I started by notifying my out-of-town family and friends that the disease had recurred. The support and encouragement I got from both near and far away was unbelievable. My Buddy was a rock. I knew he hurt just as much as I did throughout this whole nightmare. I felt blessed and lucky to have him and all the family and friends in this great time of need. My sister and brothers were devastated. My in-laws were wonderful as usual. My employer advised me I could work whenever I wanted. Everyone was very supportive, and offered to help me in any way I needed.*

Like most of the others, Lisann had someone she wanted to protect from hearing the bad news.

> *I could not tell my mother I had the recurrence because I did not have the heart and strength to explain it to her on the telephone, and not being there to hold her hand for her sake and my sake.*

In the ensuing time, as Lisann shared her distress with family and friends, she wrestled with trying to find some meaning in what was happening to her.

> *I cried and cried alone and in front of people. I felt cheated once again. I felt I was a good and honest person, and yet, was being punished somehow. I had to talk to myself daily and convince myself that "this too shall pass," and that I was going to get better with the treatment. Indeed, my faith kept me going. I felt I was going to be fine. God was really testing me again to see whether I could take it.*

Like Lisann, Barbara Ragland heard about her recurrence at work. Although her surgeon had already told her he thought the two lesions she'd found on the old surgery site were malignant, Barbara had still held out hope that he was wrong. It was hard to believe that the cancer had actually come back after nineteen years.

> *I sat for a moment at my desk and tried to catch my breath. I remember I was shaking. Then I walked in to tell my supervisor in the next office. I had a few moments in which my voice started shaking and I cried for a little bit. Since there wasn't really anything anyone could do, I went back to my office and tried to resume working but my mind was a blur.*

Divorced since her primary diagnosis in 1974, when support groups for breast cancer hadn't even existed, this time she determined to reach out.

> *I told everyone: family, friends, faculty and students that I worked with. For some reason, the burden seems lighter by not keeping things pent up inside. I've always been straightforward with my family and I think it is a comfort to them knowing I'm not withholding information from them.*

> *With fellow workers, I wanted them to know directly from me, not from whispering around the edges trying to find out what my situation was. I also preferred that they know I was away from work for a scan or doctor's appointment—not for a vacation. I found so much caring and compassion from students and faculty. Some would make a point to come in and just give me a hug or to tell me they were praying for me. This was a support group—certainly not a group who had "been there," but a group that really was concerned.*

At the time of her primary diagnosis, Barbara had sought support from her church. Church elders had joined her in prayer at her bedside before a second biopsy, and hailed the benign results as a miracle. As a single mother and sole support of her three children, she had prayed then that she would live long enough for her youngest, then five years old, to reach age eighteen.

> *Everyone knew of this prayer. When my son turned eighteen, we all rejoiced and I have thanked God ever since for allowing this to happen. I taught Sunday School for the next eleven years. When the cancer recurred, my youngest was twenty-five. Although I was absolutely crushed with the news, one of my first thoughts was that I had lived seven years past the time I had prayed for and was determined to live. If I beat this thing before, I know there's a good chance I can again.*

Penny Lebow knew just what she needed after the impact of discussing her treatment with her oncologist.

I remember being in the doctor's office at the treatment conference, trying to hold a stiff upper lip so I could grasp everything being said, although having moments of panic overwhelm me. After leaving, I remember going to our car with Mark, knowing I needed to cry and knowing Mark did too, but unable to do it with the abandon I needed in the car. The only thought I had was about my closest friend, Leora, who lived and worked nearby, imagining her big warm arms around me, creating a safe space to let go. I called her up immediately and went to her house where I related the news and we all cried together.

For Pam Hiebert, the diagnosis of recurrence provoked an existential crisis.

On the day the surgeon said metastasis, I experienced the lowest and most frighteningly intense Thursday night I have ever felt in my entire life. I stood at the living room window and stared out onto the street below for hours. I groped desperately for understanding. I remember trying to rationalize, thinking how people with AIDS were actually worse off than me. I remember thinking about all the people who have lived on this earth and how everyone eventually died. I remember the beginnings of my own awareness that I would also die.

From that awareness came a spiritual awakening that would transform Pam's experience of her illness.

It was at this darkest hour of my life that I found spirit. She rose in me like a mother protecting her young. It was in this darkest hour that I began to formulate my own battle. I let go of what I had been holding and began to plan how I would die—but die a warrior's death—I would lay claim to this diagnosis and I would launch war. I would die a death befitting a warrior, an amazon, a goddess of fire and sword. I would name my dying and lay claim to its process. I mentally moved through a spirit world of basic survival.

The need for connection with and support of the women's community she and Sylvan were part of came next.

It was at this time that I called forth my hair-cutting ceremony to prepare for battle. To strip my body clean. To disengage from earthly burden. To prepare my body for engagement of the enemy.

Many women elect to shave their heads before their chemotherapy-induced hair loss begins. Not only does it reduce the mess from falling hair, but it also exerts a measure of control, which becomes a vital part of coping. Drawing her friends close to her, Pam created a moving ritual, transforming a loss filled with fear into a challenging engagement.

> Our living room was filled with women from all walks of life. Word had gotten around that I was holding a hair-cutting ceremony and all women were invited. Many women from the choir, some from work, some from my church came. I was the warrior Queen, sitting at the head, perched upon my royal throne. I spread a blanket before me with all the trinkets of my past. People had brought things too, a stuffed kangaroo, feathers, crystals, transformation stones. I talked of battle and shedding my skin. Each woman in the room in turn arose, came toward me, and cut a piece of my long straight hair. Then it was shaved along the sides and the back and pulled into one giant long mohawk. I dipped my finger in a bowl of silver glitter and drew streaks of warrior's paint across my face, vowing to fight to the finish in whatever battle was set before me.

Bob Stafford felt a need for ritual as well. By the time Bob went to see the oncologist, he had already inferred, from what his internist had said, that his breast cancer had recurred in his hip.

> I decided to do something special that day. My wife wanted to go with me to the oncologist to hear the news. On the way I stopped at the church of a pastor friend. We told him where we were going and why. I then asked him if he would do a wedding ceremony for my wife and I there and then. Unbeknownst to her I had bought her a ring and wanted to redo my marriage vows to her. The church was beautiful because it was decorated for Christmas and there were more flowers then than when we were first married. My pastor friend's wife served as our witness.

Later, they were able to talk about what lay ahead.

> My wife's biggest concern was whether I would be around to help get our two children through high school. Our son was 10 and our daughter 13 at the time. We were at an emotional crossroads, facing terminal cancer and celebrating the renewing of our marriage vows. It didn't matter if you laughed or cried because you had reason for both.

After an ultrasound test confirmed that there was a mass on her ovary, Lucie Bergmann-Shuster and her husband, Cy, decided nevertheless to continue their plans for Thanksgiving with out-of-town friends. The surgeon's appointment would be on Monday; and there was the weekend to get through. But they hoped for their enduring connection with the natural world to uplift them and grant them some peace.

During a long, boring stretch of road on their way towards Yosemite National Park, well known as a hunting ground for hawks, Cy and Lucie were keeping an eye out for birds of prey.

> Suddenly, a hawk dived at our windshield, veering off a few feet before impact. It sent chills down our spines and no sooner did our suddenly jangled beings recover, than yet another bird of prey crossed the windshield again only a few feet away from the moving car. It was as though the two flight patterns were making a sign of a cross in our path. My husband and I looked at each other in amazement and I said, "I think the spirit world is trying to tell us something." After a long silence, I said to Cy, "I think that perhaps the hawks are my spirit beings after all. Why else would they come so close to me at this loaded and uncertain time in my life?"

> We all got to go for hike in Big Trees to look at the majestic sequoias. The ancient, giant trees allow for a serenity and peaceful acceptance of timelessness within a world of decay while heralding new growth in musty, pine-scented peat. Both of us savored the greater calm and let it carry us through to the Monday doctor appointment.

Then, three days before the exploratory surgery that would give Lucie a definitive answer about an ovarian mass found in her scans, Lucie and Cy were unexpectedly invited by friends to help them check out a sailboat they were thinking of buying.

> It was a little miracle of finding joy in unexpected places and the prospect of the sail helped us both getting past Saturday. That Sunday, the weather which had been iffy and overcast most of the week with occasional showers, turned magically warm with just the right kind of wind to allow the testing of all the major sails, of which there were many since this was a yacht racing sloop. It felt so good for me to know that my body was still there for me and vital while trimming the sheets for this big 50-foot vessel. In the course of the sail, I told my friend June that I would be going

*in for surgery and that it might very well be cancer and if so, that I might
not live very much longer, so I thanked her for this wonderful moment in
time to be sailing without worry on this absolutely gorgeous day on the
Monterey Bay.*

*While our friends, the prospective buyers, negotiated around the next
step in the business transaction with the broker, my husband and I took in
the waning light of the day, the scent of the salt air and the calming ache
of our bodies as our feet accustomed themselves to solid ground. We knew
we would sleep well this coming night having cherished the day both with
our minds and our bodies.*

I do not want this dance

For each of these people, this was the beginning of an ongoing adjustment
process that included a search for meaning within the experience, as well as
an attempt to regain mastery over the recurrence and over life in general. If
you had spoken to any of them a week or two after their diagnoses, resilience might be one of the last words they would have used to describe themselves. Nevertheless, as they moved from shock and grief to the first steps of
coping, resiliency was much in evidence.

RS Lazarus and S. Folkman, researchers in coping theory,[5] distinguish
between what they term "emotion-focused coping," a process of inner recon-
ciliation where the person is able to alter the meaning of the situation, and
"problem-focused coping," which defines the problem and its possible external solutions, weighs alternatives, works to change environmental stressors
and expectations, and learns new skills and behaviors. Throughout the
book, we'll see inner and outer processes working in tandem, for both are
crucial.

This chapter has looked primarily at "emotion-focused coping" in the early
days following a diagnosis of recurrent breast cancer. In each of the stories
above, an initial emotional and spiritual crisis moves toward some degree of
resolution through an inner or outer action. Most of the time, these actions
are related to the bonds between people and to some kind of spiritual or creative connection.

For Glenn, joining the Internet Discussion List and expressing his deep love
for his wife there in poetry and prose helped him connect with others and
sustained his strength in supporting her. Lisann's reaching out to friends and

family, and grappling with her religious beliefs, brought her through the worst of her despair. As a woman alone, Barbara's decision to reveal her situation to friends at work and in her church, as well as her family, made her feel cared about, and allowed her to perceive the intervening years since her primary diagnosis with gratitude, rather than bitterness. Penny and Mark knew that they needed to grieve with their friends. Pam's hair-cutting ceremony surrounded by her community of women provided her with a means to reframe her upcoming struggle in terms that gave her optimism and strength. Through renewing their marriage vows in the church where their wedding had been, Bob affirmed that he would be there for his wife, Sherry, and their children as long as he was able. Lucie and her husband, Cy, passed the difficult time before test results and surgery by seeking restoration and spiritual connection in the woods and on the water, in the natural world they loved, and in each other.

All of these people moved past the shock and grief of diagnosis to do something to regain the control they had lost, or to seek a deeper contact with others or with their own sources of personal meaning. By doing so, each took a first step in the direction of coping and acceptance.

When Pam Hiebert's tumor markers were on the rise for the second time, after her bone mets had successfully been controlled for over three years, she wrote these lines:

> *I cannot run, I know that from the last encounter.*
> *There is no defense, but to seek to pass through.*
> *My pulse is strong, the months I have spent in healing*
> *Are to be tested now.*
>
> *I do not want this encounter, this unwelcome second half*
> *Stalking me—stinging me with pain, tearing at me,*
> *Ripping my years away—*
>
> *I do not want this dance.*

CHAPTER 5

The Problem of Knowledge

Doctors, Information-Seeking and Statistics

KNOWLEDGE AND DISCLOSURE are often a mixed blessing for someone with a life-threatening illness. While accurate information can inform and protect, ensuring the best available care, at the same time, reading and hearing the cold, hard details can be painful at times for patients and their families.

This chapter explores the issues raised concerning disclosure by physicians, and the pitfalls and benefits of doing your own medical research. As an information seeker, it's important for you to understand the emotional fall-out often provoked by knowledge and prepare for it by finding ways of putting what you learn into perspective. This chapter shares some ideas and advice about how to do this, from published authors who have researched their cancers as well as from the patients interviewed for this book.

I want to know, but...

> I told Sherry, my wife, that next month I enter the "maybe more" phase of prognosis. Last June when I laid in the emergency room, I was faced with having a pulmonary angiogram done, putting a wire up a vein in my groin into my lungs to see if I had blood clots in my lungs. It was something I had questions about doing. Trying to encourage me, the doctor in charge came in and said he had talked with my oncologist about my situation. Then he said, "Dr. T said that you have a good six months at least, probably a year, and maybe more."

Although he no longer had expectations for a cure, and knew that his tumor markers were again on the rise, Bob Stafford felt stunned, hearing these blunt words. Depending upon how they are interpreted, such predictions often have a profound impact on a patient's morale.

He robbed me of hope in trying to encourage me. He set the mental time limits in my mind. Even though I refuse to believe them, they sneak into my mind and say, "Time is short...." Hope is vital to the patient, the victor. It is what is robbed from them by the medical community, their family and friends every time they don't believe in the life ahead.

Issues of information-seeking and disclosure—especially with regard to prognosis—are of vital importance to anyone dealing with metastatic breast cancer. For Bob Stafford, this secondhand news from his oncologist felt intensely personal in its impact. Yet this particular moment of unwitting revelation points also to larger social trends that every cancer patient would do well to consider.

Well within the memory of most people who have cancer, attitudes in medicine about revealing diagnoses and prognoses have made a complete turnaround, from euphemisms and concealment to unvarnished reality, clinically delivered. This is true for both physicians and patients.

In 1961, 90 percent of physicians surveyed said that they preferred not to tell a patient of a cancer diagnosis. By 1977, a complete reversal of attitude had taken place: 97 percent of university hospital medical staff said that their preference was for telling patients a cancer diagnosis. While citing the influence of medical school and hospital training in this change, the authors of this study cautioned, "Physicians are still basing their policies on emotion-laden personal conviction rather than the outcome of properly designed scientific studies."[1]

Patients have changed in their attitudes as well. In a 1980 survey of 256 cancer patients, Dr. Barrie Cassileth found that patients' attitudes were in line with "the contemporary standard of informed and active involvement." Younger patients preferred the participatory, informed role, while older patients preferred the older, non-participatory model.[2] According to a Harris poll in 1982, 96 percent of Americans wanted to be told if they had cancer, and 85 percent wanted a "realistic estimate" of how long they had to live if their type of cancer "usually leads to death in less than a year."[3]

Most of the people I interviewed felt this way, too. Barb Pender wrote:

The relationship that I have had with Dr. M is one of honesty. I have told him on numerous occasions that I want him to tell me when the prognosis does not look good, when my time is limited, and I have stressed that

I honor honesty above all values when dealing with my cancer. He has been wonderful to me and I have always felt blessed to have a doctor that treated me as a flesh-and-blood woman rather than a file on his desk— and I hope that when the time comes that he might have to be brutally honest that I will remember my own words to him.

It isn't easy for a patient or a physician to go against the prevailing social beliefs, however. In a thoughtful essay in *the New England Journal of Medicine*, Dr. George Annas observed:

A culture's general attitude toward death strongly influences what information about their prognosis will be provided to terminally ill patients. In our culture, with its unprecedented life expectancy, we tend to deny death altogether and celebrate new forms of medical technology designed to forestall death. In this context, it is not surprising that physicians often conceal prognostic information from their patients, just as most physicians once refused to use the word "cancer." But concealment of prognosis from patients near death makes them feel abandoned and makes physicians feel estranged.[4]

These honest conversations can be agonizing. After some weeks of increasing pain, Kathy Stone wrote her friends on the Breast Cancer Discussion List that she'd been to see her oncologist.

*He told me today that he needed to be up front with me and tell me my prognosis didn't look good at all...that the best he could do was try to keep one step ahead of the cancer and it was getting harder and harder to do and I should be aware that time was running out. I'm not sure if that statement made me **really mad** or put me into a scared as hell mode...I just know I came away feeling lost...and angry...and **not about to give up**. I might be shaking in my boots, but my boots are going to keep walking and maybe even kick some butt.*

A flurry of messages came in response, most questioning the competence and wisdom of her doctor. Realizing she'd given the wrong impression, Kathy responded:

*I wasn't angry with the doctor for him telling me there wasn't much they could do anymore except treat the pain...I **asked** him for an answer, so I expected him to be honest with me...I wanted to know what he thought my prognosis was so I could make decisions and choices. No one*

likes to think about there being that answer of "nothing else can be done."
It's easy to get mad at the messenger.

PJ Hagler has spoken about her prognosis with her doctor on a number of occasions:

> *Dr. Nick and I have been able to honestly discuss the few choices we*
> *both have in the treatment left open to us. I luckily still have a few options*
> *left open to me. When I started on Taxol we had this type of discussion.*
> *My question was, "What is an unrealistic expectation of long life. If the*
> *Taxol were to work, how much of a future can I hope for?" Well, my Dr.*
> *Nick is not one to be cornered into a time limit on life. He said he sets no*
> *limits. His intention is to get a year at a time. He told me when he signed*
> *my paper for a handicap sticker for my car that he never thought he*
> *would get to sign two of those in my case. The sticker is good for two*
> *years and he thought one would be my limit, when we started this adven-*
> *ture. I've told him I'm not afraid to die, I'm just not through living yet. I*
> *know that I will not have another 10 years probably but I could get lucky.*
> *I don't live with the idea that I might not be here tomorrow or next week*
> *or even next year. I still plan for the future. Mike and I talk about retire-*
> *ment days. But, realistically I also talk about when or if I'm not here. And*
> *I'm okay with that. I have an inner peace about my death.*

By the time PJ wrote these words, she'd been dealing with breast cancer for fourteen years, and metastatic disease for five. Clearly, coming to a state of acceptance is a result of a long, ongoing process. The patient with metastatic disease is presented with many opportunities to absorb bad news and learn to go on from there. Not everyone is fortunate enough to have the compassionate medical care, emotional support and inner resilience to do so.

The literature of medical disclosure contains stories of patients who die immediately after being told of a terminal prognosis. Anecdotally, at least, bad news can kill. "In a lot of cases, it causes people to just give up," says Marc Schoen, director of the Psychoimmune Program at Cedars-Sinai Medical Center in Los Angeles. But not all patients react this way, he says. "The flip side is the people who respond by saying, 'I'll show you.' It ignites them. It's just the motivation they need to fight."[5]

In an article with the provocative title of "Words as Scalpels," Dr. SJ Reiser writes:

The widespread belief among doctors that the revelation of threatening news causes patients considerable anguish and seriously erodes the prospect of maintaining their hope encouraged a policy of concealment for many centuries.... Advocates point out that candor can be beneficial and is favored by many patients, and that a policy of concealment usually fails to work, tends to place stress on patients by constraining discussion of anxieties generated by vague or implicit knowledge of the true situation, and exerts a damaging effect on trust in the medical relationship.[6]

Will I die, doctor? How long do I have?

Whether you decided to ask it or not, the first question in your mind after recovering from the shock of hearing your breast cancer has metastasized is most likely: Will I die from this disease, and if so, when? It is part of human nature to believe that knowing an outcome with certainty, no matter how glum, is better than living with uncertainty. And if time is short, you may want to know so that you can rearrange your priorities and tackle the unfinished business of your life while you are still feeling well enough to do so. Knowing how serious a cancer diagnosis is can also play a vital role in determining treatment decisions, as will be clear later on.

It becomes crucial, therefore, to consider the problems associated with disclosure of information, prognosis and statistics. What you are told, what you discover for yourself and the way you make sense of this information about your illness will determine a great deal of your day-to-day quality of life, for it affects everything concerning the disease: your attitude toward treatment and the treatment choices you make; your feelings of hope; the plans and priorities you decide upon; the way you connect with your friends and family; and the way the future appears to you.

You would not be reading this book if you were not an information seeker, so it may seem to you that simple truth is best. You want all the information the doctors have, and to be helped to understand it as best you can. But the truth is never simple, and the way it is delivered and interpreted can make a real difference.

In fact, the way in which a treatment is presented to you may well affect the choice you make, and you may not even be aware of this influence. An ingenious experiment in medical decision-making presented the same surgery outcome statistics to patients, but in two different ways. The lung cancer patients in this study were given a statistic to help them make a decision between surgery and radiation treatment. For every 100 men undergoing lung surgery, one group was told, statistics showed that ninety would live through the post-operative period, and thirty-four would be alive at the end of five years. The other group was told that, given the same 100 men having surgery, ten would die during the post-operative period, and sixty-six would be dead by the end of five years. Though the information was the same, surgery appeared far less attractive as an option to those who received the mortality statistics versus the survival statistics.[7] This is called the "framing effect," and was surprisingly just as pronounced with physicians as with patients. The only antidote to such subtle persuasions is awareness of the bias and having a variety of information sources.

There are other common errors of reasoning that most of us make. Risk, for example, is often misperceived categorically, with little distinction made between high- and low-risk situations. Risk is risk to us—a unified concept, with no shades of gray. Hence the fear of airplane travel, statistically far more safe than automobile travel, that follows an airliner crash. Because of this tendency, people often devalue a treatment that will lessen the odds (decreasing risk)—often the only achievable goal in cancer treatment—seeing this as relatively unimportant by comparison with their quest for what the authors of this study call the "enchanting appeal of zero risk."

In her counseling of metastatic breast cancer patients considering high-dose chemotherapy, Memorial Sloan-Kettering social worker Rosalind Kleban finds that these women are often strongly attracted to the notion that this rigorous treatment carries both the possibility of cure, however remote, and the appeal of liberation from continuous treatment, even if for a limited time. "They do see it as 'this will be it and I will not have to be in treatment any more.' In order to go through this, women have convinced themselves that this will do it." Although it may be equally effective, conventional treatment offers the much less appealing alternative of continuous treatment. "Approaching it as chronic is much more difficult, unless they are willing to be a bit more open," says Kleban.

Pam Hiebert describes how difficult it was for her to process information after her diagnosis in February of 1993.

> *I was frantic those first several months trying to make sense of what I was being told: "You need to get your affairs in order," and "Stage IV Breast Cancer has a life expectancy of around two years." I found myself very angry deep down and profoundly frustrated at all the outside advice that was coming to me (try this, try that), while no one would talk to me about dying, about death, about what it was like and how I could prepare.*

Bare information about prognosis and statistics delivered in the context of hurried medical consultations is often brutal in its emotional impact.

> *Coming in to the medical system with such a bad prognosis meant having it hammered home repeatedly that I was likely to go fast. No one in the medical field seemed anxious to give much encouragement. My oncologist raised the greatest hope when he demonstrated his willingness to go at this aggressively and challenged me to stay the course. He also admitted to me privately that he could not produce a cure but that he would stay with me in whatever lay before me.*

Long time patient advocate and writer Norman Cousins, noted for his iconoclastic views on the practice of medicine, argued that doctors have a responsibility to do far more than convey information.

> *All of us have been intimidated by illness. We've had our attention fixed on problems and not on possibilities, and we tend to become paralyzed by the fear. If a patient leaves the physician's office in a state of emotional devastation, then the environment for effective treatment has been impaired. The physician who volunteers a terminal date, for example, or allows himself to be pressured into allowing a terminal date may actually be putting a hex on the patient. You can perceive a dilemma: a patient must not be fooled, but on the other hand, a patient in a state of utter despair and depression may have very little inclination for going on with treatment.*

In his view, communication is crucial. "The patient has the right to know, and the physician has the obligation to inform," Cousins said. But a good doctor learns to be expert in "rounding out the corners of truth. A serious diagnosis can be communicated as a challenge rather than as a verdict."[8]

Compassionate physicians are acutely aware of the impact of this kind of information, and strive to be sensitive to it—and certainly it was this impulse, at least in part, that led to the belief that concealing diagnosis and prognosis was appropriate during the era of the paternalistic physician and passive patient. Many doctors are reluctant to quote mortality rates or statistics on survival time to patients, preferring to tell them, rightly, that no one can know for sure how long a particular patient will live, and that mortality statistics are based on large groups, and are to be used to weigh decisions about treatment, not as predictors of individual life expectancy. They will explain that since you are an individual, there is simply no way to predict, with any certainty, whether you will be in the larger group that will succumb to breast cancer within the predicted period of time, or the smaller group that lives for many years with it as a chronic disease, or even survives to die of other causes. While initially frustrated, many patients are ultimately able to transform this uncertainty into an opportunity for hope.

No one I interviewed demonstrated this more clearly than Caren Buffum, in her response to a member of the Breast Cancer Discussion List who inquired about mortality rates for metastatic disease.

> Sorry, but I don't trust statistics. Even my doctor looks me in the eye and says, "You are not a statistic." He has explained to me that the medical community uses statistics for decision making (you know, like one uses odds at the race track), but I'm curious why you want to know the "true" numbers. It will not tell you what is true about you. I don't offer this as a criticism, but rather as an encouragement. By surviving 10 years after my mastectomy, I am proving the statistics "correct" (the ones that say something like 86 percent of Stage I node-negative patients will survive 10 years or more). What that statistic doesn't tell you is that not all of those survivors will be disease-free and will survive to year 11. Now take another statistic—I won't give you the exact number because it may have a negative effect on someone reading this—but since my recurrence, I have survived more than twice as long as the average survivor. If I had believed that statistic, I would have been a basket case several years ago. If you are trying to get a fix on your "odds," I suggest you assume you are the best case scenario, the far end of the bell curve, the one that always does better than the odds. If evidence should then prove otherwise, you can deal with that when it comes. I believe in getting all the information I can where it will help me make educated decisions and create understanding about my medical situation. But I shy away from statistics that just give me numbers to fix my thoughts on—numbers that give me "averages." I'm not average.

But there are many who don't want to be shielded by their doctors and who may see even the above discussion as a continuation of an unwanted medical paternalism. These people are likely to come across the statistics in their own research of medical sources, just as I did when I was newly diagnosed with primary breast cancer, without anyone there to help them interpret what they read.

Sue Tokuyama is one of the many I interviewed willing to pay the price that this sort of knowledge exacts:

> *I've heard of women who find out they have cancer, find a doctor and then do everything that doctor says, without discussion. They need some kind of authority figure in which to trust their lives. Once that is done, there is no need, in their view, for further deliberation.*

> *Then, there's the feisty kind, (I offer myself as an example), for whom no amount of information is too much, no authority figure is too exalted to call "Chuck."*

Information from whatever source, whether from physicians, medical references or other patients, can be disturbing as well as enlightening, for a number of reasons. Even when correctly interpreted, charts and tables may have a negative emotional impact at first. They can make a human struggle with illness seem coldly clinical. Reading morbidity and mortality figures on the printed page can be a chilling experience, especially in the beginning. However necessary this information may be, it's reasonable to expect and prepare for this emotional response. Glenn Clabo wrote wistfully about what he learned concerning his wife Barb's Stage IV disease and its bleak prognosis:

> *I sometimes envy the less inquisitive when it comes to some things. Maybe not knowing is easier when you come to this point of the process. I sure don't recommend that anyone actually read a pathology report. Just let the doctor explain it. The printed words make it all too real.*

Misinterpretation of statistics is particularly problematic for the do-it-yourself researcher poring over medical texts and journal articles. Some cautionary thoughts about the nature of statistics are in order. "We cannot do what the public thinks we can do with statistics," says Dr. Joanne Lynn, an expert statistician at Dartmouth Medical School. "People think they are going to get something that maps out their life plan, rather than something that is more like the odds. They think that doctors have a real clue, and they don't."[9]

We've all known people who have far outlived expectations, and a few who survived despite terrible odds. Greg Anderson, founder of the Cancer Conquerors Foundation, is convinced that statistics have no place in a prognosis. "Statistics are almost always interpreted negatively," said Anderson who, at 45, received a diagnosis of lung cancer in 1984 and was told he had about thirty days to live. But Anderson found literature on lung cancer that put his chances of beating the disease at five percent. "At first I was hugely depressed. Then, as I thought about it, it made me decide to do everything I could to be in that five percent. But most people don't make it that far. Most get bogged down in despair."[10]

One of the most intelligent perspectives on interpreting cancer statistics comes from an essay written by the Harvard evolutionary biologist Stephen Jay Gould entitled "The Median is Not the Message."[11] When Gould was diagnosed in 1982 with a rare and deadly abdominal cancer known as mesothelioma, his doctor told him that there was "nothing really worth reading" in the medical literature. Undeterred, he did a library computer search on his disease. "I realized with a gulp why my doctor had offered that humane advice," Gould wrote. "The literature couldn't have been more brutally clear: mesothelioma is incurable, with a median mortality of only eight months after discovery."

Most people, unschooled in statistics, would think that this meant that they had only eight months to live. As a scientist, Gould knew better. The median, the measure of central tendency used in this example, describes that point in a distribution that separates the cases in half. Half the people lived fewer than eight months, and half lived for a longer time. Like the mean (average) or mode (most common score), the median is only an abstraction. Yet we tend to see it as the one essential truth to be extracted from that statistic. "We still carry the historical baggage of a Platonic heritage that seeks sharp essences and definite boundaries," he explains, adding that we tend to see the mean and median as "the hard realities, and the variation that permits their calculation as a set of transient and imperfect measurements of this hidden essence." In fact, the opposite is true. "All evolutionary biologists know that variation itself is nature's only irreducible essence. Variation is the hard reality."

Now that he knew that half the people with his disease would live longer than eight months, Gould set about determining the shape of the distributional curve, and in fact found it was what statisticians call "right skewed," meaning that some patients lived on for many years. Why not he? Just as important, the statistics had been based on conventional treatment. With a new experimental protocol and the best medical care, he might well outlive even the best predictions. "I had obtained," Gould concluded, "in all probability, the most precious of all possible gifts in the circumstances—substantial time." Fourteen years later, Gould considers himself a survivor.

If you research the studies on treatment of metastatic disease, you are likely to encounter the same problems. Because statistics in cancer treatment look at factors like partial and complete remissions over a number of years, the published research literature for metastatic breast cancer will always, by its nature, be a few years behind the best current available treatments. Thus, your odds are likely to be an improvement over what you read in the studies. It is important to keep this in mind.

For further information on how to go about researching your illness, see Appendix B, *Resources*.

Doing it yourself

As with anything else, there are risks and benefits to researching your own disease. Steve Dunn, who had metastatic cancer that carried only a four percent chance of survival, clarifies the pros and cons to researching the medical literature on his website.[12]

In favor of doing your own research are the following factors, according to Dunn:

- Since not every cancer doctor can be entirely up to date on the latest treatments and findings for the more than 100 kinds of cancer, and you have the time and certainly the motivation to research yours in depth, you may actually discover something important he or she isn't aware of.

- The very process of researching is empowering, in that it permits you to feel you are doing something constructive to combat the disease and may help you to cope emotionally far better than you might if you handed these decisions over to your doctors.

- Some treatments for advanced breast cancer are still controversial, for example, the various forms of high-dose chemotherapy with stem cell or bone marrow rescue. The more you know, and the more you understand about what is not yet known and the risks you are taking, the more rational and informed a decision you will be able to make.

"If you are an HMO member," Dunn rightly points out, "you have special reason to do some research. The less care an HMO gives, and the less often it refers patients outside their network, the more profit the HMO makes. In my experience, HMOs are particularly unlikely to tell their patients about promising new treatments or clinical trials. In this situation, a little research could save your life."

On the other hand, doing this kind of research can be difficult and intimidating for the layperson. Perhaps you have a friend or relative who could help, someone who has special expertise in reading and interpreting medical journals. For some of the people I interviewed, it was the spouse or partner who undertook the medical research. Whoever does it, this means learning both a new language and a new way of thinking, if you aren't already somewhat familiar with medicine and scientific method. It means learning to discuss these issues with physicians and assume a collaborative role in decision making. Because you aren't a doctor, there's a chance you may misinterpret what you read—although discussing what you've read with your doctor will help you make sense of it.

Having undertaken the research for his wife Mary's Stage IV breast cancer, Scott Kitterman gave this advice to a man whose mother had recently been diagnosed:

> One of the biggest things you or someone in your family can do for your mother is become an "expert" on breast cancer. While you won't know as much as the doctors do, your mother needs to know enough to have a general understanding of what is being done to her and more importantly why. There is a lot of judgment in medicine and often there is not a single obviously correct answer. When there are a range of options, the more informed your mother is, the more she will be able to control the direction her treatment goes. Learning the jargon is also a critical part of this. If you use the correct fancy words, then you must know what you are talking about and they will pay closer attention to what you say.

As I've already pointed out, reading the medical literature published for physicians means you will run across tables of mortality statistics as they apply to differing treatments and the various stages of the disease. Since the temptation will be to apply the statistics you find to your own situation, you must look carefully to see that the treatments are not outdated (with poorer results) and that you've interpreted the prognostic factors accurately. In addition, instead of the carefully screened list of side effects your doctor gives you, you will read about everything that could possibly happen as a result of the drugs you are taking, described coldly and clinically. This can be very alarming since many of the chemotherapy drugs used in advanced cancer treatment are quite toxic. Lastly, you may well find nothing new as a result of your investigations. What you discover may be just what your doctor had recommended in the first place.

This doesn't mean your efforts have been a waste of time. "You can look at this two ways," Dunn suggests. "If the prognosis is really bad, confirming it could be difficult to take. On the other hand, if the prognosis is reasonable, you can rest assured that you are indeed getting the best treatment available. In either case, knowing that your doctor is recommending the best treatment will also increase your confidence in him (or her)."

Before she could focus on information-seeking, Kim Banks discovered it was important that she first get past the early phase of shock and grief.

> Even with a caring doctor, friends and family, the bad news can be devastating. Initially, I need to have a good cry and really mourn the news for a day or two. After that I try to put it behind me. If I don't really grieve, I find I can't move forward. It's a very important healing process for me. After that, I research like a maniac on the topic! While I trust my doctor's recommendations, I know that he is busy treating all types of cancer, and new treatments are constantly appearing on the horizon. I also learn of alternative treatments that I would not have heard about through my doctor. The knowledge empowers me and provides me the comfort that I am making the right choice of treatment for me. I did a lot of research on my own, using medical journals, medical databases and a medical service that provides recent research documents. I also talked with a number of people throughout the community through my support group and with my nutritionist who specializes in treating breast cancer patients.

Solid, factual information can sometimes help to clarify what is known and begin to address the fearful fantasies that people have. Pam Hiebert admits having some pretty confused ideas of what might happen to her.

> In my wild imagination, in the beginning, I thought bone mets would lead to my rib bones dissolving as it spread (I had a lesion on my eighth rib), and death would happen when there were no ribs capable of protecting my lungs and they would collapse. It took a good listener like Ralph, a good sharp oncologist to calm me down. I desperately combed the book shelves at local book stores looking for information and finally found a newly published book about death, **How We Die**, by Dr. Sherwin B. Nuland. His clear, well written book gave me the help I needed to understand the way that cancer kills.

Carole Greene felt the same way about needing medical information.

> It's not the death or dying aspects of mets that scare me, it's the lack of understanding of what's going on now. I'm a nuts and bolts kind of patient, and my mind will not "let it rest" if I don't have some mental construct that fits what I am experiencing.

After months of undiagnosed malaise, Lucie Bergmann-Shuster took the news that the ultrasound had found a possibly malignant ovarian tumor in stride, and immediately sprang into action.

> Neither my husband nor I said much on our drive back to his place of work. I told him that I would obviously need surgery to determine malignancy and that I wanted to proceed with it quickly to get it resolved. He agreed. Meantime, I would be checking the Internet connections on ovarian cancer, particularly the NCI's PDQ. Driving home alone after I dropped off my husband, I went over in my mind on how to tackle this event.

> At home I logged on and an hour later got the reply from the NCI about ovarian cancer. Given the size of the mass, I knew instantly that should the cancer be ovarian, it would likely be at least a Stage II but possibly a Stage III or IV. I suspected that given the fuzziness around one edge of the mass, that it might be a likely Stage III. Prognosis, if cancer, was poor for a Stage III according to the NCI physicians document; a possible 13 percent chance for long term survival. In the evening I shared this info with my husband. Both he and I were solemn.

> The rest of the day I spent at my computer sharing my medical story with personal friends, family and "listies" on the Breast Cancer Discussion List. The many replies and well wishes kept me busy.... It was very

empowering to have a large informed community back me up in both my information searches and in my time of emotional need.

Often it is the husband or partner who will undertake the job of researching a patient's disease and possible treatments. Men report feeling more engaged and less helpless when they take on this role, which naturally shades into one of advocacy as well, especially during the times when the wife is hospitalized or too weak from the side effects of chemotherapy to fully manage this aspect of her care. This has been the case for Scott and Mary Kitterman.

> *How much to know is a difficult thing to balance. My wife has gotten to the point that she really can't deal with the technical details. She just wants to know the very basics: is the treatment working, how does this effect my prognosis, what are the side effects, and when do I come back. She leaves the details of arguing the specifics to me. I'm not the least bit shy and as an added bonus when the doctors get mad (and they do) they get mad at me and not at her.*

Bob Crisp also took over the information gathering increasingly as his wife, Ginger, became more ill.

> *For the most part, I've been the advocate. I'm the one who reads everything. I'm a part of nearly every conference about treatment. Her primary oncologist is one of the "if you don't ask, then I don't tell" variety. And, if you ask, then he gives vague information. I have had a couple of private conversations with him and he has been more open but still too vague for me. Interestingly, the radiation oncologist has been the most direct. He's the one who tells you what it is, whether you ask or not. So Ginger has gotten more from him than her regular oncologist. The people at the University of Arkansas Medical Center are very good. They try to find out how much you want to know and respond accordingly.*

Glenn Clabo discovered that when a husband does the research to ensure that his wife is getting the best possible care, it introduces another factor— he is in the position of possessing knowledge she doesn't have.

> *When I started researching breast cancer I knew that there was both good and bad with knowing as much as I did. I was always torn between telling Barb everything and not telling her anything. I solved this problem somewhat by not telling her anything too far ahead. I also tried to let her ask before I volunteered bad information. Never once did I correct her*

when she made positive statements, even if they were somewhat slanted in her favor. I know quite a bit about statistics and, frankly, don't believe in them when it comes to people and this type of situation. I always felt that Barb was going to do all that she could to stay alive for as long as she could, so telling her every negative didn't seem helpful. She knew what so many positive nodes meant because she had asked the questions and read about it. There was no putting much of a positive note on that news.

At the very beginning of this we sat down and decided that she needed to take time to decide the best route to take. A friend of mine and his wife who has breast cancer were swept along without time to think. They just did what the doctors suggested and were not as well informed as we wanted to be. I wanted Barb to make every decision with every bit of information I could get for her before going on. Barb always got visibly upset thinking about this time in the process. She felt that no one cared and this monster was growing too fast to let an extra hour go by. In fact, it was actually days that felt like weeks to me and I'm sure it felt like months to her. Once she started the testing she felt better and was so busy she just pushed ahead full speed.

As children of the age of medical miracles, we have a hard time accepting the notion of treatment failure—there must always be something that can be done! People making decisions about still unproven treatments for metastatic breast cancer—high-dose chemotherapy, for example, which combines relatively low percentages of efficacy with some morbidity and mortality risks—depend upon full disclosure to weigh all the issues carefully. They look to their doctors to help them untangle the benefit-risk ratio from the desperation that may drive these choices on an emotional level.

In an earlier era where cancer treatments were at best palliative, geared toward relieving pain or other symptoms, the notion of informed consent for painful and dangerous treatments with metastatic breast cancer patients was far less relevant than it is today. In recent years, however, breast cancer treatment is steadily moving toward more aggressive treatments that have more serious side effects, geared toward at least the possibility of an extended disease-free remission or even a cure. Consequently, full disclosure has become more important. How can a physician alone bear the responsibility for deciding whether or not a patient should receive a particular treatment?

In fact, the laws governing informed consent require the following, according to medical ethicist Ruth Macklin:

> Before invasive or risky procedures may be performed, the physician must disclose to the patient pertinent details about the nature and purpose of the procedure, its potential risks and benefits, and any reasonable alternatives to the recommended treatment. But it is not enough to recite a litany of facts. The patient must understand the information presented orally or in a written form. Furthermore, the patient's consent must be obtained without coercion; it must be granted voluntarily. Finally, patients from whom consent is sought must be competent, that is, have the mental capacity to grant it.[13]

Medicine is not magic—doctors are not gods

When first diagnosed with breast cancer, one of the more daunting tasks a woman must face is that of selecting a surgeon and oncologist who are competent and responsive to her needs. If she has a recurrence, the good relationship she has hopefully already established with her oncologist will stand her in good stead, at least as a point of departure.

In their book, *Breast Cancer: The Complete Guide*, Drs. Yashar Hirshaut and Peter Pressman write about why it can be important to seek at least a second opinion, even if your relationship with your initial oncologist has been a good one. "Even if all you want is the reassurance of a fresh evaluation, you should certainly get more than one opinion. It makes sense to reevaluate the work of the people who were responsible for your care and to consider alternatives." Drs. Hirshaut and Pressman go on to advise that since treating recurrent breast cancer requires special expertise, your treating physician— ideally head of your "treatment team"—should: 1) have treated many patients with metastatic breast cancer, 2) approach treating the disease in a "vigorous" fashion, as an "impassioned advocate, determined to secure the best results for you," and 3) act as an expert diagnostician, whose knowledge is always up to date, keeping up with the constantly changing treatments and discoveries in the field, and whose method is patient and meticulous.[14]

Like many others, Pat Leach learned the hard way about how important a second opinion can be:

> If I hadn't gotten a second opinion after initial diagnosis, I would have had extensive surgery and a doctor who intimidated me and I didn't really trust. I was so confused and scared at first, that I was willing to do whatever he said. Thank God for my friend Ruth, who had heard a group of doctors from Boston give a talk. I went to see them and immediately felt more confident, less scared, felt I was doing the best I could for myself. I've had other second opinions to confirm treatment options and never regretted doing it. I went back to the old doctor for the treatment.

For Bob and Ginger Crisp, as for many others, the most important part of this effort came at the beginning of treatment:

> We were careful to obtain second opinions at the start. However, once we had assembled a team, then it was not so much about getting second opinions as agreement from the team. In our case, it included a local oncologist, a local radiation oncologist and an oncology surgeon (who did Ginger's surgeries), the chemo oncologist, and the head of BMT (bone marrow transplant) where Ginger was treated.

It's difficult to make any hard and fast pronouncements about what personal qualities of an oncologist are likely to make a particular patient feel at ease. Some people prize their doctor's compassionate, friendly manner; others are more comfortable with a more formal, professional stance. Some expect their doctors to show a great deal of concern for how they are managing the cancer in their lives, while others relate to their oncologist as a specialist, preferring to seek their emotional support elsewhere. Some like an authoritative, take-charge manner, while others prefer more of an equal relationship, where their participation in decision-making is freely elicited, and a real give-and-take ensues.

There are some factors, however, that are universally appreciated: doctors who spend enough unhurried time; who freely share, when asked, their own reasoning process and expertise on treatment decisions; who are open to questions, no matter how technical on the one hand, or uninformed on the other; who treat family members with consideration; and who are available in a reasonable time frame both during and outside of office hours. And, of course, everyone wants the results of tests delivered as soon as possible. Delays, whether waiting for test results, scheduled appointments, second opinions or consultations, are particularly maddening for people coping with metastatic breast cancer, and serve to raise already heightened anxiety levels still further.

Sometimes, when test results get lost in administrative limbo, or other promised events fail to materialize in a timely way, women or their advocates must act assertively to ensure the best care and confront physicians who may be unresponsive to their needs.

It's difficult for many women to confront doctors on whom they feel dependent. Often it takes time to muster the courage. Kathy Stone wrote to the Breast Cancer Discussion List about her growing frustration with her doctor, and was encouraged to discuss her concerns with him.

> *Tomorrow when I have my weekly oncologist visit I need to get things straight between the doctor and myself. I don't think he realizes how unhappy I am with some of the ways he responds to me or my situation. I don't expect him to change much, but I am hoping that he will at least acknowledge the fact that I have some reasonable complaints and try to reach some sort of method to solve them.*

Clearly, she was not going into this meeting with confidence that this discussion would resolve much. "I have made yet another list," Kathy wrote. "Hopefully I will follow through and make sure we discuss the important topics before I am casually dismissed once again for another week." Her next message was triumphant, however.

> *I kept my courage and backbone and spoke to my oncologist about unacceptable behavior and attitudes from some of his office staff. About them not following up, leaving me hanging and even lying about simple things... him not reviewing my records before coming into the exam room, and my gut feeling that "the left hand didn't know what the right hand was doing" at times. He apologized, said he would try harder to make me feel more comfortable and he would speak with his staff (mainly office manager) about miscommunications. I could tell he was embarrassed and surprised...but I kept my cool...didn't get mad and treated the subject as something I was "owed" as a patient of his. I know he took the message to heart, because after my visit, he called the head oncology nurse at the hospital and spoke to her about it and asked if she had ever heard of me being unhappy or if she had ever heard of other patients being unhappy. Of course she has heard a lot and told him so. Maybe things will change.*

As she approached the high-dose chemotherapy treatment she was counting on, yet dreading, Nancy Gilpatrick found herself increasingly upset with her oncologist.

> *I've just been realizing my doctor isn't very accessible to me. I get good information from the radiation oncologist, who will talk with me for 45 minutes. My medical oncologist sends her nurse, whom I happen to like and connect with, instead of herself. I decided last Friday when I realized this that I would confront her when I go in tomorrow. I don't feel like I can change doctors at this point and I don't want to. The office is a good and peaceful place. I am going to tell her that it is unacceptable to me to pay the money when it is the nurse who gives me my care. I want her to talk with me, even if it's as simple as acknowledging my presence when I'm in the treatment room and she is walking the hall. I basically think she—who is near my age—is scared by my breast cancer. If it can happen to me, it can happen to her. I think medical professionals say to themselves, "Oh, that can't happen to me, I get mammograms," or, "I'm educated," or, "I'm rich and she's poor," or whatever. They make themselves separate from us. With me she's having a harder time. No one seems to really want to deal with the fact they think I'm going to die from this disease due to its resistance to radiation and chemo (so far). Anyway, I'm angry and I'm going to let her know that.*

The following story makes clear just how important it is to consult a physician you like and trust. When Sharon Multhauf's recurrence to bone was first diagnosed, she had been seeing an oncologist for follow-up who had been assigned by her managed care system. Her detailed account of what happened then is a classic example of poor communication between doctor and patient.

> *On December 28, 1994, Lloyd and I waited in the exam room for my most unfavorite oncologist to come in. This woman is very cold and matter-of-fact. She seems not to know how to smile, and she doesn't deal in hopefulness. She walked in and sat down, opened my chart, and proceeded to ask me how I was doing. I said I didn't want to talk about anything else right now until I knew what the bone scan report said. She hadn't received a typed copy yet, but went out to the office and listened to the dictated report on the internal phone system. She returned to tell me that there were "two things going on," at which I stiffened. She rattled off*

the places where I had always known I had arthritis, and then said that there were areas of uptake in the sacrum, pelvis and hip that were "highly suggestive of metastatic disease."

Further tests were scheduled, including an MRI. It was two weeks later, on a day Sharon now calls "Black Tuesday," that the diagnosis was confirmed. Sharon had been telling herself it was possible the initial tests had been mistaken, or that if they were confirmed, she still had a chance to somehow find a cure for this recurrence. These hopes evaporated during the consultation.

This office visit held no pleasantries. We cut to the results, and they were bad. She read the conclusions in the report and we asked to see the films. She had them with her (she knew what to expect from us by now), and she showed us the areas of arthritis and, by contrast, the areas of metastasis.

Again, Lloyd and I held tight to one another's hands, and we continued to question: What kind of result was likely from the tamoxifen? What kind of symptoms could I expect? We did not ask how long I had to live. I knew I didn't want to get that answer from any doctor right now—especially from her. We asked what would follow if the hormones failed. She said I would take chemo, starting with CAF and moving on to others. I asked her how long I would need to be on chemo, and she said, "The rest of your life." I hated that answer. She wasn't going to allow me any shred of hope for a cure, was she? Lloyd asked what new investigative treatments we might look into, and she replied, "Like what?" That made him mad, because he felt she should be leading us, not the other way around. He said, "Like bone marrow transplant," which we had only barely begun to know about. The oncologist replied, "She wouldn't be eligible for that, because she has cancer in her bones." In the months to come, when I learned about peripheral stem cell replacement, I felt very annoyed that this doctor had not responded with information about how I might be helped, rather than dismissing Lloyd's question so offhandedly.

A fact-based and rationally motivated person herself, in this situation Sharon was stunned by this doctor's coldness.

After all this, the oncologist asked me where I was having pain. The words that came out of my mouth summed up the mood of the moment. I said, "In my heart." She didn't know what to say, so she went on to the next question.

This discordance between a patient's concerns, which are only partly expressed by her physical symptoms, and the physician's focus on diagnosis and treatment, highlighted here by this disturbing example, is a problem that is to some extent inherent in any consultation of this kind. In his book *At the Will of the Body*, medical sociologist Arthur Frank makes the important distinction between disease, a bodily process, and illness, which is our total experience of living with a disease.

> *Medical treatment is designed to make everyone believe that only the disease—what is measurable and mechanical—can be discussed. Talking to doctors always makes me conscious of what I am not supposed to say. Thus I am particularly silent when I have been given bad news. I know I am supposed to ask only about the disease, but what I feel is the illness. The questions I want to ask about my life are not allowed, not speakable, not even thinkable. The gap between what I feel and what I feel allowed to say widens and deepens and swallows my voice.*[15]

The stories that follow detail the qualities some people particularly appreciate in their physicians. After her liver metastases had failed to respond to Adriamycin, Mary D'Angelo agreed to seek a second opinion at a well-known cancer center. It was after this visit that Mary finally realized that her friends who had been advising her to seek a new oncologist were right.

> *Charlie and I were in a panic state, thinking what are we going to do? When we saw Dr. H., everything changed. Here was this lovely young doctor who said, "You know, I looked at your scan and I don't think that these are new tumors." He didn't think that there were many more tumors, but that it was the way the scan was taken.*
>
> *My first doctor had cancer himself, and I couldn't deal with the idea that the person trying to save me was dying. I also felt that he had not been vigilant, and that he really didn't know what he was doing. There had been many instances of that which I overlooked, because I thought he was taking care of me well. But I always felt, after that first time of seeing Dr. H., that there was lots of hope. He encouraged me that way, although he was always bluntly honest, which I like and want. He said, "Make no mistake about it, you are going to die of breast cancer." Which was fine, because I thought, well, this is an honest person. But he said also, "I don't know when. It depends, but there are lots of treatments, and*

we'll put you on tamoxifen." I thought, what? That tiny little half-an-aspirin sized pill? That everyone is taking prophylactically? I'm going to take this for a disease that's supposed to kill me in three months, when the most deadly chemo did nothing? But I said, okay. I'll try it.

PJ Hagler describes feelings of loyalty to her doctor.

> *My oncologist wants to know everything about me and my care. He has made Mike and me a part of his team. I have had him and only him for over six years. I'm never passed to anyone else. He even walks me into the chemo room for treatments. I have his home phone number and he has called me at home. I get all the time I need to talk to him before a treatment and every ten days during treatment. I have all my needles changed in my port every Friday by his nurse. I have all my chemo treatments in his office. I always have the same nurse do all my needle changes, blood work and chemo treatments. Since 1991 they have been like a part of my family. I trust them and feel I could tell them anything and I have a pact with my oncologist that he will be honest with me and let me know exactly where I stand. He has looked at my file, which is huge, before I come into the room and he knows the results of my blood work which I have had a week before my seeing him. We feel like a team trying to get me well.*

Sensitivity is a door that swings both ways. Patients like Lucie Bergmann-Shuster are quite aware of the stresses their doctors are under, and will often strive to make their tasks easier.

> *I am very grateful to the oncologists who stick to their profession. It is tough for them to see patients diminish as the disease progresses and takes over. I try to cheer my oncologist up with my still vivacious being, even when I report problems.*

In this spirit, Lucie transformed having a Port-a-cath implanted—a subcutaneous port used to administer her chemotherapy and draw blood without further damaging her veins—by engaging her sense of curiosity and comedy. By focusing on this procedure as a mere "chore," as she decided to see this minor surgery, she was able to release some of her anxiety.

> *Everything went smoothly. I had my head covered so couldn't see anything but I could hear the chatter. At one point, my surgeon asked to do an extra fastening suture and then jestingly she said to me, "That will*

be five bucks extra," and then asked me to shift my left arm under my body and tilt the chest up some more. In no time at all, it was done. In fact, it was done 15 minutes early, so I asked for a rebate on the five bucks extra charge on the stitches. I was awake and cheerful as I watched the resident's bloodied hands apply the last of the dressing to hold the catheter in place. Everybody was in a good mood at a job well done and expeditiously. The orderly came and wheeled me out and without much further ado, my husband joined me beside the gurney, grinning from ear to ear.

After we got settled in the oncology ward, my husband explained his happy face. Dr. Kate had come out to the family waiting area in her scrubs and sternly shook Cy's hands saying, "she is gonna live." At first his jaw dropped and then he nearly roared, but given the other folks in the room he suppressed his laughter to a mere chuckle. Dr. Kate winked at him with that leprechaun charm of hers and then left. Both hubby and I are of the opinion that, whenever possible, one should have fun doing whatever job or chore we do. Knowing that Dr. Kate was of like disposition made us feel more than comforted and rather special to be included and privy to such personal jest. A woman after my own heart I would say, doing the best she can with joy and spunk.

Kim Banks also worries about expecting godlike powers from doctors, fearing that this will encourage even more unreality in an already distorted relationship.

We all want to be treated by caring, competent doctors. I'm a perfect example—I did not return to an oncologist who was considered an expert on breast cancer, simply because I felt like I was being treated like a number. I believe our confidence in our doctors can affect how well we tolerate and respond to treatment. The mind is a powerful thing—and I wanted that power reinforcing my treatment in my fight against this disease.

I think we have to remember that doctors are people, too, and are under an inordinate amount of stress. They are taught in medical school that they must appear knowledgeable and confident at all times. Maybe your doctor cries when he sees a patient crying, and feels that allowing a patient to observe that would lower their confidence in him. I can't imagine what it would be like to be the person that has to break the news to a

person that they have cancer. It must also be incredibly difficult to prac-
tice in a field where the tools against the disease cause so much pain and
often are not effective. I could imagine having many bad days if I were in
my oncologist's shoes.

As we've seen throughout this chapter, the problems of knowledge and responsibility weigh heavily on the shoulders of all who must deal with a life-threatening illness: patients, families and physicians. From some years of experience in acting as an advocate on behalf of sick relatives and dealing with the medical profession, Scott Kitterman speaks with a certain authority when he says:

> *The proper role of a doctor is to inform you, educate you and guide*
> *you to make reasonable decisions. He is not there to sit on high and*
> *inform you about what is going to happen to you next. This imposes a dif-*
> *ficult burden on both patients and doctors. As patients, and their loved*
> *ones, it is incumbent on us to learn enough to understand what is going*
> *on and participate intelligently in the decision-making process. Doctors*
> *must be willing to be open with us and, in addition to fully informing us*
> *about the details of our situation, help us with that education process.*

Glenn Clabo found himself waiting with his wife, Barb, for the results of yet another MRI. Symptoms of dizziness and left-sided weakness had marred her recovery barely two months after completing her high-dose chemo with stem cell transplant. Yet, for all the fear his knowledge brought, Glenn never wished that he'd known less about the disease, or about Barb's prognosis.

> *The bottom line? Tell me everything there is to know...the good, the*
> *bad, the scary...everything. Don't let me live in denial and allow me to*
> *take for granted that those things I cherish most will be there in my mind's*
> *future. Make me realize that now is when that thought of love and appre-*
> *ciation should be expressed. That touch, smile, look that I used to put off*
> *needs to happen now. Don't take that away by giving me a false sense of*
> *hope that it's okay to put it off until tomorrow.*

> *The hope will always be for a tomorrow...but we all need to be made*
> *aware that tomorrow may never come. Please don't hold back informa-*
> *tion to make it easier on me now. It's more important that I know all the*
> *possibilities, so I'll not regret what I didn't do when I had the chance. We*
> *all have too many regrets to live with as it is. Don't we?*

CHAPTER 6

Medical Treatments and Choices

TREATMENTS FOR METASTATIC DISEASE are fraught with complexities and contradictory interpretations, and are not easy for a lay person to evaluate. For these reasons, this chapter has been difficult to conceptualize and to write. You may find some of the information here hard going at times. Still, it's important to persist, despite the confusing options and concepts. Through understanding the choices open to you, and why they are recommended, you can clarify your own treatment philosophy. By learning as much as you can about recent advances in treatment, as they apply to your specific situation, you can help your medical team secure for you the best, most appropriate treatment for your disease.

In the spirit of clarity, this chapter will first look at where to seek a current overview of medical information on the standard treatment of metastatic breast cancer, then at the kinds of drugs and other methods used for treatment and the ways in which physicians balance the effectiveness of these drugs against the cancer versus their toxicity for the patient. A new section on emerging treatments and the promise and hope of molecular biology has been added for this edition, with more about clinical trials. Discussing the treatment philosophies that go into deciding how aggressively to treat your cancer, and the part you play in those decisions, leads into an exploration of treatment controversies, using high-dose chemotherapy as a prime example. And finally, some patients will talk about how they arrived at their own treatment decisions and how they felt about these decisions after the fact.

An overview of medical approaches

The current medical reality is that no single treatment or combination of treatments will cure metastatic breast cancer. Breast cancer is, however, among the most *treatable* of solid tumors. That's important to remember.

Thus, the aim in treatment is to convert a fatal disease to a chronic one. According to Dr. Eric P. Winer, writing in the professional journal *Oncology,* "More treatment options exist for patients with metastatic breast cancer than for most patients with cancer."[1]

There are treatments that can potentially buy you time—often many years. And there are some treatments that are controversial—doctors don't know yet if they offer a chance of cure or if they even extend life. As with any rule, there are exceptions; a few people appear to survive metastatic breast cancer beyond all odds and reason. By the time you are reading this, there may well be some medical advance that will offer you the possibility of an even longer life span, during which a cure might become available.

As you read this, bear in mind that continuous refinements in current treatments are always being tested, fine-tuned and put into practice. Because this field of knowledge is constantly changing, and because each case is unique, this chapter will only attempt to discuss the available treatments in the broadest of terms, and survey the emerging new therapies in clinical trials, placing the real focus on what you need to know and find out to be able to make informed treatment choices.

An excellent place to start looking is the National Cancer Institute's Physicians Data Query (PDQ) cancer database, now widely available to patients by telephone, fax, e-mail and on the World Wide Web (see Appendix B, *Resources*, for details). As described on the web site, this database "contains peer-reviewed summaries on cancer treatment, screening, prevention, and supportive care; a registry of approximately 1,600 open and 9,500 closed cancer clinical trials from around the world; and directories of physicians, genetic counselors and organizations that provide cancer care."[2]

These peer-reviewed statements are available in two versions, both of which are prepared and reviewed by physicians who specialize in this area. First, there are documents for patients and the general public written in easy-to-understand terms. It's a good idea to start here, and to review the general information provided about the disease, its treatment and managing side effects. Then, if you wish, you can go on to the much more useful detailed (and candid) summaries of current state-of-the-art treatment information compiled for physicians and health professionals, complete with recent references to medical journals, allowing you to review relevant abstracts. Materials for this section always come from publications that are peer-reviewed, meaning that they must withstand the high standards for inclusion set by the research and clinical community of doctors working in this field of oncology. The Health Professionals cancer information summaries are updated monthly, and are an excellent jumping-off place for your research. Bear in mind, please, that because of the intended readership, prognostic information is sometimes presented in ways that may seem brutally frank. Obviously, the NCI is aware that many patients read these statements, so they issue the following disclaimer: "This information is intended for use by doctors and other health care professionals. If you are a cancer patient, your doctor can explain how it applies to you, or you can call the Cancer Information Service at 1-800-422-6237."

Another good source, written in language for the layperson, is the second edition of *Dr. Susan Love's Breast Book*,[3] which includes two chapters on dealing with metastatic disease, the first an explanation of the disease, the second on available treatments. Hirshaut and Pressman's *Breast Cancer: The Complete Guide* also offers a clearly explained chapter on recurrence.[4]

"Unlike researchers, I am not looking for a broadly applicable treatment regimen," wrote Mary Kitterman's husband, Scott, making an important distinction. "I've got one particular case I am especially concerned about." If you make the decision to inform yourself thoroughly on the relevant treatment and disease information, as opposed to relying on your physicians' recommendations alone, what you really need is the most up-to-date *specific* information upon which to base your decision, including relevant clinical trials. These specifics will enable you to function in partnership with your doctors when it comes to decisions about treatment. Certainly, you'll discover additional questions, theories and treatments to bring to your oncologist's attention. Bear in mind that it is sometimes very difficult to extrapolate to an individual situation from reading published research or reports on ongoing clinical trials. While confusing at first, second opinions, as discussed in the last chapter, can be an important way to confirm a decision, introduce new information, or clarify treatment controversies.

While much of the medical information is available without cost online or through medical libraries and other sources, another option may be to turn to one or more of the commercial for-profit database search services who can take the details of your situation, search the literature and prepare a report for you. This may or may not be worth the expenditure of funds, as Beverly

Zakarian, Director of CAN ACT, cautioned in *The Activist Cancer Patient: How to Take Charge of Your Treatment*:

> The more difficult and individual medical conditions are, the less likely there is to be a large body of information available. Ironically, that's when treatment choices must be most artful. In these situations, it's more important than ever to have a skilled and experienced oncologist who can incorporate the complexities into a personal treatment plan. A computer search might offer intelligent new options to consider because it can tap extensive files of possibly helpful information. Remember that the largest number of reports in the medical literature concentrate on treatment for primary occurrence of the commonest cancers. And recurrences can be very individual, complicated by a person's poorer health after treatment or metastasis to distant sites and difficult organs.[5]

Drugs

Many different kinds of drugs can be used to treat metastatic breast cancer and relieve its symptoms. The specific treatment selected will depend on whether or not the tumor is hormone positive, various other indicators revealed by testing or the pathologist's report, what drugs have been tried before, and the treatment philosophy of the patient and doctor. Drugs can be grouped into three general types:

- **Cytotoxic drugs** kill cancer cells and can be considered poisons. When delivered systemically, they harm all rapidly dividing cells, not only cancer cells. This accounts for side effects like bone marrow suppression (lowered blood counts) as well as hair loss, and a variety of gastrointestinal symptoms. These drugs work by interfering with different aspects of a cancer cell's ability to reproduce, and so they are often used in combination with one another for maximum effect, and to circumvent drug resistance. They include alkylating agents, antimetabolites, taxanes, vinca alkaloids and antibiotics, to mention the most common types of cytotoxic agents. Common drugs in these categories include: cyclophosphamide (Cytoxan), methotrexate, doxorubicin (Adriamycin, Doxil), 5 fluorouracil (5-FU), vincristine, paclitaxel (Taxol), docetaxel (Taxotere), vinorelbine (Navelbine), thiotepa, melphalan (L-PAM), cisplatin (Platinol) and others. For generic names, brand names and manufacturers of these and other drugs, see Appendix C, *Common Drugs in Use with Metastatic Breast Cancer*.

- **Hormonal drugs** can retard the growth of cancer cells by changing the hormonal environment of the cancer itself. Many cancers of the breast, even after they metastasize, remain hormone-sensitive or hormone-dependent for their growth, having receptors on the tumor cell's surface that respond to these substances. Oral hormones or hormonal antagonists, like tamoxifen (Nolvadex), an anti-estrogen; megestrol acetate (Megace), a progestogen; anastrozole (Arimidex), an oral aromatase inhibitor that inhibits estrogen production in the adrenal glands; prednisone or decadron, both adrenocorticoids; halotestin, an androgen or male hormone, and others are commonly used to treat metastatic disease still responsive to these substances. Less frequently, hormonal methods also include surgical, radiological or chemical ablation, which means that some of the endocrine glands are removed or prevented from functioning. Oophorectomy, surgical removal of the ovaries, is being recommended more frequently for younger women.

- **Experimental treatments**, such as biological response modifiers, growth hormones, antibodies, vaccines, and many other innovative approaches are being used in combination with chemotherapy to stimulate the immune system or to affect cellular repair in novel ways. In addition, already approved drugs are in clinical trials for use in new combinations and circumstances. Dozens of clinical trials are under way, at varying stages of completion. This edition of this book includes a new section later in this chapter touching on some of the more promising avenues of research.

Surgery and radiation

Although they are among the most effective tools in primary breast cancer, surgery and radiation are both treatment methods that provide local control of disease. Thus their role in controlling a disease that by definition has become regional or systemic is somewhat more limited, and most often involves palliative, or non-curative, care.

However, surgery continues to play a significant role in metastatic breast cancer. Surgical biopsies are often performed, as well as surgery to implant devices like ports to deliver chemotherapy and ease blood draws, or implanted pumps to permit pain relief medications to reach affected areas.

Bones of the arm, shoulder, leg, pelvis and spine that have broken due to osteolytic bone metastases can be repaired and pinned, maintaining function and relieving pain. Bob Stafford was able to have a broken femur pinned so he could walk again, and Sandra Yandell had parts of her spine replaced.

Occasionally, depending upon the metastatic site, it will be possible for a surgeon to "debulk" or even rid a patient of measurable breast cancer metastasis by removing all or part of an isolated tumor from a part of the body that won't be damaged by the surgery. Lucie Bergmann-Shuster, for example, had tumors that had spread to her ovaries removed, as well as some of the cancer that had metastasized to other areas of her abdomen. Sometimes an isolated tumor in the liver or lung can be removed. This type of surgery generally doesn't halt the spread of cancer altogether in metastatic patients, but it can lessen the "tumor burden" in the body, and possibly make treatment more effective.

A minor surgical procedure, performed at the bedside, is often used to control malignant pleural effusion, where the area around the lungs repeatedly fills with fluid containing cancer cells, causing shortness of breath and making frequent drainage necessary. A process called "sclerosing" can often resolve this problem, greatly increasing a patient's quality of life. A chest tube is inserted by a surgeon to drain the pleural area, and the lung is allowed to expand over a day or more. Then a sclerosing agent, usually an antibiotic like tetracycline or bleomycin, is instilled to close the space where fluid collects. PJ Hagler had this process successfully performed.

Radiation is also widely utilized in metastatic disease. It serves a different function than in primary breast cancer, where cure is the goal and radiation is used to destroy any residual tumor left after lumpectomy or mastectomy. The goal of radiation in metastatic disease is palliative, to control the disease by relieving symptoms such as pain, pressure on vital organs, or neurological problems. Patients who receive radiation therapy for relief of symptoms usually undergo a course of daily treatments for one to four weeks. Strategies for offering one or two higher dose treatments to stop the growth of bone metastases, instead of a lower-dose "fractionated" series, have been utilized in other countries, and may find acceptance in the United States.

After consulting with a radiation oncologist, the patient goes into a simulator room so treatment can be planned. The field to be irradiated is marked with permanent marker and possibly tattoos, which enables the technicians to align the patient properly each time. The actual treatments last only a minute or two each day and are painless.

The most common use of radiation in metastatic disease is to relieve pain from bone metastases. The majority of metastatic breast-cancer patients will eventually develop metastases to the bone, and radiation is very effective in easing the pain. The patient's response helps determine how long treatment will last. Once sufficient doses have been given to alleviate the pain, it is less likely that the cancer will return to the same area.

Radiation is also used to relieve symptoms in other parts of the body, and the side effects depend on which areas are being treated. When the bones are targeted, there are usually side effects only when sensitive organs are included in the treatment field. Treatment to the chest area, for example, may cause some nausea and lung scarring, and possible damage to the heart. Radiation to the brain often causes drowsiness and disorientation, although mental function returns to normal after a short time. Cortisone medication to reduce swelling and prevent seizures is given along with radiation to the brain. Skin recurrences may be treated with chest-wall radiation, which causes skin reactions and possible lung scarring. Radiation to the head and neck can cause a dry mouth, difficulty in swallowing, changes in taste, and earaches, while treatments to the stomach and abdomen can cause nausea and diarrhea. Fatigue is a common reaction to any kind of radiation, and reddening or irritation of the skin is also frequently encountered. Your doctor can prescribe creams or other medication to help relieve most symptoms.

Here are the experiences of two women who had radiation to common metastatic sites. Sharon Multhauf described her reactions to a course of radiation she had to control an enlarging tumor in her sacrum, or lower back, which was beginning to exert pressure on a nerve and cause loss of sensation as well as pain.

> I knew that I would need to choose my food carefully to minimize the intestinal effect of the radiation, so I faithfully followed the dietary guidelines provided by the doctor. But even with all my precautions, it took only a few days for bowel distress to hit, and it got worse as the weeks wore on. (I hate to think what it would have been like if I had not been so careful.) I also took good care of my skin, yet still ended up with some painful

burns, which sent me on a shopping trip for "boxer" style underwear with no elastic at the legs. And, of course, I got very tired from the daily treatments, so I didn't try to accomplish much during that time. I had my treatments in the morning and I took a long nap every afternoon.

When the need for this treatment arose, my husband and I had plans in place for a European vacation. After much consideration, we decided to go ahead with a shorter, less ambitious trip, and that was a powerful motivation for me during my treatment. Even though the discomfort worsened each week, I was able to leave three days after the end of treatment, and I tolerated the flight, in part because of the comfortable business class accommodations we had splurged on. The first week of the journey, I had to keep a slow pace and eat carefully, but soon I found that I was able to do more of what I wanted to do each day without serious limitations.

Barb Pender describes her experience with radiation for skin metastases:

My nodules looked like very small boils and they began in the surgical armpit. I underwent 34 out of 36 radiation treatments and they still were developing fast and furiously. My radiation oncologist took me off the last two treatments and felt there was nothing more he could do—but the treatments seemed to have a post-radiation effect because the nodules began to disappear. During treatment, the radiated area became very leathery looking and under the arm the skin was so burnt it was black. That has all gone away now. I did find myself a little tired, but I managed to still go to work. Within a couple months my skin was softer than normal because it was "new" skin.

Some years later, Barb had visual problems that stemmed from small metastases in the back of one of her eyes that turned out to be peppered throughout her brain. Again, radiation was proposed.

I had 14 radiation treatments covering the whole brain and including the backs of both eyes. Because of the sensitivity of the area being radiated, they made a mask for me. These masks are plastic mesh that bolts to a table so you cannot move your head. The treatments are very quick so I did not feel claustrophobic at all. I found a wonderful aloe cream to put on my head so that my scalp would be spared a lot of the *redness. The area of the head where I used the cream just looked like I had been out in the sun. Not realizing the radiation was hitting behind my ears, I neglected to put the cream there. Needless to say they got oozy like a very bad sunburn. I did lose my hair again.*

Though scans showed most of the lesions had receded or disappeared, about nine months later more episodes of dizziness and headaches indicated that two of Barb's metastatic sites were growing again. She then underwent one of the new targeted radiation therapies developed to treat hard-to-reach metastases—three-dimensional stereotactic computer imaging technology, sometimes known as "gamma knife," in which beams of radiation intersect within the brain to precisely target tumors in areas inaccessible to surgery.

The mask for this was more of a tightly form-fitted mesh mask. There is more of a set-up involved with the stereotactic procedure, and I did end up experiencing some claustrophobic anxiety toward the end. The techs were wonderful though...they just freed me from the mask and let me sit up for a few minutes. It was all I needed to be able to finish up.

Standard treatments

The standard medical treatments for recurrent breast cancer may be found in the PDQ cancer information summary for breast cancer. (The synopsis that follows, however, might be somewhat outdated by the time you read this, so check the most recent PDQ.) Standard treatments will differ, depending on whether the cancer still shows evidence of having a large number of hormone receptors—and according to prior treatments and when in the disease progression the treatment is given.

As of this writing, standard first-line treatment (first treatment following recurrence) for hormone-receptor positive, or unknown hormonal status, metastatic disease is tamoxifen (Nolvadex), especially if visceral disease (to the liver and other organs) is not present. For pre-menopausal patients, oophorectomy (surgical removal of the ovaries) is an option that is sometimes recommended. When the cancer comes back, further hormonal therapies are usually tried as second-line treatments.

It's worth pointing out that those who tested hormone-receptor positive on first diagnosis do not necessarily remain so—and vice versa, though more rarely, which probably raises the question of false-negative testing in the first place. Consequently, a later biopsy can provide useful information. In one study, in fact, 36 percent of estrogen-receptor positive tumors following first diagnosis were no longer positive at the time of recurrence. If estrogen-receptor (ER) and progesterone-receptor (PR) status is unknown or positive, then the site(s) of recurrence, disease-free interval, response to previous treatment, and menopausal status will all be additional factors in selecting further treatment.

When a second hormone treatment fails, many oncologists will move on to chemotherapy, since there is less chance of a third hormonal treatment being effective. Sometimes, however, hormones may be successfully reintroduced after a period of ten months or more post-relapse. As noted earlier, radiation treatment for isolated bone metastases, especially to alleviate pain or prevent fracture, is standard therapy, concurrent with hormonal treatment and/or chemotherapy. Surgery for localized or visceral recurrence is also considered standard, although it is often not possible, because of the location or the fact that the disease is already widely disseminated.

When the recurrent tumor is known to be ER- and PR- negative (where there are only a very small number or no estrogen and progesterone receptors found on the cancer cells), however, chemotherapy is usually the first option to be considered. The PDQ statement refers to five equivalent combination first-line chemotherapies, each with supporting research, as standard treatment. These are CMF, CAF, CA, CMFP, and CMFVP, which are various combinations of the following six drugs:

C = cyclophosphamide (Cytoxan)
M = methotrexate
A = doxorubicin (Adriamycin)
F = 5-fluorouracil
V = vincristine
P = prednisone

Caution is expressed about the cardiotoxicity of Adriamycin, its potential to damage the heart and cause congestive heart failure if the maximum dose is exceeded. A new drug, dexrazoxane (Zinecard), has recently been introduced that appears to reduce this risk. While not yet generally included as standard treatment, one recent promising new first-line treatment emerging from Phase III clinical trials involves combining Adriamycin with Taxol. Safer, less toxic formulations of anthracyclines are becoming available, as discussed later in this chapter.

People dealing with osteolytic metastases to the bone, which render bones fragile and can lead to weakening and fractures, should consider a course of bisphosphonates. Clinical trials have shown that pamidronate (Aredia) and clodronate in such patients leads to a decrease in skeletal problems. External-beam radiation therapy to areas of bone and tumors in soft tissue may be recommended both to control pain and control local disease.

Unfortunately, over time, each drug or combination of drugs, whether hormonal (affecting the growth rate of the cancer) or cytotoxic (chemotherapy that kills the cancer cells) eventually fails as the surviving cancer cells mutate to become resistant to these drugs. Thus, the best chance for complete response, or remission, is usually the first round of treatments, called first-line, with diminishing returns usually occurring for courses of treatment following relapse, second-line, third-line and so forth. If there's progression of disease, the tumor is said to be "refractory," but the PDQ goes on to say that paclitaxel (Taxol) and docetaxel (Taxotere) have given good second-line responses, albeit with significant toxicity, with response rates in various studies (complete and partial) ranging from 6 percent to 57 percent of the patients treated. A relatively new drug, vinorelbine (Navelbine) is cited as having some good success as a second- or third-line treatment.

Applying standard treatment to your own medical situation

What does all this mean? If you underwent chemotherapy after your primary diagnosis, referred to as "adjuvant" treatment, the chemotherapy drugs you received then are likely to play a role in determining the drug or combination of drugs your oncologist will recommend as first-line treatment for metastatic disease. Remaining cancer cells in your body may have become resistant to the drugs you were given when you were first treated, so new drugs that are most likely to be active against the tumor will probably be used. If enough time has elapsed since your adjuvant treatment, however, the same drugs may have regained their effectiveness. If you have not had prior chemotherapy, or are Stage IV at primary diagnosis, you may be offered CMF or CAF as first-line treatment for metastatic disease, since these combinations of drugs have proven activity against breast cancer. High-dose chemotherapy with autologous stem cell rescue as an option is discussed later in this chapter, at some length.

As noted above, if your tumor has a high number of receptors to estrogen and/or progesterone, commonly referred to as ER- and/or PR-positive, this means that its growth is still, at least in part, modulated by these hormones. This is a favorable indicator, because it means that your treatment for metastatic disease is likely to begin with, and certainly will include, hormonal treatments like tamoxifen. This anti-estrogen is relatively non-toxic and is used in the adjuvant setting with newly diagnosed patients. In a significant number of women with positive hormone receptors, tamoxifen slows, stops or even regresses tumor growth for a period of a few to many months, even years.

Eventually, though, this treatment is likely to stop working. Usually, at this time, another hormonal treatment will be tried, such as Arimidex, an aromatase inhibitor, or Megace, a form of progesterone. Other hormonal drugs may follow, beginning with the least toxic and most effective. Women with slow-growing tumors high in hormone receptors who have good responses to these treatments have been maintained for years on hormonal manipulation, with good quality of life. Sometimes doctors will "rest" patients on hormones between chemotherapy treatments. Dr. Susan Love writes,

> When the tumor does show up again, sometimes just stopping a drug can give a secondary response. It seems that whatever we do to change the hormonal environment helps throw a cancer's growth off and stop it for a while. If we continually change the environment around the cancer, we can keep putting people into remission for a long time.[6]

In treating you, your doctor's goal is always to maximize effectiveness, while minimizing toxicity. Weighing this balance, taking into account quality of life and other personal values, along with potential treatment effectiveness, will be a vital consideration for you throughout your treatment for metastatic breast cancer. You are in charge of these choices, whatever your doctors recommend—and the more active a role you take in decision-making, the better you are likely to feel about it, whatever the outcome. Clearly, there's a learning process involved, as you discover more about your disease and the possible treatments, their risks and benefits, and as you clarify your own priorities. There are no right answers that apply to every patient, but there will be right answers for you at given points in time. You, your family, and your physicians will seek them out, together. Those answers, however, are likely to change as the disease progresses and the treatments offered become more problematic in terms of probable efficacy versus toxicity.

Since your history is individual, your treatment should be designed by an expert team of physicians in careful and thorough consultation with you. While no single form of treatment has emerged as most effective in treating metastatic breast cancer overall, there may well be a clear preference for a specific treatment in your case. Differing combinations of old and new drugs are constantly being tested, and the results of these clinical trials are used to refine the treatments offered.

As we have pointed out before, at the time of this writing, no drug or combination of drugs has shown proven efficacy in completely curing or eradicating metastatic disease. In most cases, it is not clear whether one regimen versus another even prolongs life; such is the variability of response. But that doesn't mean these drugs are not effective overall. Remember: Metastatic breast cancer is a treatable disease. Whatever controversies you may encounter about one treatment being superior to another, the basic theory behind both hormonal treatments and combination chemotherapy has been proven sound, repeatedly tested in large clinical trials over many years. And the particular drug combinations you will be given have demonstrated effectiveness in a significant percentage of patients in these trials. Will they benefit every patient? Unfortunately not.

Dr. Samuel Waxman, medical oncologist and researcher at Mt. Sinai Medical Center in New York, puts it this way:

> You don't know if a patient will respond until you try. All of these treatments are based on the concept of using combinations of non cross-resistant drugs, each of which has shown activity in killing or inhibiting breast cancer cells in the laboratory, in animals, and in the clinic. If you put them together, there should be more than additive effects and a more potent clinical response. That's the whole basis of combination chemotherapy—using non cross-resistant drugs with different mechanisms of action, and drugs that come with differing toxicities so that their use is tolerable.

The problem is this: tumors are not homogeneous (all of one kind of cell), but heterogeneous, meaning that in any tumor, there are many kinds of cancer cells, all at different points in their growth cycles. Breast cancer cells that survive chemotherapy drugs react by mutating to increasingly resistant forms. Hormone-insensitive cells eventually dominate. Eventually, most cancers become both hormone- and chemo-resistant—or, as doctors call it, "refractory." This is why it is said that the first course of treatment is likely to be the most effective—because more of the cancer cells are sensitive to the chemotherapy drugs at this point.

Some intriguing research has been done with in vitro chemo-sensitivity testing, where a sample of your tumor cells can be tested in the laboratory to determine the most effective drugs in vitro (literally, "in glass"). As of this writing, these findings are not yet fully conclusive and have not been widely used in clinical applications. This promising area of inquiry, with its potential of sparing metastatic cancer patients the toxicity of drugs not likely to be effective for them, is well worth keeping a careful eye on. References to this type of testing can be found in Appendix B.

Until this technique, or one like it, is perfected and widely used, your doctor won't really know if a drug or combination of drugs will work for you until it is tried. This is quite literally a trial-and-error process, where your doctors, on the basis of clinical studies of other breast cancer patients, and what they know of your individual case, will try to recommend the most active, least toxic treatment for your cancer. Periodically, scans, tumor marker tests or other measurements of the impact of the treatment will be done to assess whether this regimen should be continued, or another one tried.

You and your doctor: Finding a shared treatment philosophy

In oncology today, as in so many other areas of medicine, there are significant controversies that give rise to real differences in treatment philosophy. Since it is your life and ultimately your choice, these differences in philosophy are vitally important to you.

Some doctors believe that treatment for metastatic breast cancer must be palliative, in the sense that since it cannot cure, controlling the spread of disease, relieving symptoms and restoring patients to as normal a life as possible for as long as possible ought to be the primary goals. Quality of life is of paramount concern.

Others disagree passionately, arguing that doctors who stress palliative care are "giving up" on their patients prematurely, and that the newer, very aggressive treatments can significantly prolong lives, and even offer cures in a few cases. To them, the increased short- and long-term side effects seem a worthwhile price to pay for a chance at an extended remission or even cure.

Clearly, personality factors come into play as well—both yours and your doctor's. A good relationship with an oncologist ought to be a little like any good partnership, where there's a need for mutual respect, a shared philosophy of treatment and open communication. If you're a cautious person by nature, a risk-taking, clinical-trial minded oncologist may make you very uneasy. Conversely, if it's important to you to leave no stone unturned in your search for effective treatments, dealing with a conservative oncologist, who stresses palliation, may prove frustrating.

The best doctors listen carefully to their patients' wants and needs, and tailor their own approach accordingly. Dr. Samuel Waxman explained how he approaches his patients with metastatic disease:

> You have to hear a person. Some people want to go the whole route, and even in their last breath be on an experimental program. Others will say, "If you can't really do anything for me, then just make me comfortable." Others say, "Doc, I don't want to go through hell. If you can do something without putting me through hell, and there's a chance, then do that. But don't put me through hell." I feel this is true not only with cancer but with any disease, that everyone has a right to tell you what they want, and it's your obligation as a physician to respect that. Most people will more or less tell you what their position is.

Though there are clearly some guidelines and indications, it's likely that you will discover that no one really knows in advance exactly what the best ongoing treatments for you are likely to be. If you consult several different oncologists, especially if they are practicing at different institutions, it is likely you will receive differing recommendations. In the absence of definitive answers from clinical trials, these controversies in ideology are inevitable. One doctor may want to put you on hormones, another may want to add combination chemotherapy to the hormonal treatment, still another may suggest you might be a candidate for high-dose chemotherapy. This doesn't mean that your doctors don't know what they're talking about, but only that, given the available information, they have drawn different conclusions about how to proceed.

It won't always be this confusing, of course. There are many situations for which consensus does exist, where the choice is straightforward, for example, the use of radiation to treat isolated bone metastases, or the use of surgery to remove isolated loco-regional masses. These are both excellent, proven treatment methods. Radiation for bone metastases reduces pain, stops tumor growth and can prevent broken bones.

Also, the standard first-line conservative treatment for metastatic breast cancer has now incorporated intensive multi-agent chemotherapy with growth factor support (which protects the patient from infection by stimulating the bone marrow to produce white cells). So-called "induction" chemotherapy, often given in preparation for high-dose chemotherapy (with stem cell transplant), is similar to this kind of intensive standard regimen. What this often means is that you have some time, while undergoing treatment, to carefully weigh all options for this important decision. It is also very possible that your particular situation, as it develops, will argue for one approach over another.

Confusing and disturbing as conflicting recommendations may be, they also suggest that control over your treatment is in your hands, and that the choice, ultimately, is yours to make. Until there is, at last, some sort of treatment consensus about metastatic breast cancer in general, it makes sense that you should pursue discovering what is the best treatment for *you*. This leaves you free to look within yourself and ask some hard questions, based on the information you've gathered, your values, your family and support network, your tolerance for pain and discomfort, your willingness to risk a gamble. When you make yourself familiar with your doctor's approach and become mindful of your own wishes, the way ahead will begin to seem clearer, step by step.

Keeping current with new and experimental treatments

In the ongoing struggle for control of the disease, new treatments are constantly being introduced into clinical trials. In the last several years, breast cancer research has been burgeoning, spurred in part by the influx of government research funding that advocates from the National Breast Cancer Coalition and other organizations have fought so hard to win since 1992.

Basic cancer research begun a quarter century ago has accelerated understanding of the mechanism of cancers on a cellular level. Many innovative treatment methods are just beginning to flow from these new developments, as well as further refinements of conventional drugs. Now that more energy is being expended in genetic and molecular biology research, there is every reason to believe that within the next few years, sophisticated new methods that are targeted (only to cancer cells) rather than systemic (affecting normal body cells)—and thus less toxic—will be found to further prolong life for those with metastatic breast cancer. Some of the more exciting new developments are touched upon in the section, "What's new?" later in the chapter.

Because this field is rapidly evolving, it makes good sense, when you discover your breast cancer has metastasized, or when the disease progresses further, to devote some real time and effort to researching the state of what is currently known about treatment for your specific situation. As we've pointed out elsewhere, having a spouse, friend or family member do the research for you can work just as well. There may well be new clinical trials for which you are eligible. There may be innovative treatments unpublished as yet in the literature, or not yet widely known, that your doctor may not even be aware of.

Those who do participate in clinical trials perform an invaluable service, advancing and refining knowledge in the field of oncology that will eventually help other patients. The National Alliance of Breast Cancer Organizations (NABCO), in collaboration with the National Cancer Institute, estimates the rate of breast cancer patients receiving treatment in clinical trials at about 5 percent. This very low level of participation is thought to have slowed the rate of progress in treating the disease successfully. Why more women do not take part has to do with limitations on research funding, as well as with public and physician attitudes and barriers erected by the health care system. NABCO speculates that certain misunderstandings perpetuate the low participation rate:

> By law, all clinical trials must include safeguards to protect patients. Trials must be reviewed by both the sponsoring institutions and the medical community for patient safety and scientific merit. Trials sponsored by the National Cancer Institute (NCI) are required to meet extensive ethical standards of the National Institutes of Health (NIH).

Participants in a clinical trial must give their informed consent based on extensive, understandable information and explanation, and may withdraw from a trial at any time. Patient information is kept strictly confidential.

Most health plans do not cover experimental treatments or the associated doctor and hospital costs. However, TRICARE/CHAMPUS, the Department of Defense health program, has agreed to reimburse members who participate in NCI clinical trials. The NCI along with the American Society of Clinical Oncology (ASCO) and advocates are working with government and private health providers to insure coverage of patient participation in high quality peer-reviewed clinical trials.[7]

In a clinical trial, drugs are first tested for dosage and efficacy, and then the best available treatment is compared with one or more experimental treatments that have already been tested in the laboratory and on patients to determine levels of toxicity. Phase III clinical trials are often done at multiple treatment sites so that enough patients can be enrolled to make the findings valid. There are usually strict requirements for acceptance, and extra testing and record keeping is done for evaluating progress. The treatment protocols, both standard and experimental, are designed by experts in the field, based on the latest findings. Patients are closely monitored for symptoms and side effects, so medical care is generally excellent. If possible, the study is "blind," so that raised expectations of the experimental treatment don't confound the findings. So that the results can be scientifically valid, patients are typically randomly assigned by a computer to the different study groups, or "arms." This is the best way to rule out differences in outcome that may be due to other factors. Sometimes, in smaller studies, patients are matched or "case controlled" instead, so that very similar case histories can be compared.

Ask your oncologist to suggest clinical trials that may be relevant to your case, the National Cancer Institute suggests, since he or she is likely to have access to trial information. But be prepared to take a lot of the initiative yourself in investigating and researching possibilities. While most doctors are happy to do so, some may hesitate about losing their patients to a clinical trial team. Others may be biased toward research at their own institutions. Also, oncologists treating patients with many different kinds of cancer may not have the time or inclination to research all available trials, and may be aware only of the higher-profile trials.

Since clinical trials often take years to enroll enough patients and demonstrate results, sometimes ethical problems result when it begins to look as if an experimental drug will be more or less beneficial, or sometimes even harmful, than the standard treatment with which it is being compared. If the protocol being tested involves currently available substances, women will often elect not to join a clinical trial, in which they run a fifty-fifty chance (sometimes less, if there is more than one experimental arm of the study) of being randomized *not* to receive the drug. Instead, if the drug is already approved for other uses, they may try to find a doctor who will treat them independently. This has happened in recent years with the proliferation of off-trial use of high-dose chemotherapy with stem cell transplant, discussed later in this chapter.

Clinical trials advance medical knowledge, and they also benefit patients. Women who participate in clinical trials do so in part because they know that the knowledge gained will help others, ultimately, and also because this is one way of getting state-of-the-art treatment, observation and care. Most importantly, they choose to participate because they hope to gain access to experimental treatments at least as good as the best standard care for their stage of disease. In her book *The Activist Cancer Patient*, Beverly Zakarian advises a commonsense approach. Forget the popular myth of trial participants as "guinea pigs," she says:

> There is only one important question: Are YOUR best interests served by participating in a clinical trial? Because a clinical trial is, practically speaking, just another treatment option, you should evaluate the information and make treatment choices the same way you would if it were not a trial.[8]

As stated earlier, the NCI CancerNet Service on the Internet is a good place to look for experimental treatments currently in clinical trials, as is the Centerwatch Clinical Trials Listing Service. Both web sites explain the nature of clinical trials.[9] For further sources of information on how to find clinical trials and evaluate them, see Appendix B.

Clinical trials: A closer look

"The new drug development process is lengthy, risky and costly," reports Joseph A. DiMasi, of the Center for the Study of Drug Development at Tufts University, Boston.[10] Typically, a new chemical substance under consideration will go through five separate stages of review.

- **Early research and pre-clinical testing** are the first two stages of reviewing a new drug. Before a drug company can test a drug on people, it must first experiment in the laboratory on cultured tumor cell lines, and on live animals, usually mice implanted with human tumors. These studies will attempt to measure toxicity and determine if the new substance demonstrates chemical properties that might be useful as a drug. When a drug shows promise in vitro, where agents are tested on cell cultures, and in animal studies, the drug company will then file an "investigational new drug application" with the FDA for permission to begin human experiments. The FDA has 30 days to approve or deny the application. Human clinical trials normally have three successive phases.

- **Phase I** trials, using small numbers of human patient volunteers, usually 40 to 80, determine how the body handles the drug, and what safe levels are for its use. Different doses are tested (dose escalation) and in some cases tumor response is also assessed.

- **Phase II** studies done on a larger group, usually between 100 and 300 patient volunteers, evaluate the drug's effectiveness and look for side effects. All patients are likely to receive the treatment at this level, unlike a Phase III trial, in which patients are randomly assigned to experimental and control groups. A drug moves on to Phase III trials if it shows clear clinical efficacy.

- **Phase III** studies are usually multi-center, large-scale trials involving 1,000 to 3,000 volunteers. These are randomized trials, in which an experimental group that receives the test drug is compared with another group that receives standard treatment to confirm effectiveness and monitor reactions to long-term use. Sometimes, more than one experimental group is used, where each "arm" may look at a different dosage or different combination of drugs.

  Optimally, although this is not always possible, neither the researchers nor the patients know who is receiving the experimental drug. This "double blind" process rules out the so-called placebo effect, a known and measurable phenomenon in which physiological responses to a drug may be influenced, at least temporarily, by belief (or lack of belief) in the efficacy of a substance. These trials, in which the new treatment is compared with the best proven treatments, are considered the "gold standard" of clinical research, because they control best for possible "confounding" variables, other factors besides the experimental treatment that may explain differences between the two groups. Phase III trials typically last for several years, and refine knowledge concerning the drug's effectiveness and side effects.

When a drug successfully completes Phase III testing, the pharmaceutical company may request FDA approval so that it can market the drug. If the company produces at least two trials showing both safety and efficacy, it may file a "new drug application" for permission to market the drug.

As you can see, this is a thorough, exhaustive and expensive process. According to Dr. DiMasi, for every 5,000 compounds evaluated in early research phase, only five actually moved to clinical trials last year. And of those five, he says, only one will eventually be licensed by the FDA.

Activists have frequently worked with the FDA and the National Cancer Institute to "fast track" the research process, and make promising drugs in clinical trials available for compassionate use outside of trials. Because supplies of drugs are often severely limited before approval, patient lotteries have had to be used, as they were with the monoclonal antibody Herceptin.

What's new?

The year since this book's first publication has proved to be something of a watershed in cancer research—characterized by as much hype as hope. Tamoxifen prevention trials claimed that the drug prevented 45 percent of breast cancer cases in high-risk women, but no one was sure for how long, or at what cost. Nobel laureate James Watson, discoverer of the structure of DNA, allegedly predicted a cure for cancer within two years—then told the media he'd never made that claim. One biotechnology company's stocks soared, then plummeted, as overblown reports about new drugs were swiftly punctured. The media ran headlines that took anxious cancer patients on a roller coaster ride from desperation to breathless expectancy and back to despair, as they discovered that the "magic bullet" anti-angiogenesis drugs touted by media and eager biotech companies had yet to be tested on humans, or even synthesized in quantities sufficient for human testing.

"Everybody is waiting for the cure," said Donald Coffey, a physician treating prostate cancer patients at Johns Hopkins. "All sorts of overhype and craziness are going on."[11]

But the truth behind the hype is that a revolution of sorts does seem to be unfolding in laboratories and clinics around the world. Scientists are working on a cellular level, manipulating genes and molecules, learning how to turn on and off the chemical switches that directly or indirectly control cell growth and proliferation. Details of how cancer cells divide and grow uncontrollably are at last being deciphered. "We have learned as much about cancer cells and advanced as far in the last 10 years as we have in computers," Coffey said. "We just can't believe the progress—it's exploding on us."

"When President Nixon declared war on cancer back in 1970, there was a lot of excitement and a lot of money available, but the science and technology were very primitive. It was like being given a book to read without an alphabet," said researcher Dennis Slamon, of the Revlon/UCLA Women's Cancer Research Program, from whose laboratory the new breast cancer drug Herceptin has emerged. "But once molecular biology and biotechnology came on line, once we were able to sequence genes, clone genes, and understand their function, we finally had an alphabet." The old cancer treatment paradigm of throwing in a "hand grenade," hoping that you kill more bad cells than good, is at last becoming outdated, Slamon believes, to be replaced by what he terms "the great hope and promise of molecular biology."[12]

"The black box that was the cancer cell has been opened," agrees Bert Vogelstein, a genetics expert at Johns Hopkins. "As researchers, we feel a tremendous amount of hope, probably for the first time in the history of cancer treatment."[13]

Others are less enthusiastic. British researcher Ian Tannock wrote in a recent *Lancet* supplement:

> At cancer meetings, excitement surrounds the sessions on molecular oncology, and its application in biological and genetically based therapy. Sessions on surgery, radiation therapy, and chemotherapy are quiet by comparison. Patients and their support groups want to hear about gene therapy and immune-mediated biological therapy. There is disbelief when

I try to convey gently the sad truth that in 1998 the impact of gene-based therapy is zero and of biological treatment is minimal. For the next few years, cancer management outside the context of a clinical trial will continue to be based almost entirely on surgery, radiation therapy, and systemic treatment with chemotherapy or hormones.[14]

"The techniques of molecular biology have revolutionised our basic understanding of human cancer," echoes researcher David Lane, original discoverer of the p53 tumor suppressor gene. "Yet to date this knowledge explosion has failed to bring radical across-the-board improvements in patients' care, creating a sense of frustration in the clinical community and in the public at large."

Lane points out that a quarter of a century has passed since specific genetic changes in human oncogenes were first identified, marking the beginnings of the molecular biological approach to the study of cancer. What will the next twenty-five years bring?

Twenty-five years from now we will be able to determine accurately, before treatment, the probability of a suitable therapeutic or palliative response in the individual tumour in the individual patient. In twenty-five years' time we will have developed a new generation of cheap and effective treatments for cancer that are not toxic to normal cellular components and that accurately target either the specific genetic defects in the tumour being treated or target the specific physiological state of the tumour and its interaction with the surrounding stroma.

Looking at the nearer future, Lane predicts that, "Molecular biology has the capacity to deliver thousands of such specific inhibitors over the next decade."[15]

Even ten years feels like a lifetime to someone with metastatic breast cancer—as it may well be. There are no promises here. It remains to be seen if the new treatments now being tested will be of benefit to you, even if you are able to gain access to them through clinical trials or through the expanded access programs for compassionate use that many drug companies have instituted. But some of them are already here, today, and more will be by the time you read this. So it makes good sense to inform yourself, and to hang on for the emotional ride that new hopes—and some inevitable new disappointments—are bound to provide. Let's take a look at some of the more promising developments on the immediate horizon.

Improvements in conventional treatments

"I'd love to put radiation and chemotherapy out of business, but it's not happening any time soon," says Dr. John Mendelsohn, oncologist and president of the M.D. Anderson Cancer Center. "We're still going to need all the help we can get, at least over the next five to ten years."[16]

Many of the newer therapies, such as the monoclonal antibody Herceptin, awaiting final approval by the FDA as of this writing, have been shown in clinical trials to work far better in conjunction with chemotherapy than alone.

Improvements and refinements are constantly being made in chemotherapy drugs, alone and in new combinations, and in the ways in which chemotherapy drugs are administered, making them less harmful to the rest of the body.

One example is the efficacy of dexrazoxane (Zinecard) in preventing or reducing the incidence and severity of the potentially damaging affects of Adriamycin on the heart. Another is the liposomal anthracyclines that have been developed to enclose toxic drugs in an "envelope" of protective lipids (fats) and thus protect other parts of the body. Anthracyclines in clinical trials, including liposomal daunorubicin, liposomal anamycin, and liposomal doxorubicin (to be approved and marketed under the names Doxil and Evacet), are demonstrating much lower toxicity profiles than are found with conventional formulations. Clinical trials have shown that liposomal doxorubicin reduces the cardiotoxicity sometimes associated with conventional doxorubicin (Adriamycin), as well as reducing nausea and vomiting, mouth sores, fever and infection.

Chemo-embolization is a method of delivering chemotherapy drugs directly to liver metastases via infusion through implanted tubes. It can be used in selected, otherwise healthy patients who have encapsulated, hypervascular tumors. In trials, this technique has shown reduced toxicity with higher doses of chemotherapy and has produced results superior to systemic chemotherapy. Lisann Charland, with a tumor in her liver and minimal disease elsewhere, had this treatment done at Stanford over three years ago as of this writing, and continues to be stable.

A new process called photo-dynamic therapy (PDT), involving the administration of drugs which can kill tumors when activated by light without hurting healthy surrounding tissue, is currently in clinical trials to treat surface skin lesions in breast cancer. PDT destroys cancerous cells by using fixed-frequency laser light to activate photosensitizing drugs which accumulate more readily and persist longer in cancer cells than in other body cells. Injected by vein, and timed precisely, these photosensitizing drugs work by releasing quantities of an active form of oxygen which destroys the cancer.

In early 1998, the FDA approved capecitabine (Xeloda), a new oral fluoropyrimidine carbamate, and the first oral tumor-activated anticancer drug that has an effect mainly at the site of the tumor rather than in normal tissues. In tumors, Xeloda becomes fluourouracil (5-FU), a known effective chemotherapy agent. In Phase II clinical trials, Xeloda was able to reduce tumors by at least half in a quarter of heavily pre-treated patients. This oral drug is likely to replace the 5-FU continuous administration pumps late stage patients have been using, with better tolerance, fewer side effects and more convenience.

Among the newer chemotherapy agents in clinical trials are the anthrapyrazoles, similar to anthracyclines like doxorubicin, of which losoxantrone is the most promising, as well as teloxantrone, piroxantrone and CI-958. Other thymidylate synthase inhibitors being tested besides capecitabine (see Xeloda, above) are Raltritrexed, Uracil/tegafur, SI and others. A number of antifolates, of which edatrexate appears to be the most promising, are under investigation. New vinca alkaloids, similar to vinorelbine, are under evaluation, as is at least one new taxane, similar to paclitaxel and docetaxel. A new drug called miltefosine (a hexadecylphosphocholine) has been approved in Europe and is under current use as a topical agent for local recurrences of breast cancer. Analogues of camptothecin such as irinotecan (CPT-11), topotecan and 9-AC are being studied.

A number of aromatase inhibitors are being tested similar to anastrozole (Arimidex), which is already widely in use, among them letrozole (Femara), approved for advanced breast cancer in 1997, and vorozole, which has been submitted for FDA approval. Other hormonal treatments under investigation include mifepristone, onaprisone, toremifene, droloxifene and other antiestrogens and antiprogestins. The role of the newly approved estrogen antagonist raloxifene (Evista) in advanced cancer is under investigation.

Drugs that work to strengthen bone loss can act as palliative agents for patients dealing with bone metastases. Among these are bisphosphonates, pamidronate (Aredia), clodronate and Strontium-89.

Vitally important to patients undergoing treatment are the drugs Zofran, Kytril, and a new drug called Anzamet, which have been effective in preventing or greatly decreasing treatment-induced nausea and vomiting. The widespread use of these drugs has made effective chemotherapy treatment possible for many patients previously unable to tolerate its debilitating effects, and has dramatically improved quality of life for almost all people receiving chemotherapy.

Refinements are not only being made to specific chemotherapy drugs and regimens, but to the theoretical models and hypotheses that support their use, emphasizing a need for new strategies. In an article entitled "Evolving Concepts in the Systemic Drug Therapy of Breast Cancer," Dr. Larry Norton, a breast cancer oncologist and researcher from Memorial Sloan-Kettering Cancer Center in New York City, admits that, "It is possible that further understanding of the natural history of tumors will enable better treatments to be developed." In advanced cancer, "dose intensity" strategies like high-dose chemotherapy have shown clear limitations, even when apparent complete responses are achieved, thus "throwing doubt on the assertion that optimal cytotoxic therapy can kill all tumor cells." Other approaches are sorely needed, Norton believes:

> This will require a better understanding of the molecular biology of breast cancer and the ability to predict and assess the sensitivity of individual patient's tumors to individual therapies. Furthering our understanding of the biology and behavior of tumor cells may lead to significant improvements in the long-term prognosis for patients with early and advanced breast cancer.[17]

The new targeted biological therapies

Since every cancer is composed of many different types of cells, each responding to different kinds of growth factors and other signals, the specifically targeted cancer treatments of the future are likely to be complex mixtures of chemicals, individually tailored to each individual tumor type—a far cry from today's less specific chemotherapies that have an impact on all rapidly dividing cells in the body. While these newer substances don't usually kill all cancer cells, they produce their therapeutic results with minimal side effects, potentially turning the cancer into a manageable, chronic illness that may be prevented from progressing.

Gene therapy

In cancerous tumors, genes that normally keep cell growth in check become damaged and no longer are able to function. Over fifty of these mutated genes have been identified in a variety of cancers, and these fall for the most part into three major classes: oncogenes, tumor suppresser genes and mutated reparative genes. Oncogenes control cell growth, and are mutant versions of normal genes. According to pharmaceutical researchers Allen Oliff, Jackson B. Gibbs and Frank McCormick, an oncogene "stimulates cell progression through the cell cycle—the sequence of events in which a cell gets larger, replicates its DNA and divides, passing a complete set of genes to each daughter cell."[18] Tumor suppressor genes normally prevent the growth of malignancies, acting as a kind of brake on cell growth and progression. "Many cancers result from the loss or malfunction of the key regulatory proteins that these genes encode," state Oliff, Gibbs and McCormick. The third type of cancer-related gene, mutated reparative genes, governs the repair and replication of DNA. Without these reparatory mechanisms, the researchers write, "the chances that a damaged gene will be repaired fall drastically, and the likelihood rises that the damage will ultimately be transmitted to the cell's progeny as a permanent mutation." The first two types of genes have diverse functions in growth regulation, differentiation and programmed cell death. Mutated reparative genes have a more indirect role in cancer growth, according to an article on cancer genetics in *Lancet*: "These genes are involved in DNA repair and in maintaining the integrity of the genome in the face of DNA-damaging agents, such as ionizing radiation."[19]

More than half of all cancer patients (and probably a third of breast cancer patients) share a mutation in the p53 gene, which suppresses tumor growth. "Often called the guardian of the genome," according to researchers Oliff, Gibbs and McCormick, "it prevents replication of damaged DNA in normal cells and promotes suicide, or apoptosis, of cells with abnormal DNA."[20] Researchers are working on creating viruses carrying healthy tumor-suppressor genes that can actually "infect" cancer cells. Using the adenovirus that causes the common cold, they inactivate the cold virus by deleting the gene causing its replication process and slipping the p53 gene into its place. In early testing, the introduction of healthy p53 genes in cancer patients has shown some ability to stop tumor growth and even cause some tumors to decrease in size—although there have been problems delivering the virus to all areas of tumor.

Tests have begun on another such gene, known as E1A, in women with cancer of the breast or ovaries. Stem cells infused with the MDR (multi-drug-resistant) gene are being used in conjunction with high-dose chemotherapy in an attempt to circumvent the drug resistance that makes most such procedures fail.

Another genetic therapy in early stages of clinical trials is based on a growth-signaling oncogene known to researchers as RAS, present in about 30 percent of breast cancers and even more common in pancreatic, colon and lung cancers. This gene, when active, tells cells to divide repeatedly. A number of drug companies are currently working on RAS inhibitors, which some investigators feel may show even more promise than the anti-HER-2/neu drugs discussed in the next section.

Monoclonal antibodies

Researchers have found that growth factors and their receptors play a key regulatory role in cell proliferation and oncogenesis. Monoclonal antibodies target certain proteins on the surface or on the nucleus of the cancer cells to block certain key sites, interfering with a tumor's ability to absorb the growth factors it needs from the bloodstream.

Herceptin (anti-HER-2/neu humanized monoclonal antibody) is likely to be the first of the new gene-based therapies for use in breast cancer to make it to the market. Herceptin targets the HER-2/neu protein, produced in excess amounts in some women with breast cancer. Over-expressors of this substance, about 30 percent of women with breast cancer, have too many copies of the HER-2/neu oncogene, which makes a protein that helps send the signal for cells to divide. In clinical trials with heavily pre-treated metastatic breast cancer patients, both as a single agent and more effectively in combination with Adriamycin or Taxol, Herceptin has shown some effectiveness against this particular breast cancer cell mutation, which tends to be aggressive, hard to treat, and resistant to hormonal manipulation. When it works, as it seems to with a significant minority of over-expressors, it has prolonged the time to tumor progression by a few months to several years. Its side effects have been relatively mild, with flu-like symptoms in the early treatments, and some reversible cardiotoxicity in combination with Adriamycin and Taxol. At the time of this writing, this drug is expected to become available as early as late 1998. In the next years, HER-2/neu testing may become a routine part of the staging process for newly diagnosed breast cancer patients, and Herceptin may well have a role to play in adjuvant treatment.

Other antibodies in development target other growth factors. Antibodies for epidermal growth factor (EGF) are currently being tested in head and neck cancers, and a drug known as SU101, which targets platelet-derived growth factor (PDGF), has shown good response in glioblastoma, a particularly deadly brain cancer.

Vaccines and immunotherapy

Cancers are extremely clever at evading the body's immune defenses. Researchers experimenting with dozens of "personalized" vaccines made from antigens taken from a patient's own tumor cells are trying to provoke an immune response whereby the patient's white blood cells would be induced to attack the cancer. Trials with melanoma patients have already shown favorable results with this relatively non-toxic approach. "We plan to kick-start the immune system," says Dr. Brian Czerniecki, of the University of Pennsylvania's School of Medicine.[21] There and at Stanford, vaccines are being made from rare, star-shaped "dentritic" white blood cells, which alert the immune system to the presence of cancer. The potential problem with this approach stems from the fact that tumor cells have many different kinds of mutations, each of which would have to be identified and targeted. Currently in clinical trials is a vaccine against breast cancer polypeptide MUC-1, linked with agents that stimulate the immune system. Vaccines against RAS and p53 oncogenes are also being tested, and an antibody-linked vaccine called TriAb has shown immune activity in heavily pre-treated metastatic breast cancer patients against the HMFG antigen, present in the breast cancer cells.

Since cancer has the ability to evade the body's own immune system, augmenting immune response is another possible approach. Biological response modifiers like Interleukin-2 have been used to stimulate the immune system. Because patients receiving allogenic (donor) transplants following high-dose chemotherapy often seem to do better despite graft-versus-host-disease

(GVHD—a frequent and troublesome side-effect of donor transplants), a few researchers are now experimenting with inducing low-grade GVHD in people who've undergone autologous stem cell transplants, reasoning that an immune system stimulated by GVHD might be more likely to search out and destroy cancer cells as well.

Trying to induce an immune response specific to cancer is painstaking, complex, and frustrating work. Lloyd Old, an immunology researcher at Memorial Sloan-Kettering Cancer Center, puts the task into perspective:

> Despite the great hope of immunotherapy, a dark cloud hangs over all our attempts to control cancer by immune mechanisms. Cancer cells are masters of deceit and disguise—veritable Houdinis that can readily alter themselves to evade immunologic recognition and attack.
>
> Perhaps these therapies will yield cures—the universal objective of cancer researchers, health care providers and, of course, patients. A more achievable aim, though, may be developing therapies that can change the nature of cancer from a progressive and lethal disease to one that can be controlled throughout a long life. That result would be less than ideal, but it could make a world of difference for many afflicted with tumors not readily treatable today.[22]

Anti-angiogenesis factors

To grow beyond the size of a small pea, all solid tumors require their own blood supply to deliver nutrients. Tumors thus have to force the construction of special blood vessels. To accomplish this, they secrete substances that stimulate blood vessel growth in neighboring tissue, inducing the nearest blood vessels to grow new branches in their direction, a process known as angiogenesis. Judah Folkman, whose research group at Children's Hospital Medical Center of Harvard Medical School has been researching angiogenesis since the 1970s, describes what happens then:

> Once neovascularization occurs, hundreds of new capillaries converge on the tiny tumor; each vessel soon has a thick coat of rapidly dividing tumor cells. Some of these cells are not angiogenic but are nonetheless sustained by capillaries recruited by neighboring cells. Now the tumor can expand rapidly—in a matter of months, the mass may reach one cubic centimeter in size and contain around one billion tumor cells.[23]

In 1992, clinical testing began with the first anti-angiogenic drug, known as TNP-470. Dozens of substances are currently being tested that block angiogenesis, although some chemicals identified as anti-angiogenic, like interferon, have proved too weak to produce significant effects in highly malignant tumors. These drugs work in a radically different way than other cancer therapies, Folkman emphasizes:

> Antiangiogenic therapy, in contrast to many other therapeutic approaches, does not aim to destroy tumors. Instead, by limiting their blood supply, it attempts to shrink tumors and prevent them from growing. Antiangiogenic drugs stop new vessels from forming around a tumor and break up the existing network of abnormal capillaries that feeds the cancerous mass.

Prior to the 1998 conference of the American Society of Clinical Oncology, Folkman and his research group received enormous but premature media attention for dramatic results in experiments in mice. He hopes to have his drugs, endostatin and angiostatin, in human trials within a year or two. Among the nine anti-angiogenic substances currently being tested in clinical trials with breast cancer patients are Marimastat, SU5416, Neovastat, Combretastatin, squalamine, TNP-470, and thalidomide—the same drug whose anti-angiogenic capacity produced birth defects when it was used during pregnancy. One company is working on development of a "tumor homing peptide" that links to the anti-cancer drug doxorubicin in a compound called THP-dox, and—the company claims—finds and destroys developing blood vessels in tumors.

Other new targeted therapies in clinical trials

Anti-metastatic factors are directed at enzymes that help cancer cells enter the bloodstream, dissolve tissue and move through capillary walls. An enzyme called telomerase, necessary to cancer cells so that they can keep on dividing, has been isolated, and researchers are working on telomerase-blockers that will force cancer cells to age and die like normal cells. So-called "antisense" molecules have been developed to replace strings of DNA that tell oncogenes to produce growth-promoting proteins.

Retinoids like 4HPR, which are derivatives of Vitamin A, can induce a process called apoptosis, or programmed cell death, in cancer cells. Some retinoids have actually been able to induce a reversal of the process by which cancer cells become undifferentiated, or less like normal cells. This differentiation therapy has proved effective in some kinds of leukemia, and is beginning to be used in solid tumors. A new retinoid known as Targretin (bexarotene), already in trials for lymphoma, lung and other cancers, has demonstrated tumor regression in tamoxifen-resistant tumors in animals and will soon be in clinical trials with advanced breast cancer patients.

Since cancer clearly involves something gone wrong in the normal genetic controls over cellular processes, such as growth, it's a good bet that many of the keys to future successful treatments will be found through genetic research. On the Internet, the NCI CancerNet Service offers a good place to look for experimental treatments currently in clinical trials, as does the Centerwatch Clinical Trials Listing Service. Both web sites explain the nature of clinical trials.[24] Look in Appendix B for further information on clinical trials and how to find them.

Many of the people interviewed for this book found out about new forms of treatment from other patients participating in the Breast Cancer Listserv on the Internet. Online discussion groups are often an excellent place to find out information concerning treatments not yet widely known in the oncology community. Although they don't have an oncologist's expertise, of course, well-informed patients who keep up with the medical literature will often find out about new drugs, or new uses and combinations of older drugs, before their oncologists do. Information about how to subscribe to and participate in the Breast Cancer Listserv discussion group is listed in Appendix B under Listservs.

A treatment controversy: High-dose chemotherapy

Treatment controversies are likely to make you feel profoundly uneasy. You may even avoid seeking another opinion for fear of being overwhelmed with contradictory information and advice. Whom should you trust? It's quite hard enough dealing with a life-threatening illness, but to also find that your doctors don't agree on treatment is even more disquieting. You are not alone in feeling this way. Jeff Belkora, a volunteer decision consultant at the Community Breast Health Project of Palo Alto, advises breast cancer patients that:

> Not running into controversy in breast cancer may be a sign that you
> need to gather more information! Although the lack of consensus about

how to treat breast cancer can be frightening, at least researchers,
clinicians and patients are experimenting with new techniques and
procedures, and generating "controversy." From their experiences and
learning, you can strive to craft a strategy that you believe makes the
most sense for you. But be prepared to make commitments: You will have
to choose who and what to believe, and who and what to ignore. This may
be difficult, for while no one has found a breast cancer treatment that
dominates all others on every dimension, people do have favorites, and
they tend to advocate them with passion. Each may appear convincing,
even as they are contradictory. That's why you need time to analyze
everything in a way that's comfortable for you. Aim to be comfortable and
clear about the reasoning behind every breast cancer decision you make.[25]

Currently, the most dramatic and urgent controversy in the treatment of metastatic breast cancer exists between physicians who believe that a very
aggressive approach early in the progress of metastatic disease raises the possibility for long-term remission or even cure, and those who adhere to the
more conservative intensive standard treatments and who feel that until
definitive results confirm the efficacy of high-dose chemotherapy, the procedure itself is too toxic to routinely offer to patients.

Since there is clearly some dose-response ratio with chemotherapy, in recent
years there has been a trend toward the use of very aggressive treatment protocols, generally in patients under fifty with no other significant complicat-
ing health problems. This section will focus on one of these major controversies, involving the use of high-dose chemotherapy (HDC) with bone marrow
or stem cell support (sometimes called "transplant" or "rescue") with metastatic breast cancer patients.

You should be aware that this chapter, while it goes into some detail on this
issue, is not intended to provide a full or substantive sense of the treatment
issues involved with HDC, but only a feeling for the nature and complexity
of this controversy. If you are considering this treatment, think of this as a
jumping-off place for your investigations. If you are not a candidate for this
treatment, read it for the sense it may give you of how physicians, scientists
and patients work to resolve an important treatment controversy, as well as
some of the less obvious confounding variables that come into play, concerning the economics and politics of health care choices.

While this procedure is often referred to in popular and professional literature by differing initials and names—for example, as autologous bone marrow transplant (ABMT), or peripheral stem-cell transplant or rescue (PSCT; SCR)—this book will refer to this treatment simply as high-dose chemotherapy, or HDC. HDC will thus be differentiated from *intensive* chemotherapy regimens which do not require stem-cell or bone-marrow rescue for treatment survival, but for which growth factors like granulocyte colony stimulating Factor, or G-CSF (Neupogen) that stimulate white blood cell production in the bone marrow are frequently required.

HDC involves the use of very high doses of varying combinations of standard chemotherapy drugs that would be fatal to the blood-cell-producing bone marrow without reinfusion of the patient's own previously harvested and frozen stem cells (the immature cells from the peripheral blood that form white and red cells and platelets) or bone marrow. The use of the patient's own stem cells, rather than those from a donor, is why this kind of transplant is called autologous. This treatment usually, though not invariably, follows an "induction" period where the "tumor burden" (amount of measurable cancer) is reduced through an intensive chemotherapy regimen. This also enables doctors to make sure the tumor is still sensitive to chemotherapy before the high doses are given, almost always a precondition for HDC.

The proponents of HDC believe that "hitting it hard" with high-dose chemotherapy, before the cancer has had a chance to become resistant to treatment, confers the best possibility of treatment success, at least for a subset of younger, otherwise healthy patients whose tumors are chemo-sensitive, who have limited disease and who can withstand the side effects. Depending on the drugs, dosage levels, general health and specific responses, the acute and delayed side effects of HDC may include, but are not limited to, nausea and vomiting, diarrhea, mouth and intestinal ulcers, bone marrow depression (leukopenia, thrombocytopenia, hemolytic anemia), anaphylaxis, peripheral neuropathy, lung damage, hearing loss, cardiac toxicity, acute infections, and a number of less common but serious symptoms like renal dysfunction, hepatic veno-occlusive disease, hemorrhagic cystitis and secondary cancers. High-dose chemotherapy means these drugs are given in doses from 3 to 31 times their standard dosage level, depending upon the combination.

The National Cancer Institute figures say that, according to the Autologous Blood and Marrow Transplant Registry-North America, the number of women with breast cancer receiving HDC grew from an estimated 522 in

1989 to 4,000 in 1994. "About one-third of all stem cell transplants reported to the Registry in 1992 were for breast cancer, making it the most common cancer being treated with this therapy."[26] By 1995, 6,000 cases had been reported to the Registry,[27] and it was estimated by the Registry director that the actual number of HDC procedures for breast cancer was twice that number.[28]

There is no question that HDC produces more complete and partial remissions following the treatment, and this has led to great excitement and enthusiasm. There are reports of women doing very well, with no apparent disease, for several years following the treatment, but there are more reports of relapses within a few months, and a few reports of long-term bone marrow suppression and other side effects that are troublesome and even life-threatening. A certain small percentage of patients die from the toxicity of the procedure itself. While yet unproven, this treatment is being widely offered, with the vast majority of HDCs occurring outside of clinical trials, and covered by health insurance, despite resistance on the part of insurers. A significant number of court cases against insurers have been won by patients seeking this treatment. Reasons for the difficulty in enrolling patients in clinical trials are attributable both to physician and patient reluctance. According to the Women's Health Network:

> *Physicians have been reluctant to encourage their patients to enter these studies, and women themselves have balked at becoming study participants for a number of reasons. Experimental drugs require regulatory oversight that limits access to treatment only through clinical trials, but experimental medical procedures do not have this requirement. To the extent that patients can afford experimental procedures, they probably can find physicians who will provide the treatment outside of a clinical trial. Women are turning down clinical trials because they are afraid that they could be randomized to conventional chemotherapy rather than HDC with ABMT/BCT. Furthermore, it is often in the physician's and hospital's financial interest to offer the more aggressive treatment to patients who can pay for treatment (HDC with ABMT/BCT costs range from $50,000 to $200,000) or are insured for the procedure. Seven states now mandate insurance carrier coverage of HDC with ABMT/BCT for citizens, as does the U.S. for federal workers.[29]*

It appears that the safety of the treatment has increased considerably over the past few years, as treatment centers have refined their techniques and precautionary measures, with published figures varying from 5 percent to up to 17 percent for treatment-related "early deaths," occurring up to a month following treatment. According to the North American Bone Marrow Transplant Registry, treatment-related mortality during the first 100 days following HDC has dropped from 22 percent in 1989 to 5 percent in 1995.[30] During the same six-year period of decreasing mortality, however, the percentage of patients receiving HDC who had metastatic breast cancer (as opposed to high-risk primary breast cancer) decreased from 93 percent to 50 percent, with a corresponding increase from 7 percent to 50 percent in high-risk patients who had loco-regional disease.[31] So it's likely that fewer very sick patients with extensive pretreatment—who would certainly be more at risk for adverse affects of HDC—received the HDC at the end of the period under question.

"Based on the recent studies, the mortality for this treatment has decreased substantially in the past few years," concurs oncologist Craig Henderson from the University of California, San Francisco. "However, it's not clear that high-dose chemotherapy with ABMT is the best treatment for any group of patients, that it will cure any patient that would not be cured by other treatments, or that it will prolong survival to a greater extent than commonly used conventional dose chemotherapy."[32]

Dr. Karen Antman, Chief of Medical Oncology at Columbia Presbyterian Medical Center in New York City, urges careful patient selection. Patients with advanced refractory disease are not likely to benefit from the procedure, she warns, but goes on to say that of those untreated, chemo-sensitive patients who do achieve a complete response (CR), "A quarter to a half of those achieving CR have no evidence of progression with follow-up intervals of two to four years in trials at multiple institutions."[33]

Dr. Gabriel Hortobagyi, of the MD Anderson Cancer Center at the University of Texas, reviewing a decade of Phase I and II trials of "dose intensification" (yet another term used for HDC), writes:

> *Results from these trials suggest that dose intensification with hemopoietic support markedly improves overall response rates and consistently results in complete remission rates approaching 50 percent in patients with previously untreated metastatic breast cancer. Although no study has demonstrated an improvement in median survival, several investigators suggest that 15 percent to 25 percent of patients treated with*

dose-intensive therapies remain in unmaintained remission 2 to 5 years after the procedure. It is uncertain whether this apparently reproducible group of long-term survivors is related to the beneficial effect of high-dose chemotherapy or to the extraordinary patient selection process undertaken in high-dose chemotherapy programs.[34]

To try to answer this question, Dr. Hortobagyi and his colleagues reviewed a series of studies at M.D. Anderson, of 1,581 metastatic breast cancer patients who had been treated with doxorubicin-based conventional chemotherapy before 1982, so that they could look at long-term results. Among the 263 who achieved a complete response, nearly 19 percent remained in complete remission five years later (3 percent of the total number of patients). In many respects this group, identified as having a much better prognosis, perfectly matched the group of patients who meet the stringent selection criteria required by the trials for HDC. Not surprisingly, their outcomes were also similar.[35]

But for doctors and patients to gain a really accurate sense of the relative effectiveness of HDC in relation to standard intensive chemotherapy, historical controls are not conclusive evidence. Women must be randomly assigned either to the experimental treatment or to the comparison treatment, which must be the best conventional standard-dose chemotherapy available. There are three current well-designed, randomized, controlled trials investigating HDC, both in women with metastatic breast cancer and in very high-risk Stage II/III primary breast cancer patients who have more than ten lymph nodes showing signs of cancer or who have inflammatory breast cancer. These multi-center trials, taking place throughout the country, have had considerable initial difficulties with enrollment, but expect, before the year 2000, to provide some real answers. It is likely that by the time you read this, more will have been clarified about which patients can actually be helped by this treatment, and which may do better or as well with conventional treatments with far less toxicity.

Some oncologists, like Dr. Yashar Hirshaut, have seen a number of their metastatic patients do remarkably well and go on to have extended disease-free remissions.

The best results are obtained when we hit hard with the initial treatment after a recurrence, so as to destroy as much of the disease as we can—and, if possible, all of it. If, despite our best efforts, the cancer again recurs, it may be because it has become resistant to the drugs in use. We may be able to prevent such a development by alternating different forms of chemotherapy or by refining the use of such techniques as bone-marrow transplant, placing the first and primary emphasis, whenever possible, on trying for cure. We attempt to accomplish that goal with a minimum of disruption of life of the patient but with the understanding that when we are dealing with an aggressive cancer, we must act aggressively.[36]

Other oncologists are concerned that the toxicity of HDC leaves the majority of women who are not helped by this treatment with fewer options when their cancer recurs. Dismayed at the widespread marketing of HDC outside of clinical trials, they still consider this aggressive treatment highly experimental in the metastatic setting. Dr. Samuel Waxman, oncologist and researcher at Mt. Sinai Medical Center in New York City, maintains that:

Statistics show that there should be a 50 to 60 percent response rate with breast cancer with conventional chemotherapy, 70 percent with intensive chemotherapy, and maybe 80 percent with high-dose chemotherapy with stem-cell support. I don't think there's any doubt that marrow- and stem-cell supported high-dose chemotherapy can give you a better response rate. I just don't know if that translates into more time.

Like many other cancer doctors, Waxman believes it is possible to get equal results with far less toxicity by "playing out" differing treatment combinations, trying to outwit the cancer by ingenious combinations of drugs.

There's an art to this as well as a science. There are many effective chemotherapy protocols and ways of manipulating hormones. We can rest a person on hormones and then return her to chemotherapy. If you just bring a woman in and shoot from the hip with high-dose chemotherapy, it does not insure improved survival. Sure, there's evidence that the more chemotherapy you give, the more cancer cells you're going to kill. But that doesn't mean you're going to cure the patient, because it's very difficult to totally eradicate cancer once it is in some recurrent form. Cancer cells are impervious to drugs at given times in the cell cycle and, unlike normal cells, have an innate drug resistance, or rapidly acquire it because of their genetic instability.

To date, only one randomized, controlled study has been published, involving 90 patients in South Africa.[37] This study demonstrated an impressive complete or partial remission in nearly 95 percent of patients receiving HDC (as opposed to 53 percent in the sub-optimal standard-dose treatment arm) and indicated that 20 percent of patients had extended remissions of two years. While the conventional treatment arm was less than state-of-the-art intensive chemotherapy, the results in the HDC treatment arm were seen as encouraging.

At a 1995 oncology conference, a summary review of HDC results to date was presented, citing a number of small studies done over the prior decade, which seemed to indicate the importance of patient selection in determining success, and citing a few long-term survivors as possible evidence of efficacy.

> *Subsequent studies of HDCT in patients with Stage IV breast cancer were designed to maximize the response with a doxorubicin-based induction regimen prior to high-dose consolidation. Several published studies obtained similar results, i.e., 15–20 percent progression-free survival at greater than 2 years. Whether remission induction prior to HDCT improves disease-free survival remains to be determined in prospective randomized trials. It is unclear whether there are specific subsets of Stage IV patients more likely to benefit from HDCT than others. The most promising area of study in breast cancer is in patients with high-risk primary disease. Phase II data for patients with greater than 10 axillary lymph nodes shows 64 percent disease-free survival at 5 years.*[38]

How is a patient to know which treatment to select, if there aren't relevant studies available yet? In the absence of more controlled, randomized studies providing a direct comparison, a meta-analysis of treatment studies can be used to provide a broader basis for decision-making, though no definitive conclusions can as yet be drawn.

Published in 1996, such a meta-analysis was done by the World Health Organization affiliate ECRI, comparing 49 uncontrolled studies, involving 1,017 metastatic breast cancer patients treated with HDC, with 35 studies of 4,889 patients with similar characteristics treated with standard-dose chemotherapy regimens. This constitutes the most comprehensive review of the available data on HDC until that point.

The ECRI meta-analysis came to a number of striking conclusions. According to this study, the initial higher response rate to HDC appears to have little or no effect on disease progression and longevity, and may instead be related to favorable treatment selection, since chemo-insensitive patients were routinely screened out of HDC studies. While some subgroups may indeed do better with HDC, there is no way of identifying these patients for sure, and thus protecting other patients from the significant toxicity and mortality risk of the treatment. Most important, published studies actually appeared to show higher and longer disease-free and overall survival rates for standard-dose chemotherapies. Even in the case of the one randomized South African HDC trial mentioned above, ECRI lists seven published trials where survival was equal or better with standard-dose therapies.[39]

In early 1998, an extensive review of the medical literature of HDC for breast cancer appeared in the February edition of the *Journal of the National Cancer Institute*. This review article's excellent bibliography culls out the important research articles from the hundreds that have been published to date, and would be valuable for this alone even if it did not also offer other important insights. The physicians who wrote this review, JoAnne Zujewski, Anita Nelson and Jeffrey Abrams, came to many of the same conclusions that ECRI had. Existing studies, they found, showed:

> *The median survival (with HDC) is similar to that of historic controls, and a small percentage of persons remain disease-free three to five years after therapy. It is this small percentage of persons (the "tail on the curve") who remain disease-free that has led to the enthusiasm for this procedure.*

They also found that the patient selection that is central to HDC is crucial, leading to overestimation of results by those who have interpreted the Phase II studies over-optimistically. In reviewing the largest study of historic controls (mentioned earlier in this section), done at MD Anderson,[40] they make the point that:

> *The authors estimated that 65 percent to 75 percent of patients eligible for conventional-dose chemotherapy programs would not be candidates for HDC/ASCR programs. This rigorous selection process would be expected to identify a subgroup of patients with a better prognosis. Indeed, in this analysis, patients potentially eligible for HDC/ASCR did have higher overall response rates, higher complete response rates, and a median response rate that was 65 percent longer than patients treated with the same doxorubicin-containing regimen in conventional doses.*

Zujewski and her colleagues conclude:

> *Despite the frequency with which this procedure is performed, the role of HDC/ASCR in the treatment of breast cancer remains undefined. Given the limitations of available data, it is somewhat surprising that thousands of women have undergone HDC/ASCR for the treatment of breast cancer. Perhaps physicians are not as familiar with the limitations of the data as one might presume.[41]*

Developments continue. In August 1998, a randomized study of HDC in ninety-seven high-risk breast cancer patients from Holland was published in the British medical journal, *Lancet*. With a median follow-up period of just over four years, the overall and relapse-free survival in this study showed "no significant difference between the patients on conventional therapy, and those on high-dose therapy." Although the results await confirmation by larger randomized studies still in progress, the authors conclude:

> *High dose therapy is associated with substantial cost and acute toxic effects, but also has potentially irreversible long-term effects. Until the benefit of this therapy is substantiated by large-scale Phase III trials, high-dose chemotherapy should not be used in the adjuvant treatment of breast cancer, apart from in randomized studies.[42]*

Taking a chance on life: How people decide

Given the toxicity and risks of HDC, and the fact that the research findings are still equivocal, why do doctors recommend it and younger women continue to decide on this treatment in such large numbers? The simple answer is that we don't base our choices solely on science, on proof of a treatment, or on lack of proof. Breast cancer patient Bill Sherman put it this way:

> *How do we "know" anything we do will save our life? I don't think we do. We gather as much information as possible and make a "leap of faith" and hope/pray we made the right decision that will be beneficial for us. I have learned there are no right answers that apply to all of us and although we all have breast cancer, it is still very much an individual disease and the responsibility for how we attack it is very much an individual decision. The bottom line: I have to do what I decide is best for me with no guarantees of the outcome.*

A provocative study conducted at a London hospital, published in the *British Medical Journal* in 1990, compared attitudes about chemotherapy choices among cancer patients, doctors and nurses, and the general public. When asked if they would undergo a hypothetical aggressive chemotherapy treatment, given a relatively low percentage chance of cure, of prolonging life or of palliation of symptoms, the study, even when repeated, found that health professionals and the general public felt they would require a 50 percent chance of cure to undergo the treatment, while many cancer patients were willing to undergo treatment for a one percent chance of cure. Cancer patients said they would undergo treatment if it might give them one more year of life, while health professionals and the general public said it would only be worthwhile if it conferred two to five years of extended life. Finally, patients said they'd risk the treatment for only a 10 percent chance at palliation of symptoms, while health professionals and the public said that they'd require 75 percent chance of palliation. "Patients with cancer are much more likely to opt for radical treatment with minimal chance of benefit than people who do not have cancer, including medical and nursing professionals."[43] Much more on the thorny and complicated issue of treatment choices will be discussed in Chapter 11, *Final Gifts*, in the section on end-of-life decision-making.

A 1995 mail survey by the Soper Research firm, jointly sponsored by the National Alliance of Breast Cancer Organizations, Y-Me Breast Cancer Organization of Chicago and the Susan G. Komen Foundation, asked 1,500 women with metastatic breast cancer about their treatment choices. Of the 256 women who responded, over half said that it was they, not their doctors, who took the lead in selecting treatment. More than three quarters said that side effects and quality-of-life issues were far less important than tumor response to treatment. And nearly half felt that the main encouragement of chemotherapy was the preservation of hope. "This came as a surprise to many of us, who expected some desire for balance between aggressive therapy and quality of life," said Michelle Melin, Director of Patient Services for Y-ME. "But we found many women willing to pursue very aggressive therapy continuously until there were no more options."[44]

It is obvious that both doctors and patients pay attention to anecdotal information along the way, even though, as everyone knows, your second cousin Mabel's friend's case is of no statistical value in predicting your own treatment outcome. If you know someone with metastatic breast cancer in long-term remission following HDC, this is likely to color your decision. Conversely, if someone you know has died or been disabled from the treatment, this is bound to make you wary. Dr. John Winberg, of the Foundation for Informed Medical Decision-Making, puts it this way:

> There is a lot of raw information out there that simply is almost all case reports of individual patients, and in the epidemiologic literature case reports get the lowest grade of all, in terms of validity, because they do not have a control group, they do not have a balanced statistical evaluation. So the idea basically is to inform the patient in detail about the different outcomes associated with the different treatments, and at the same time to make it clear that the decision ultimately depends on the patient's own view of the situation, the patient's own preferences. There is no single right answer which the doctor can prescribe.

The doctor who recommends high-dose chemotherapy to you may well have known a few patients who've had excellent results, with no apparent, or minimal, lasting side effects. The hope is that the remissions enjoyed by up to 20 percent of patients receiving the treatment will prove to be very long-lasting. To many younger, otherwise healthy patients, this treatment seems like a risk well worth taking. One caution, however: Physicians associated with a bone-marrow or stem-cell transplant program may not be the most objective or unbiased parties for you to consult in evaluating the advisability of going this route. Doctors are human, too, and it's only human nature to believe in the treatment they offer patients. And medicine, let's not forget, is becoming more and more a bottom line driven business. It's wise to pursue an objective second option from an oncologist unaffiliated with a transplant program before making your decision.

Examining the way people make treatment decisions, and even the nature of hope itself, may shed some light on why people decide as they do, and how you can find your way to your own best decision. Sound medical research is one important basis for our decisions, but it is far from the only factor we take into account when making our choices. Cancer researchers, physicians and patients often have radically different perspectives, as the two studies cited above suggest. Michael Lerner, director of Commonweal, a California health and environmental research institute, and cofounder of Common-weal's Cancer Help program, has been studying medical decision-making his whole professional life, and discusses it at length in the preface of his book *Choices in Healing*:

> Cancer researchers, like all scientists, often do their work best by a constant process of doubting whether promising results from a new study are actually correct or not. That healthy process of doubt leads them to check and recheck every study. They have nothing to lose and everything to gain by living in a research culture that emphasizes the primacy of doubt. Their goal is to contribute to the formulation of lasting true statements about the biomedical nature and treatment of cancer.
>
> People with cancer are fundamentally in a different situation. To begin with, the time perspective of cancer patients is different. They are more interested than cancer researchers in treatment possibilities that offer some hope during the time defined by their particular disease.[45]

By analogy, as Lerner points out, the cancer patient is rather like a government policy maker faced with a national emergency, say an environmental crisis. She must make an immediate decision on the basis of incomplete information and uncertain outcomes. Her scientific advisors have an important role to play—they must tell her what is known about the crisis, what is not known, what would clearly lead to disaster in the face of current knowledge, and what risk levels may be involved with other courses of action. "The policy maker then decides on a course of action based on considerations that are often entirely extraneous to the scientific argument," Lerner points out. "The policy maker decides for the nation just as the cancer patient must decide for himself."

Reflections on treatment choices

Cancer patients sometimes talk about an inner acquiescence to treatment, a combination of acceptance, resignation and hopefulness that enables them to withstand the side effects and uncertainty that go along with chemotherapy. The choices made for or against HDC, with its quality of being a high stakes gamble, only magnify the sensitive, personal nature of every cancer patient's choice of whether or not to seek treatment.

When all was said and done, most of the people I interviewed felt they had made the best decisions for themselves, at the time—whatever their choices had been, and whatever the outcome. Over and over again, they emphasized the importance of the following factors:

- Getting all the relevant information.

- Understanding the treatment goals and process as fully as possible.

- Considering the risks and benefits of treatment in relation to the possible outcomes, including a full awareness of potential side effects.

- Gathering other medical opinions.

- Talking with other patients, and spouses or partners.

- Developing a sense of real trust in the treatment team, particularly in the primary oncologist.

- Then turning inward to make the best decision they could.

A certain empowerment, psychologically beneficial in itself, is inherent in this kind of decision-making process. It's altogether possible, of course, that people rationalize their decisions, whatever they are. Having no regrets is important for emotional well-being, but for the people I interviewed, this seemed to depend far more on having gone through a reasonable decision-making process than on whether or not the outcome was the one desired.

Monica Driver, a high-risk primary breast cancer patient, at first agreed to HDC, and cited the reasons for her choice:

> Factors that influenced my decision? The notion of "hit it hard before it becomes resistant" made sense to me (some old biologist-type training there) and to my husband. My husband and I agreed with Susan Love's notion that a research protocol can be a good way to get treatment. The local MDs were enthusiastic about the particular study I was being offered. Obviously, much of this was personal and specific to our own situation. But that's how I/we decided.

After her stem cells were harvested and her induction chemotherapy was underway, Monica began to have doubts, and decided to consult a psychiatrist who had worked with many breast cancer patients. Monica explored her feelings:

> For a long time the most pressing argument for going forward with HDC, other than to stay alive for my family, was to psychologically avoid any "What ifs" or "If onlys" should cancer return. I could comfortably say, "Well, I did everything I could to lick the beast and it was just not meant

to be." This does make some sense, but it seems a backdoor means of making a decision.

Do I do the practical, expected thing and try to possibly prolong my life via HDC while both risking long-term side effects and giving up a number of months for recovery, or do I kick over the traces and live to the fullest now while I feel physically able to do so? She (the psychiatrist) described this as living with joie de vivre. I have always been the practical caregiver type, thinking of everyone before myself. Now that I have accepted the fact that my life may not be open-ended, I feel like kicking over the traces and really letting my hair down (that doesn't mean a whole lot as I only have half an inch to let down, but you know what I mean). She did not help with the decision, but I felt better for having discussed it and for being understood. It was also the first time that I had admitted, even to myself, to a basically selfish desire to live fully in what time I have left. I think if I were younger, had young children, or felt sicker, this would be an easier decision. I don't look forward to the HDC/ SCT itself, but that is not what holds me back. It is the loss of time and the possible long-term quality-of-life problems. When I read about others who go through HDC/SCT and then have recurrences so soon afterwards, I falter.

It wasn't easy to maintain her decision to forego the HDC in favor of conventional chemotherapy. Monica experienced a great deal of pressure from her physicians:

It is hard to buck the tide, go against the advice of multiple doctors, and to decide something which "might" shorten your life. The doctors even attempt to lay guilt trips on you. When I told the first oncologist that I was hesitating (she strongly advised HDC/SCT), she said, "Well, if you could see the rapidity with which your cells are dividing you wouldn't hesitate for a minute." She said this in front of my husband, which added to the pressure on me because then he wanted me to do the HDC and I felt guilty not to be treated more aggressively for "his" sake. This whole thing is horrible. Doctors at BMT centers spend hours with you, often 3 to 4 hours with more than one doctor at a time—where else would a doctor spend so much time with you? It can only mean that they want and need you in their unit.

Ultimately, her husband fully supported her decision, and Monica went on to seek two courses of intensive chemotherapy as a substitute for the HDC. She is grateful for the fact that unrelated health concerns which made it impossible for her to take the most common drug used for HDC caused her to research the issues more thoroughly than she might have.

> *If I had not had to shop around for someone who would treat me off study, I might have been swept into HDC after 4 rounds of CA and not had time to explore not only my options, but my own heart.*

Monica has found a way to live comfortably with her choice, and even to redefine courage, as in this message to another woman who was wrestling with the same decision:

> *One thing I think you should know, and that is that the opposite decision can be made out of love also. Out of love you can decide not to fight further. Everyone is different, and clinging to the last vestige of life is not always right. You are not a hero just because you fight against all odds. Don't for a minute think that if you decide not to go forward with the most aggressive treatment that you are any less a hero.*

As the husband of a Stage IV breast cancer patient, Glenn Clabo thought a great deal about his wife having chosen HDC. Following her decision, he wrote:

> *I've read the theories, opinions, thoughts and feelings about amount versus success. I'm not comfortable with the less may be better attitude. I'm too scared to say more is better.... I defer to the doc and Barb's wishes. She's my love, but it's her life. I guess this comes down to Barb's wish to do the most she can while healthy enough to make it through. I have my concerns with all the long-term possibilities, including...what if nothing is done? She has put her head down and said, let's give it hell. I'll continue to pass the info and support her through whatever she decides to do.*

After his wife had undergone the treatment and was recovering well, Glenn found a discussion on the pros and cons of HDC on the Breast Cancer Listserv agonizing to read:

> *For those that question the cost and success of this.... Don't you realize without focus there is no hope? Without hope, what's next? Does someone like Barb wait and take her chances that she'll be here if this is proven*

*years from now? What else can her decision be based on but hope? The
desire to live.*

Breast cancer activist Karen Gray, who participated as a patient-advocate in
the preparation of the Patient Reference Guide of the ECRI meta-analysis,
responded:

> *Hope is something that anyone can have whatever the choice. It isn't
> limited to those who have HDC. Hope can always be a part of our lives
> because it isn't dependent on statistics at all. It is a state of mind entirely
> independent of one's condition in life. And if you need focus you only need
> know that there are always a residual few who end up doing well despite
> a grim prognosis. There are always the unusual cases to focus on whether
> they are taken as spontaneous remissions, miracles or whatever. They can
> serve us all as life-jackets so we don't sink into an ocean of depression.*

> *I know a number of women who choose standard intensive therapies
> and there is no difference between their being hopeful and those who did
> HDC being hopeful. Both know they're playing at a game table where
> they don't control the spin of the wheel and time alone will show the
> results.*

> *Hope is not a matter of rationality. It is a matter of inner affirma-
> tion of a future where survival and health remains one possibility—how-
> ever remote—until death closes the door to all possibilities except itself.*

Shari Kahane, also a high-risk patient, detailed the kind of questions she had
asked herself in making her decision about whether or not to undergo HDC:

> *The decision whether or not to have high-dose is a very personal one
> that only the person involved, with the help of his or her family, can
> make. There are many difficult aspects to this decision. First, do I want to
> take the risk of possibly dying from the treatment? Second, what is the
> possible benefit of this procedure? In some cases it is not known yet what
> the long-term benefits will be. Third, which chemo regimen might be most
> effective? Fourth, if I decide to do this, where should I do it? Where are the
> survival numbers the best? Fifth, what are the long-term side effects and
> am I willing to accept them?*

> *For some women, high-dose is not the right choice. They may not
> have tumors that respond well to chemo or they may be too uncomfort-*

*able with the risks of such aggressive treatment. I believe it is an
immensely personal choice that has to be made carefully and under no
pressure from either the treating physician or the patient's family. I can
only relate my own experience. When faced with a very poor prognosis
that no one disputed, I chose high-dose because I had two young children.
If I died during the procedure I wanted them to know that I had done
what felt right to me. I do have permanent side effects of nerve damage to
my hands and feet and my white blood cell count remains very low. I will
never have the energy I used to have, and still have other lingering effects
as well. My own personal belief was that the "big guns" were right for me
but may not be so for everyone. Like anything else in life, one has to
weigh the potential positives and negatives, explore all options, be as
informed as possible and then make the decision.*

Jacque Fisher, who elected to try HDC after a regional recurrence was followed by a pleural effusion, came to see her own decision-making process
this way:

*Through all of this there have been a lot of woulda, shoulda,
coulda's...those will drive you crazy. I have gone through all of the stages
of denial, acceptance, anger...fear, etc. What I have tried to do is investigate my alternatives, choose treatment, place faith in my judgment, my
doctors and God, and then turn it over to them! I try to never look back
and rethink once I have chosen my path. I aggressively fight the disease
and any kind of "acting sick." Even when I am in a "down" period...I am
convinced that all is going well...only looking back do I see how weak I
was.*

Scott Kitterman encouraged his wife, Mary, to undergo HDC as her best
choice, although they both knew that there was little chance of long-term
remission:

*I asked Mary if she'd rather bunt and maximize her chance of get-
ting on first base or swing hard and try and knock one out of the park
knowing that increased her risk of striking out. She didn't even hesitate
before saying knock one out of the park.*

For Barb Pender, too, it was not the outcome that dictated whether or not
she felt at ease with her treatment choice.

I am still here three years later—not cancer-free, mind you (it did return within the year after my second transplant), but I am still here and that is what is important to me. The BMT bought me time—time to see my son reach sixteen this year, time for my grandson to get a little older to attempt to understand illness and death, and time for my three-year-old granddaughter to know I exist. Others might say that my BMT was not successful because of the cancer returning but they are wrong! Every procedure that I undertake is a success to me by virtue that I am still alive. But please keep in mind that this is my personal experience and not everyone has the same experience. I had heard of the good stories and of the bad stories—I could only pray that mine fell somewhere in the middle and, to my surprise, it was better than I had hoped.

Not everyone is as sanguine, however, looking back. As his wife, Ginger, lost ground, Bob Crisp reflected on the state of cancer research with some bitterness:

Everyone wants to think they are taking an aggressive approach to cancer and that they can handle it. Ginger's had four surgeries, extensive radiation, several different chemo regimens, a HDC/SCR and is about to have some more radiation. The treatments have certainly been brutal and difficult. The cancer continues. Is it possible to overtreat cancer? Looking back, the answer for me is yes.

We don't need to be fighting harder; we need to be fighting smarter. After our twenty-five-year [as of April 1996] and $37 billion "war" on cancer we have: 1) 13 percent increase in cancer incidence, 2) 7 percent increase in death rate, and 3) the five-year survival is virtually unchanged. I still contend that we can't leave the research to the isolated medical community which has a proven failure record. It is time for new paradigms, starting with multi-disciplinary research teams.

As a high-risk primary breast cancer patient, Bonnie Gelbwasser continues to feel that the choices she made were right for her:

At diagnosis in early December 1993, I was told that the five-year survival rate for women with inflammatory breast cancer was 50 percent. However, my doctors also stressed at that time that with aggressive treatment and with the strides in medical research and care, I could hope to beat those odds.

So my hope was to get five or more years of life. The head of the Bone Marrow Transplant Unit at the hospital was adamant that I not view the ABMT as a cure, but rather as a chance for a longer life. That was perfectly acceptable to me. No one promised me the moon.

Sue Tokuyama felt much the same way about her HDC, but would have handled it differently on an emotional level:

Do I think the HDC/ABMT was worth it? I don't know. I just needed to do the most reasonable thing at the time, with as much intelligence as I could muster. It seemed like the best thing they had to offer. A few people on the list have flown through the process with far more grace and panache than me. My experience would be better described as an angry, awkward, profane brawl, or blind shadow-boxing.

Would I do it again? Yes. In retrospect, I wish that I had spent a couple of weeks prior to the experience creating peace inside myself.

For what it's worth, a year out—Mr. Nasty seems to be gone, or hiding well.

Whatever their treatment choices and situation, patients appreciate support for making their own decisions. Joleene Kolenburg was moved by her husband's support of her treatment choices:

My husband got a call from a friend of his from the past today who had heard about my mets to the lungs. He told Jack that his wife had a breast removed recently, had one treatment of chemo, lost her hair, and was sick and said, "No more." Went to another doctor who said she did not need any more chemo. It might kill any cancer cells, and it might not. She might get mets and she might not. And if she took chemo, she still might get mets. So she went back to work and is doing fine. I guess he wanted to talk with Jack to prove that yes, you could get mets even if you took chemo (as I did) the first time around. He quoted scripture about "the time to die," etc. Jack told him we believe that, too, but Jo (me) was a fighter and wanted to do everything she could to fight this thing, and he was with me 100 percent. It was the first time that Jack had talked at length with anyone about this and I was proud of him, and pleased that he supported my decision when talking to his friend. Jack told him that it was good that he (the friend) supported his wife's decision, just as Jack did mine. "After all, it is their life and their decision."

Kim Banks wrote of her tendency to regret treatment choices later on:

Because of my recurrence I have sometimes regretted not trying harder to take tamoxifen three years ago—I have a history of migraine headaches and the tamoxifen caused them to quadruple in intensity. Thinking back, I know now that I made the right decision for me at the time. I don't want to spend the rest of my life worrying rather than living.

Something I'd like to add: Many breast cancer patients feel pressured from family and friends, as well as themselves, to choose the most aggressive treatment. Often they don't really know what it is like to go through those treatments, nor do they understand the difference in outcomes (in many cases, negligible). I guess it's another situation where we must know ourselves and be true to ourselves. Make the decisions for our own reasons and derive comfort in knowing that we've chosen what is best for us.

CHAPTER 7

Hope and Healing for the Rest of You

Complementary Therapies

METASTATIC BREAST CANCER PATIENTS often find they need more help than their doctors can provide. To a large extent this does not derive from the failing of individual physicians, but a realistic appraisal of the limits both of medicine itself and on the time and capacities of its practitioners. The focus of increasingly complex and specialized Western medicine is on disease, and not on the needs of the whole person. This has led people, in ever-increasing numbers, to seek help from outside the medical community. This chapter discusses the importance of complementary methods and the vital role they can play in your life, as well as the qualities people have found most helpful—and unhelpful—in relationships with their doctors.

In seeking other kinds of help, it's important for you to distinguish between alternative treatments, designed to replace Western medicine, and complementary methods, which work alongside medical treatments. Many models of cancer in the popular culture involve a simplistic, blame-the-victim mentality, without understanding the harm this can cause. Metastatic breast cancer patients who turn to complementary treatments must select between many choices. Evaluating what is right for you can be difficult and confusing, and involves a process of self-discovery. Since depression and anxiety are common problems for people dealing with advanced cancer, it's also important for you to think about better ways of handling the difficult emotions that go along with coping with a long-term illness, and regaining a sense of hope and control. Support and self-help groups are discussed as an integral part of that process.

Finally, the chapter closes with a reflection on the difference between medical cure and "healing," a more inclusive concept that takes the whole person into account.

Purveyors of hope

While the vast majority of breast cancer patients undergo conventional medical treatments, many also seek out other methods for dealing with the disease and the emotional stress it causes. These diverse methods, variously termed holistic, alternative, complementary, unproven, unconventional or unorthodox, have evolved into an enormous industry in the United States. They form an integral part of a popular culture that focuses increasingly on inspirational and spiritual themes and non-medical treatments for—and explanations of—serious illness. Billions of dollars every year go into the pockets of purveyors of unconventional approaches, legitimate and otherwise. A 1991 survey showed that the number of visits to alternative medicine practitioners in the United States, an estimated 425 million, actually exceeded the visits to all primary care doctors in that year.[1]

In fact, more than half of all cancer patients participate in some form of unorthodox or unproven therapy, and three quarters of them don't tell their oncologists.[2] Techniques and ideas considered "fringe" only a few years ago are now in the mainstream, thanks to best-selling gurus like Deepak Chopra and Bernie Siegel.

Due in part to the success and popularity of anti-professional self-help groups, influenced by the 12 Step or Recovery Movement, peer cancer support groups have become common in cities and towns across the country. Both Western and Eastern traditional healing techniques like chiropractic, homeopathy, naturopathy, acupuncture and Chinese herbal medicine are enjoying revivals. Large numbers of people are becoming involved with once esoteric practices like yoga, meditation, massage therapy and Eastern movement therapies like Tai Chi and Qi Gong.

Various special diets, herbal remedies and nutritional supplementation, including megadoses of anti-oxidants and other micronutrients, are often touted as "immune system boosters" or cancer-fighting agents. These influences have influenced our media, and affected our pocketbooks and our health practices, as well as our spiritual and psychological beliefs.

Medical disillusionment and the new holistic healing movement

It is no accident that the holistic health movement, as it is sometimes called, seems to be flourishing at a time when conventional Western medicine is more beset than ever with ethical, moral and financial problems, and the public's trust in physicians and the health care system in general is at an all time low. As an aging population, most of us grew up in an era when stories of scientific breakthroughs and miraculous cures were commonplace. We've come to expect miracles and magic bullets, and it's easy to understand why. In our lifetimes, innovations in public health, antibiotics and immunization have saved millions of lives. Advances in surgical techniques have revolutionized care for many previously incurable conditions. But now, the picture has changed. It is the chronic disorders of modern life—cancer, stroke and heart disease—that are now responsible for the deaths of most Americans. For these complex diseases, there are no simple cures. And these days, the advances of medical technology, as often as not, are accompanied by grave ethical and practical concerns. End-of-life dilemmas and our collective reluctance to acknowledge and make provisions for death and dying become ever more evident.

Although there have been clear gains in the field of oncology, the bright promise of technical medicine has failed to offer up a victory in the "War against Cancer" declared thirty years ago, and we can't help but be bitterly disappointed in this failure. After all, press and the media have made it their business to whet our appetites for breakthroughs far beyond realistic possibilities. Ironically, perhaps, it is the real and remarkable advances of medicine in this century that have led to our greatly increased life expectancy—although at times it seems that we live longer only to be in worse health, and to face longer illnesses and slower deaths.

Medical ethicist Daniel Callahan writes:

> The power of modern medicine resides in its almost magical possibility of offering us a relief from biological necessity, granting us new powers to manage our fate and our destiny, presenting an image of unlimited hope, genuine knowledge and great progress.... Yet the image easily becomes an illusion and a mistake, not because it is wholly without foundation, but because it is partially and half blind.[3]

Blind, as Callahan and many others have pointed out, to certain unassailable realities, not the least of which is that the vast majority of us will die of some illness or other. Some physical limitations and inevitabilities of being human are simply beyond our control, although at times, dreaming of miracles, we tend to overlook this. We are not just complex machines that can always be repaired, a metaphor that dehumanizing Western medicine often appears to promote.

To the extent that conventional medicine has failed to embrace a fuller, more person-oriented sense of healing and becomes increasingly—and of necessity—specialized and disease-focused, patients will continue to look elsewhere for the help they need. This is probably inevitable, and not necessarily a failure of medicine; it is rather a realistic reaction to how overblown our expectations of medicine had become in the latter half of the century, as well as a reflection of how vast the field of medical knowledge has become. As Bonnie Blair O'Connor, a community medicine specialist and ethnographer, writes, "Conventional medicine does not and cannot provide everything that people need in order to cope with all aspects of the experience of illness."[4]

As suggested elsewhere, disappointments with the quality of medical care are many and legion. Nowhere is this more evident, or more poignant, than within the relationship between doctor and patient, particularly in dealing with late-stage cancer. A shocking number of oncologists seem unable or unwilling to remain emotionally engaged and encouraging with their patients who are dealing with metastatic cancer. In a recent article, entitled "Words That Heal, Words That Harm,"[5] published by the National Coalition for Cancer Survivorship, Dr. Elizabeth Clark examined the impact of doctors' words on patients.

> *We know that words are capable of wounding, perhaps because we expect so much of them. We also know that words can provide comfort and hope, and perhaps have the capacity to heal. At NCCS, we recognize the power of a medical professional's words and the emotional impact— positive or negative—that a statement can have on an individual.*

According to Clark, particularly wounding statements from physicians were those that:

- suggested lack of control over the disease

- were trite or took the form of platitudes

- compared survivors to others or to statistics
- disregarded feelings and concerns
- were cold or cynical
- indicated continuing support was conditional
- destroyed hope

By contrast, doctor's words that cancer survivors found most helpful:

- were proactive and empowering
- reframed the problem more clearly and positively
- normalized the cancer experience
- acknowledged individual differences
- validated feelings and concerns
- showed genuineness and compassion
- assured continuing support
- conveyed hope

Doctors: A love-hate relationship

A candid conversation among breast cancer survivors about which qualities they liked least and appreciated most in their physicians mentioned a number of specific behaviors that serve to illustrate the generalizations above. Here, in their own words, is a compilation of their responses. First, the dislikes:

I hate it when doctors...

- *talk down to you because you can't possibly understand the technical stuff.*
- *don't do a rigorous and thorough job and miss things.*
- *order $200 worth of blood tests and don't even tell you what they tested or why. And don't give you the test results.*
- *don't mention the consequences of some choices or exaggerate the consequences of the choice they don't want you to make.*

- *don't tell me and my husband the truth about the extent of my disease—only telling us that "if this happens, it is very bad." I don't want or need a doctor that hides my condition behind gentle words—tell me the truth, tell me the facts and let me go forward.*

- *discourage information gathering and research. My first oncologist told me not to read anything because it would scare me. While little that I read spoke to Stage IV Breast Cancer, I am a librarian and researcher. To tell me not to read and research this horror I was confronted with was like telling me not to breathe. But if I had followed his treatment suggestions, I probably wouldn't be breathing now.*

- *patronize me, or tell me not to worry. I have a fatal disease. Who are they kidding?*

- *are insensitive to the way they discuss and share information. My doctor had the nerve to do a very short, very fast exam, look at my pathology report and say to me, "You have 11 of 14 lymph nodes positive. Chances are the cancer will come back in 2 to 3 years and depending on where it comes back we won't be able to do anything for you. Now what kind of chemo should we try?"*

- *denigrate the treatment decisions my other oncologist and I have made. Yes, I chose a BMT/PSCT. Yes, it isn't a perfect treatment and I have side effects as a result. But I am still here and that was more than what he could offer me in the beginning.*

- *treat me like a disease, rather than a human being.*

- *introduce the student doctors in a cursory fashion, then ask if I would mind them being there while I am being examined, and then talk to the students about me as if I am not in the room. I don't like it when I meet the doctor and call him "Dr. Smith," but he calls me "Lynne."*

- *think their time is more valuable than mine. When they make me wait for them and don't even bother to apologize. I am a working mother of two—why do some doctors think they can keep you waiting for two hours in the waiting room and then try to rush through your exam and questions just because they are behind schedule?*

- treat me like I'm a piece of meat on an assembly line. In this category, I would place interminable waits in treatment rooms after being told it will just be a few minutes. Or being clothed in a skimpy and undignified paper gown. Or when doctors try doing exams without first giving you a gown and the privacy to change. Or doctors who overbook or try to squeeze too many patients into one day.

- don't return my phone calls or they return the phone call only the next day.

These same women, however, were also quick to point out the qualities in physicians they most prized:

I love it when doctors...

- *take me and my condition seriously, are truthful with me and do a thorough and meticulous job.*

- *are competent and up to date with the latest in medical research, clinical trials and technology. I love doctors who have had excellent training, have excellent intellectual skills* **and** *who remain open-minded, realizing that they don't already know everything, that medicine is an art as well as a science and that new data and ways of thinking might have something to offer.*

- *don't patronize me but explain how they think, answer my questions and don't assume that I am too dumb to understand. A good doctor listens. Not just hears, but listens! Answers questions straightforwardly, involves me in the game plan, i.e., "This is what I recommend. What are your thoughts on this?" I love doctors who don't feel threatened by my many questions and my wanting to have a say in my treatment.*

- *remember to call me with the test results and quickly. This shows that they care what happens to me. Sometimes my oncologist will call me days after my appointments, tests and treatment to ask how I'm doing or to follow up on a concern or question I may have asked.*

- *respect my opinions as well as their own. I also love that we have had agreements and disagreements and we always leave each other feeling good about the exchange. I know because I make* sure to ask him if everything is okay between us after we have had a disagreement. It has only happened two or three times, but yesterday with no disagreement at all, it was he who asked me if I was happy with my visit.

- *treat me like a person*—not an inconvenience or another annoyance. My oncologist asks me about my sons, my husband and is truly concerned about us as a family living with cancer. I like it that she told me what she would do if she were me, not to make me choose a particular treatment, but to let me know that as a young mother and wife herself, she understood my concerns for my children and my husband in light of my disease.

- *remember who I am and why I am there to see them,* when they take some time getting to know me, to find out something about the rest of my life and share a little about their interests outside of medicine. Good doctors understand that each patient is unique, and brings his or her own background, experiences, and secret fears into the mix.

- *pay attention to providing their patients with human dignity,* shown by such 'extras' as a small changing room off their exam room, roomy cloth gowns, a staff who treats you with worth, knocking on the door before entering the exam room, conducting the "talking" part of an exam in street clothes. My doctor allowed me to dress before she gave me the results. I faced the worst news in my life in my own clothes. Not in a skimpy gown with a hole down the back. I love it when doctors prioritize and let you know it. I don't mind waiting when I know the doc is taking the time to deal with another patient's crisis. It lets me know that if I have a crisis he will take the time to deal with mine.

- *are considerate of and sensitive to my feelings.* On two occasions (while dealing with a cancer diagnosis and dealing with a miscarriage) I had surgeons who did not at all rush through the news, didn't let me rush through the news, and gave me time and space to absorb what they were telling me, have an emotional reaction and **then** ask my questions. My surgeon squeezed my hand when he was telling me I had cancer, rather than distancing himself. I love being touched, one human to another.

- *enter their profession in order to be healers. I know they're given all sorts of abuse and harassment throughout medical school until they often come out bitter and cynical—but most still have the heart of a healer if you look for and encourage it.*

In the era before modern medicine, physicians knew that hope, comfort and caring were among the most important tools they had to offer. Is it any wonder that patients seek other kinds of help in droves when their own doctors fail to appreciate these crucial human needs? The lack of compassion in much of modern medicine is psychiatrist David Spiegel's largest concern:

We don't have a health care system but rather a disease cure system. The public believes and many doctors behave as if most illnesses are curable... The expectation of cure has led to an explosion of invasive, expensive and often risky interventions that have at best marginal effects on survival. We have focused too much on diseases and too little on the people who have the diseases.

Most Americans die of chronic and progressive illnesses: heart disease, stroke and cancer. Cure is the exception, not the rule. What these patients need is health caring. Compassionate care should help people live with illness by relieving suffering, managing symptoms and coping with the uncertainty and fear of further illness.[6]

Complementary therapies: A feeling of control and choice

You want to feel cared for, and you want to feel there is always something that can be done, that there is hope and help for you, no matter how serious your condition. A feeling of being in control of your experience—becoming, in the current parlance, "empowered"—is probably important to you, as it is to many other cancer patients. While the outcome of your treatments and the ultimate course of your disease may be unknowable, the sense that you do have control over your own responses and choices matters a great deal. Using various complementary treatments is one important way in which the people I interviewed were able to accomplish this.

Joining a support group, seeking a therapist or counselor's help, learning self-hypnosis for pain control, or other methods to reduce stress and achieve feelings of peace and transcendence, renewing and strengthening your spiritual beliefs through prayer, meditation, involvement with temple or church, seeking out a massage therapist or yoga instructor, making dietary changes—these and other similar health-promoting choices can be extraordinarily helpful in coping with your illness. Each person will make her own choices from the ever-expanding menu of options, but it is almost always helpful to see yourself as being in charge and to encourage those helping you to see you as a whole person.

But it is not always easy to select other kinds of help from the bewildering array available. Like other metastatic cancer patients, you've probably been besieged with information from well-meaning friends and family members about alternative and complementary treatments. It's likely that you have already heard enthusiastic anecdotal reports of someone's cousin who went to a clinic in Mexico with incurable cancer and now is perfectly well again. Or that a friend of a friend's terminal disease is now in remission, thanks to a special diet. Or that your cancer is caused by intestinal parasites, negative thoughts and emotions, high power lines, dairy products, a passive personality, food preservatives, a devastating personal loss, an imbalance of Chi, or energy—the list goes on and on.

A visit to any New Age bookstore or a look at the bulletin board or on the shelves of a health food emporium will yield literally dozens of remedies and unconventional theories and treatments for cancer, from shark cartilage to Essaic tea, from acupuncture to Qi Gong, from visualization to affirmations. As I wrote this, a message appeared on the Breast Cancer Discussion List from a man claiming his wife's "golf ball" sized breast tumor and liver metastases had been 100 percent cured with a combination of Essaic tea, a "light frequency gun" and something referred to as "colloidal silver."

What have you got to lose? your friends may ask. Your cancer has returned or spread, and conventional medical treatment has obviously failed to provide a cure. You can't help feeling a sense of bitter disappointment. With advancing illness your sense of knowing what is right for you may well have been undermined. You may feel out of control, for the moment at least, and are looking for some way to regain a sense of hope.

Consumed with the panic that often accompanies dealing with advanced cancer, you may not be able to easily answer the question of just what it is that would make you feel better and more in control—emotionally, let alone physically. You may no longer quite trust yourself to know what you want, or what you "should" be doing. This may be new territory for you—and, as you soon discover if you look, there's a vast marketplace of books, tapes, herbs, remedies, practitioners and clinics out there waiting to satisfy this need and prey upon your desperation.

This is the point at which you are most vulnerable to a sort of "grasping at straws." In the face of feelings of desperation and despair, literature and testimonials that promise miraculous cures may come to have a nearly irresistible allure. It will come as no news to you that some promoters of alternative treatments depend on the desperation of cancer patients who turn to them as purveyors of hope. Let the buyer beware.

Some doctors are trying to help patients make sense of the options. Holistic physician Dr. James Gordon, director of the Center for Mind-Body Studies in Washington, issues a strong call for the integration of complementary methods of healing into the practice of medicine.

> *Much of what we have tended to regard as peripheral or trivial must become central: the therapeutic use of nutrition, exercise and relaxation; the mobilization of the mind to alter and transform itself and the body; group support. Techniques that are fundamental to the healing systems of other culture—like acupuncture and yoga—should be fully integrated into our own. Alternative approaches, nourished on our own soil yet largely scorned by the medical establishment—herbalism, chiropractic and prayer among them—should once again be considered as members of the family of official medicine.*

> *This open-minded, integrated approach grows out of a sense of the origins and dimensions of our present health care crisis. It in turn must be predicated on profound changes in the kind of care we pay for: our research priorities and our medical education. The key is understanding what we have lost as well as gained through our high-tech, disease-oriented medicine.*[7]

Complementary versus alternative treatments: An important distinction

It's important to understand the distinction between *complementary* treatments, which are intended to augment conventional medical care, and *alternative* treatments, which often try to force cancer patients to choose between what they offer and Western medicine, by claiming that conventional medical treatment, particularly chemotherapy and radiation, is too toxic and damaging to natural processes to be helpful.

Unscrupulous providers are eager for your business. Be on guard for simple explanations or remedies and magical cures. The methods they tout typically offer quasi-scientific models of cancer, seeing the disease as resulting from a single, simple process arising from poor diet, stress, mental outlook or environment. They hold that properly motivated cancer patients can mobilize their defenses. They will offer testimonials and case histories to "prove" this, and will justify the lack of scientific studies by claiming to be "too busy working with patients." They often claim that their easy, non-toxic methods have been rejected by the "cancer establishment." Apart from the potential damage wrought by their denial of Western medicine, some alternative methods are clearly harmful, through toxicity or other direct physical harm, as with large doses of some "natural" herbal preparations and vitamins. They may also be exploitive, by depleting needed financial resources and by raising hopes of miraculous cures.

Michael Lerner, as director of Commonweal, a California health and environmental research institute, and co-founder of Commonweal's Cancer Help program, has had occasion to counsel thousands of cancer patients about their treatment choices and to investigate many methods outside Western medicine. In his thoughtful and comprehensive book *Choices in Healing: Integrating the Best of Conventional and Complementary Approaches to Cancer*, Lerner offers a common-sense approach for patients to evaluate what is right for them.

> Among the numerous complementary methods used by cancer patients, I believe four "life-style" approaches—spiritual, psychological, nutritional and physical—provide a variety of open, ethical approaches to cancer that, carefully explored in consultation with a doctor, can be of potential benefit.

Without making rash claims for complementary treatments, Lerner's vision of the role these life-style changes can play in patients' lives is enthusiastic and encouraging:

> I have seen hundreds of people whose quality of life has been greatly improved by complementary approaches, though the course of their cancer has not dramatically changed. Thousands of women and men have

told me that prayer groups, support groups, diet, yoga, traditional Chinese medicine and other resources in various combinations have transformed their lives in the face of a life-threatening disease.

On rare occasions, I have seen spontaneous remissions in some of the most life-threatening cases. One young woman with metastatic breast cancer did what thousands of other women with breast cancer who explore complementary therapies have done. She changed her diet, took herbs and vitamins, joined a support group and developed a strong spiritual life. She has been in complete remission for several years. Her oncologist has no explanation.

More often, I have seen what seem to be examples of life extension, though without cures. An older woman with an advanced cancer had been on hospice care when her son gathered her friends from around the country for a party to celebrate her life, with her favorite music, favorite food and favorite people. After the party, her cancer unexpectedly subsided. She went off hospice care, rediscovered her passionate interest in poetry and lived another year. She wrote a book of beautiful poems, and then, when the cancer returned, acknowledged that she was ready to die.

There does seem to be a correlation between an apparent prolonging of life, or at least a profound improvement in quality of life, and a patient's development of a unique and personal reason to live.

In short, there is no single right way to fight cancer. The best general approach in my judgment is to learn what you can about the conventional therapy options, to get the best conventional treatment you can that makes sense to you, to explore complementary therapies only if they interest you and to recognize that this is uniquely your life struggle and that you are the best authority on how you want to go through it.[8]

Appendix B, *Resources*, includes a number of references to readings in the healthy life-style approaches that Lerner refers to. It's likely that you already feel drawn to one or another—or perhaps several—methods for "working on yourself." Think of this as a life-affirming project in the larger sense.

Think of what might feel healing for you at this time in your life. While there is no single right answer, there may be one or more approach that is right for *you*. Would it be finding someone to talk to who knows firsthand how you feel? Might it be spending some time every day or every week in quiet contemplation, or writing in your journal? Or taking a yoga class, or finding a good massage therapist? Or studying nutrition and learning how to prepare healthier foods?

The activities you try, and the people you consult, will be determined by your time and inclinations—and, of course, by your pocketbook. It's important to think of yourself as taking action, taking control. Think about what kinds of things you can do for yourself that would make you feel good, and cope better with your illness. A review of local resources is likely to reveal any number of opportunities for you to explore. Whatever you decide to do, enjoy yourself, and let it make a difference in your life.

Stress, personality and metaphors of illness

Surveys of breast cancer patients show that more than 40 percent believe their disease was caused, at least in part, by "stress."[9] Many women seem to develop private scenarios linking the timing of their initial diagnoses or recurrences to particularly trying life events. But while all sorts of fanciful theories abound, and have since recorded history began, it's important to remember that despite decades of research, no one has yet proven that traumatic events cause cancer or worsen prognosis, or that certain kinds of people are more cancer prone. This is not to say that there is no mind-body interaction, but only that it is likely far more complex than we yet understand—and that emotional harm can result from simplistic theories of causality, thoughtlessly applied.

As Susan Sontag has observed, "Any disease whose causality is murky, and for which treatment is ineffectual, tends to be awash in significance."[10] Sontag might have taken this observation a step further to add that in the absence of certain knowledge about a mortal illness, theories of treatment and causality also run rampant. Whether or not you feel drawn to develop your own ideas about causality, at some point, you will probably encounter someone eager to offer up his or her own theory of why you got sick.

Many cancer patients find this infuriating, feeling that they are being blamed, somehow. It may help protect you from the meddlesome impact of the know-it-alls of the world if you stop to consider that it's probably their own fears and their need to preserve protective illusions about life that underlie such judgments and overconfident beliefs. Keep that in mind when the next well-meaning relative or friend offers a panacea, or refers to the "stress" or "loss" that brought on the cancer. Clearly, these people need, for whatever reason, to feel that life is orderly and fair, that every disease has its clear causes and cures. Wouldn't we all like to believe that everyone, at least potentially, could have complete control over catastrophic events? Wouldn't it be great to know that people would be safe from cancer if only their lives were exemplary?

Current social metaphors tend to imply that cancer patients are weak or ineffectual people who have in some way participated in their disease—the so-called "Type C" personality, defined as passive, emotionally inexpressive, conforming and unassertive. "The cancer personality is regarded...with condescension, as one of life's losers," Sontag observes. It's hard for anyone in today's pop-psych, self-help American culture not to feel at least some sense of self-blame or shame over having a life-threatening illness.

Unfortunately, in reaction to these pervasive beliefs and the pernicious victim-blame that so many find wounding, cancer patients sometimes take an opposite stance, and come to see their disease and their bodies mechanistically, to see the disease process fatalistically, and look *only* to Western medicine for guidance and help. This may be nearly as problematic as the opposite extreme, because real avenues of help and hope that might be explored are then closed off.

It comes as no surprise to anyone with metastatic cancer that there's a stigma associated with the disease. Common metaphors of the disease can actually contribute to this. When cancer treatment fails or is particularly arduous, medicine's mechanical images of the body as fixable machine often yield to those of all-out war. Disease becomes the invading enemy to be fought against with the arsenal of medicine. There is much talk of heroic measures, last-ditch weapons, courageous battles. Warlike imagery plays a role in eliciting fear when cancer is conceived of as an invincible enemy, mindlessly mowing down victims in its path.

Patients themselves become objects of fear. Even those who have a non-contagious disease like cancer can evoke anxiety and nameless dread, and are often shunned rather than supported. Pediatrician and writer Perri Klass, commenting on the widespread impact of the military metaphor among medical personnel, says that patients themselves "become battlefields, lying there passively while the evil armies of pathology and the resplendent forces of modern medicine fight it out. The real problem arises because all too often the patient comes to personify the disease and, somehow, becomes the enemy."[11]

Passivity equates with feeling defeated, a victim of disease. The resulting feelings of despair and hopelessness, devastating in themselves, clearly reduce the quality of day-to-day living for all concerned, patient and family members alike.

It's important to be aware of these metaphors, for they can exert subtle influences on both how you think about your disease and how you choose your treatments. However broadly and unconsciously they are used, the value-laden metaphors of war may well not be appropriate for you. Must the definition of courage for a cancer patient always be to "fight with the weapons" of medicine? Does choosing a less-toxic treatment protocol, for instance, mean you aren't "prepared for an all-out battle?" Does choosing to discontinue treatment mean "surrender to the enemy?" Is this choice less heroic than any other? Most importantly, does someone whose illness has progressed feel a sense of shame at having been "defeated?"

Many people choose to adopt other imagery, preferring to see cancer as a journey, for example, or finding a different image that conveys other aspects of the disease experience. Jenilu Schoolman once wrote me that she had come to conceive of her body as a multi-family apartment building. Her cancer was like an unruly tenant who couldn't be evicted, but had to be kept in line and taught respect for the other inhabitants of the building.

Like many people I interviewed, Caren Buffum found meaning through keeping a journal about her experience, using this metaphor to describe the process:

> I think there is a comfort in knowing that as I slip closer to the end of my life, it is not growing smaller like a candle being burned to the bottom. That in writing my story, even if the writing only selectively captures what my life has been about, it becomes less like that candle and more like a road—though traveled on, it continues to exist behind me.

Yet, there were also times when the metaphor of war felt apt to Caren, as when she characterized her day-to-day experience with the disease:

> We are adversaries in a cold war. Cold, because were it all-out war, I would be totally absorbed in the land of the sick, engaged continually in

hard battle, my breath in gasps and the fear of being overcome ever
present. We (my illness and I) know we are engaged, and yet at home it is
business as usual—dinner on the table at 6:30, "Jeopardy" at 7. The dog
is walked and there is a small victory when he "does it" outside and not on
my beige carpet. My son is accepted at Temple U. (a breath of relief)—
then a treatment—engage the enemy—fatigue, queasiness, feelings of
insufficiency.... This visit to the trenches saps my energy. I climb out to be
greeted by my Westie's eager puppy kisses.

"I created my own republic, putting myself at the helm"

If you've read this far, it will be clear that the patients I interviewed have
chosen conventional Western medicine as central to their treatment. Yet that
was not all they did to get the help they needed. Pam Hiebert, in remission
for her bone metastases, spoke of her choices when she was first diagnosed
with Stage IV breast cancer:

> I bought books dealing with alternative care and made myself reach
> outward to find ways to ease my suffering. The political health war
> between alternative and conventional medicine left me feeling like a pawn
> as I continually felt the bias in each camp.

> I created my own republic, putting myself at the helm and the doc-
> tors as my strong advisors. All that time I continued to eat whole natural
> foods and to furnish my body with the supplements I knew it would need
> to recover from the ghastly poisons that lurked throughout my body. I
> drank quarts of water daily to flush my system and refused to wear any
> products that prevented me from sweating to release the toxins. I reeked
> of chemicals by the time all the chemo ended.

> Among the memories that stand out in my mind as I look back at
> that time, making that phone call to the osteopathic physician who had
> been treating me for lower back problems prior to the cancer diagnosis
> was significant. I wanted to let him know what was going on. He said to
> me, "Now is the time to name what is happening to you. You must take
> this and name it. If you do not, then your doctors will name this alone
> and you still will have to survive in their model." I am eternally grateful

to Dr. John. This past Christmas I wrote to him and told him I am still liv-
ing and how much positive effect his words had with me.

Later, after the chemo and surgery, I continued to experience agoniz-
ing and severe body pain. I have found a form of toning and stretching
called Pilates, that turned the process around and dramatically decreased
the extent of pain I lived with on a daily basis. (It also raised my hemo-
globin, which surprised and delighted my oncologist.) I've also read a
book by Andrew Weil, M.D., called **Spontaneous Healing***. The book is*
written with clear methods I can use for heightening my immune system. I
have made changes in my dietary patterns after reading this book. I am
doing more herbal medicinal teas (green tea and ginger) and have added
flax oil (Omega 3) to my diet. Dr. Weil has a whole chapter devoted to
tonics that boost the immune system.

I have been taking Chinese herbal medicines since my chemotherapy
and mastectomy ended and continue to believe in their added effective-
ness. Acupuncture has helped me with muscle cramps.

I've also incorporated imagery in my quest to heal, working with a
physician who taught me about symbolic imagery. I still use this imagery
to induce healing within. Now I think of this effort as inner being trans-
formation. Sylvan calls it my work, and I deeply appreciate her affirming
words.

Bob and Ginger Crisp sought help where it seemed most natural to each of
them. Ginger chose various complementary healing methods, as her husband Bob describes:

Early on Ginger would get in the hot tub every a.m. and use this as a
place for visualization. She worked hard at doing the work to mobilize the
immune system. She was against cancer support groups from the start
and has stayed that way. She felt this would be too negative for her. She
had one discussion with a naturopath who gave her a few ideas. I think it
fell into the category of "can't hurt, might help." She followed a very care-
ful diet: low-fat, lots of veggies, etc. She simply became more strict about
her diet so it was not a big change. She read some on cancer and nutri-
tion and may have picked some ideas from that. Her oncologist is
aware—indifference is probably a better description—and I think he sup-
ports some complementary treatments, not because he believes in them,

but because he knows it gives the patient a degree of control, which is good. If it were some off-the-wall or possibly harmful treatment, then I'm sure he would say something.

Like Pam Hiebert, Bob was quick to acknowledge the role that feeling in control played, not just for Ginger, but for himself as well,

> This is a part of our personalities but it plays out in different ways. I come from the knowledge is everything school and she comes from the listen to your body school. So I read everything, follow every lead, etc. She pays a lot of attention to diet, etc. She has near complete control over blood now as she will get tests, read the numbers, check how she feels and decide to get a transfusion or not. The oncologist just leaves standing orders, so we can get a test, go to hospital, get the transfusion and he won't even be informed until later. Ginger is taking CoQ-10 and bovine cartilage now. She does some regular Reiki work with a group of women trained in such stuff. She has had about all that surgery, standard chemo and radiation can provide. There are not many options left. Next is a parallel course of living life one day at a time and checking on possible alternative treatments.

Nancy Gilpatrick, diagnosed at Stage IV, spoke of the treatments she had sought out as she prepared for her high-dose chemotherapy, and also of her need for moderation in pursuing them:

> I do alternative medicine as well as conventional. I believe both have things to offer us and neither has all the answers. I am seeing a Chinese herbalist. She prescribes an herbal tea that I drink twice a day. I see an acupuncturist who is working with my pain as well as side effects. In January I worked with a native American shaman who journeyed with my body and talked specifically to the cancer cells. On the second visit he worked with the mouth sores I had. The next day they were gone. He told me that the bone mets would work the same way only it would take longer as there is more damage to the bones. I have since gotten more mets so I don't know about what he said. However, I got great peace in my work with him. His style works with mine, which is a more gentle "get the cancer out of my body" than aggressive fight visualization.
>
> I have decided to not tackle every alternative presented to me, and there have been a lot. I will do one or two things at a time. I don't want to

be a "patient"—alternative or conventional medicine. I want to live my
life, and spending it in appointments day after day isn't my idea of a way
to live and enjoy my life. Moderation is my way.

Lucie Bergmann-Shuster had sought training as an acupressure massage therapist before her recurrence, and had already made healing body work a part of her life.

> *Since the time of my mother's death, I have been getting treatments*
> *every other week and now weekly. About a month ago I arranged to have*
> *my husband get massages from the same therapist although there is noth-*
> *ing wrong with him. To me it is like a deep mini vacation in the space of*
> *one hour or less that revitalizes and recharges.*
>
> *Now would I say that this is pertinent to my cancer and how I man-*
> *age my coping? Yes and no, but I would have done it anyway, as I think*
> *everybody should, to improve quality of life. Mind you, my initial reason*
> *for going was my back, not my cancer. Getting Qi or Chi type therapy is*
> *one of those things I do—kind of like eating and pooping and sleeping and*
> *loving and exercising and being. Did I do anything I would not have con-*
> *sidered before my cancer? I don't think so, except maybe eliminating any*
> *and all processed food, especially junk food, from my diet.*

For Barb Pender, it was a chance encounter with a particularly helpful psychological technique—as well as her ongoing participation in her support group and her faith in God—that has helped to sustain her:

> *After my divorce in '86 I put myself through college. I particularly*
> *enjoyed my Psych classes. In one class in particular my instructor also*
> *used hypnosis in her counseling. She told us about "taking ourselves to*
> *another place." In class she took us to her green pasture. I have never for-*
> *gotten that class nor that experience. In fact, throughout every procedure,*
> *scan, surgery, etc., I have been able to master the art of "going to another*
> *place." Last year I had a bone scan, and a friend went with me. She*
> *watched as I was scanned—they made a calculation error and had to*
> *repeat the process. I never moved a muscle and, in fact, did not even*
> *know that the scan was repeated. The tech doing the scan was trying to*
> *apologize to me during the procedure and apparently I was ignoring him.*
> *Maureen just said, "You'll have to apologize later—she's in another*
> *place." This ability to leave my body had helped me tremendously during*

the many MRI's and scans that I have had and I would recommend it wholeheartedly to anyone!

Coping with emotions

Living with metastatic breast cancer isn't just a single crisis that you can get through with grit and determination—it's a siege that goes on and on, calling for every coping skill you possess and demanding strengths and resilience you never knew you had. There are bound to be times when you wonder if you can hold on any longer.

Pat Leach described her feelings when her cancer came back:

> *The liver tumor stayed the same—for a year. Then a CT showed slight increase in size. Panic again. I wanted to crawl in bed, cover every part of me, suck my thumb and just not have to deal with any of it.*

Lisann Charland also felt panicky when news came of another recurrence:

> *The weekend seemed endless. The helpless and morbid feelings would not go away. I had to go through the motion again—clean house—who gets what. I even talked about my funeral plans. Buddy and I used to joke and I used to tell him "hang me over the fireplace when I am gone" so I would not miss anything. This was not a joke anymore—my life was passing me by, and this could be the inevitable sooner than I expected. My mind raced in different directions and played havoc with me. It could not be happening to me again, I said.*

For Kathy Stone, it wasn't any one particular piece of bad news, but just feeling worn down by constant nausea and pain:

> *I have been so blue this week...I think it is because I want things to get better and realistically, they are probably as good as they are going to get right now...and I have to accept that and make the most of it. I'm trying...*

PJ Hagler worried that she was running out of the stamina she depended upon:

> *I'm still awful depressed. It seems like this stuff never ends. I admit that this has been such a tough year for me. I'm usually so positive and upbeat, knowing I will overcome this too. I know much of this depression*

is from the fever, low white counts, hospital stays, etc., etc. And I have had
such good news about the tumors getting smaller and the mass going
away. I have so much to be thankful for but I'm so tired of fighting. I
would just like a time of rest when I felt good.

These are common experiences for women with metastatic disease, the low times you don't get to read about in the inspirational cancer books that feature heroic determination and maintaining a positive and hopeful attitude.

If you're like most metastatic cancer patients, you have discovered that it is all too easy to become "medicalized" as you spend long hours and days in waiting and treatment rooms, being wheeled around from radiology to nuclear medicine, clad only in flimsy hospital garb, a plastic bracelet proclaiming your identity. Immersed in diagnostic tests and treatments, one simple truth often seems overlooked. Parallel to the whole process of diagnostic testing, selecting and undergoing treatments, is the *person*—you—whose life is profoundly affected by all of this. This is the reason people speak of feeling depersonalized in medical settings. This is happening to *you*, to *all* of you, not just to your physical being. Sociologist Arthur Frank, writing of his own experiences with heart disease and cancer, brings it into focus:

> *Medicine has done well with my body, and I am grateful. But doing* > *with the body is only part of what needs to be done for the person. What* > *happens when my body breaks down happens not just to that body but* > *also to my life, which is lived in that body. When the body breaks down,* > *so does the life. Even when medicine can fix the body, that doesn't always* > *put the life back together again. Medicine can diagnose and treat the* > *breakdown, but sometimes so much fear and frustration have been* > *aroused in the ill person that fixing the breakdown does not quiet them.* > *At those times the experience of illness goes beyond the limits of medi-* > *cine.[12]*

The cascade of emotional states—as you cycle through repeated diagnostic testing, treatments, remission, and the seemingly endless waiting, uncertainty and anticipation that accompanies your diagnosis—can be overwhelming at times, as the implications and realities of all this reverberate throughout your entire being. Those closest to you feel this acutely as well.

Compounding these feelings may be the sense that when you visit your oncologist, despite a careful focus on the details of disease and treatment, there's comparatively little attention paid to you—the actual person to whom all this is happening. It's easy to see how and why this can occur, and how well-meaning physicians often don't have the time—or sometimes, sadly, the inclination—to communicate with their patients on a real person-to-person basis. The compassionate and expert physician should be aware of this lack, and should encourage—or at least not discourage—a patient's wish and need for additional help—as long as this doesn't interfere with medical care. Many patients, sensing that their doctors would be dismissive or disapproving, don't tell them about the other kinds of help they seek, even when it might be important to do so.

Help for depression and anxiety

While it is not inevitable that people living with metastatic breast cancer become anxious and depressed at points during their disease and treatment, it is certainly not uncommon, especially if there is some compromise of physical functioning. Reviewing the literature on clinical depression and cancer, psychiatrist Mary Jane Massie, of Memorial Sloan-Kettering Cancer Center, found that studies showed that serious depression depended to a large extent on the degree of physical disability, ranging from 23 percent in those whose lives were least affected, to a whopping 77 percent rate of clinical depression in those most severely affected.

In addition, poorly controlled pain, symptoms of advanced disease, concurrent medical conditions and family or other personal problems—as well as treatment with a number of common cancer medications—make it far more likely that people with metastatic disease will experience depressive symptoms at some point or another.

Massie, an expert in psycho-oncology, the study of the psychological problems of cancer patients, explains:

> The normal response to hearing the diagnosis of cancer is sadness about the loss of health as well as about anticipated losses, including death. This normal response is part of a spectrum of depressive symptoms that range from normal sadness to adjustment disorder with depressed mood to major depression.

She goes on further to state that the symptoms of depression in a physically healthy person—loss of appetite and weight loss, insomnia, loss of energy and fatigue, lack of interest in normal activities, including sex—have "less value as diagnostic criteria for a cancer patient because they are common to both cancer and depression." Since cancer patients routinely show these symptoms as part of their disease or treatment, what Massie looks for, instead, is the degree of despair patients may be feeling, their feelings of hopelessness, guilt, worthlessness, as well as any suicidal thoughts.[13]

If you are experiencing *any* of these symptoms, it's important to alert your doctor immediately. Having cancer is hard enough. There is no need for you to suffer from depression as well. Help is available.

Anxiety poses similar problems of identification, according to Massie. "The normal fears and uncertainties associated with cancer of possible death, disfigurement, dependence on others, disability and disruption of new relationships are often severe." As with depression, the most common anxieties are felt in response to adverse circumstances.

> *Reactive or situational anxiety is seen at crisis or transitional points in the course of cancer, that is, at the time of diagnosis, awaiting a new treatment, prior to major surgery, on completion of lengthy treatment, and in advanced and terminal stages of illness...[when it] reflects the uncertainty of the future, the uncertainty of treatment effectiveness, the pursuit of new or alternative treatments with the fear of failing to find the right one, and the fears associated with actual poor respiratory function or chronic uncontrolled pain.[14]*

Doctors commonly try to manage their patients' reactive anxiety by offering information and support. A thorough educational preparation or "walk through" about what to expect from a treatment or surgery is an example of this effective approach. Good pain management, through pharmacologic or other methods, is also essential, for anxiety almost always accompanies unrelieved pain.

There are many non-medical techniques to relieve anxiety. You almost certainly have developed some of your own that work for you. Information seeking, distraction, exercise, reframing the crisis as a challenge, reaching out to others—these are only a few of the common coping mechanisms people use. Simple strategies are often most effective. Prepare for time spent waiting or receiving treatment. Take an interesting book on tape to doctor's appointments, or watch a video during a chemo infusion.

Studies have shown that the judicious use of minor tranquilizers, brief psychotherapy and behavioral interventions like self-hypnosis, meditation or relaxation techniques are all extremely effective, alone or in combination, to help most people cope with reactive anxiety.

But if you are suffering from anxiety that interferes with your day-to-day functioning, your sleeping or eating patterns, or results in panic attacks accompanied by feelings of dread, difficulty breathing or fear of dying, don't make the mistake of thinking you must be "strong" or "stoic." Help is readily available, in the form of effective medications, psychotherapy and behavioral methods you can learn to help control these feelings.

In the last two decades, behavioral techniques have received particular attention. These "self-regulatory strategies" to control symptoms of pain and anxiety in medical settings include self-hypnosis, meditation, guided imagery, autogenic training, progressive relaxation and biofeedback.

In the comparatively new field of behavioral medicine, research has shown that techniques like these can alter physiological and psychological functioning. "Particularly in cancer, they are now extensively applied to control psychological distress and pain," writes psychiatrist Renee Mastrovito in a psychooncology review article.[15] "Contributing to this change are an increased interest in Eastern religions and philosophies with their emphasis on self-control through meditation, an increasing emphasis on the individual's role in maintaining personal health and in actively participating in treatment and care during illness." These techniques, which derive from a variety of sources, typically involve two stages, where the patient is first guided through a cognitive activity, which will then create an altered state of awareness. An example of this kind of technique would be a "body scan," a guided imagery process that involves progressively relaxing the muscles of your entire body.

It is also true that your experience of increased physical pain can be amplified by the *meaning* it comes to have for you. For example, if you understand pain to mean that your disease may be progressing, that thought, along with the worry about what lies ahead, can lead to even more suffering and anxiety on your part. In conjunction with medical problem-solving about pain reduction, these techniques offer ways of coping not only with your physical distress, but also, more importantly, with the emotional distress of the disease and its treatment, by putting you more in control of your own emotional and thought processes.

A prime example can be found in the pioneering work of Jon Kabat-Zinn, Director of the Stress Reduction Clinic at University of Massachusetts Medical Center, who has introduced the practice of mindfulness meditation into medical settings as a way of coping with the anxiety and pain of illness. Based on Buddhist concepts, this simple but profound practice involves cultivating the ability to pay attention in the present moment, and to look deeply into oneself. It involves a willingness to look at and be with things as they are, a process Kabat-Zinn calls "embracing the full catastrophe," Zorba the Greek's term for the "poignant enormity of our life experience."

> *For me, facing the full catastrophe means finding and coming to terms with what is most human in ourselves....Catastrophe here does not mean disaster. It includes crises and disaster but also all the little things that go wrong and that add up. The phrase reminds us that life is always in flux, that everything we think is permanent is actually only temporary and constantly changing.*[16]

In many hospitals, the behavioral medicine or social work departments offer classes and groups that train patients in these techniques. Books and tapes describing these methods are also widely available. If you have not yet added one or more of these techniques to your own treatment plan, you might consider looking at Appendix B, for suggestions on where to look.

If you're like most people, what you fear most is the unknown. Contact with other patients who have already experienced a situation that scares you can often significantly reduce your anxiety, helping replace your fearful fantasies with real-life stories, which are rarely as frightening. The words on this page, and the stories you find here in this book, are also examples of a complementary strategy, one based on the belief that hearing about how other people have coped and gaining perspective on the common problems you face will help you to feel more in control. The next section will have more to say about support groups, how to find them and make use of them.

Your oncologist should be made aware of any symptoms of depression and anxiety that are more than transitory in nature. If your doctor seems to dismiss your feelings, it's important that you persist in seeking relief of your anxiety and depression, just as it is important to persist in seeking relief from physical pain. There is help for you. Medication and short-term psychotherapy, as well as a variety of other methods, can make an enormous difference. An evaluation by a psychiatrist who is expert in working with cancer patients is an excellent first step. Support groups where you have a chance to compare notes and share experiences and feelings with other patients can be invaluable as well.

Dealing with the ups and downs of illness

Many people pride themselves on their independence and self-control. Acknowledging emotional distress can be very difficult for them, as it carries with it a sense of personal failure. It's important to remember here that finding out that you need emotional help and support does not mean you are weak or that you have something wrong with you psychologically. All it means is that you are a human being in crisis—and sometimes it takes a great deal of strength to admit this and do something about it.

Many of the people I interviewed were brave enough to be honest about the despair and terror they felt at times. Barb Clabo, struggling with failed treatments over several months following a Stage IV diagnosis, was candid about her reaction after learning the treatment hadn't worked and the tumors in her liver were growing:

> Will I ever receive any good news? I kept my composure—just a few tears—and a little anger until I reached the car and then again let loose. Cried all the way home with bad news for Glenn. After arriving home I felt a feeling of being trapped. I kept pacing and crying, not knowing which way to turn. It was awful. Taxol was supposed to work. I was having such a good week of feeling good after having been feeling so bad for so long. And then this! Up and down—Up and down—It is really draining.

Then on CAF, when her tumors began finally to shrink, Barb had trouble tolerating the treatment, winding up hospitalized and in isolation. Each time, as the effects of her treatment weakened her physically, she felt as if her emotional resilience was tested to the breaking point.

> I feel like I'm slipping into the illness experience more and more, and I am so very frightened that I might disappear into it. During treatments I sometimes feel as though I am sinking in quicksand. I get in up to my neck and the last minute I get snatched out. I wonder how many times this can happen successfully without sinking all the way.

Kathy Stone was able to be philosophical about the emotional ups and downs she'd experienced in the two years since her diagnosis:

> I do know that I've shed a lot of tears, I've yelled some and even screamed with frustration.... Yes, I think it was always frustration, not rage that made me scream...and there were/are times I've felt like my heart was going to literally break in two.... I've felt suffocated trying to "hold" in tears and I've cried with all my being and soul at other times. Most of the time I attribute the tears to the medicine and the effects of chemo and the "mental" imbalance it can throw a person into. My husband and I laugh now and say it's the medicine when I'm having an especially emotional trying time...but we don't just laugh it off either...we both know that those "mental" emotional chemo times are sometimes the hardest to handle...at other times they are a welcome relief.

But then Kathy's mother died, and her own pain got out of control for awhile and there were several trips to the hospital, followed by days of depression as she struggled with her intense distaste for "being hooked" on the pain medications:

> I guess I need it for pain, I just hate the thought of being doped up all the time and I still have the nausea. The only difference is I've found myself in depression and having anxiety attacks, which is just not like me. I can hardly find a thing to smile about, and yet I have instance after instance of things I should be smiling about.... I just seem to cry most days. I hope it is the medicine and things can get worked out.... It is a very frightening feeling when it happens.

One thing that disturbed Kathy deeply was the sense of social isolation she was beginning to feel, so one night she asked Chuck to take her to a community fund-raiser for leukemia:

> I talked my husband into taking me down for just a few minutes in order to buy raffle tickets, etc., and do our part for the "cause." I guess I still want to feel a part of things. When I walked in everyone seemed really happy that I had come down, but when we said we couldn't stay, the owner of the place (someone whom I've always felt to be a good friend) turned real cold and said, "Kathy, you have become a hermit and you aren't any fun anymore...why did you even bother to get up out of your sickbed to come down...so you could make the rest of us miserable?"

...then she laughed...because she thought she was making a funny. Most of
the time, I would have laughed too, but all I could do was bite my lip, toss
my tickets on the counter and tell her I hoped we never had to change
places...she wouldn't find my spot a whole lot of fun and I left. I'm afraid I
made a fool out of myself for one thing, but more than that I was really
hurt by her remarks and that bothers me. I feel like I'm not only becom-
ing a "hermit" as she said, but I'm becoming too sensitive and I don't
want to push people out of my life and become surrounded with my
illness.

"I felt I was sicker emotionally than my psychiatric patients," confessed Pat Leach, who worked as a psychiatric nurse, looking back at the early days after her first recurrence.

A cloud hung over me, constantly. One day at work, I felt a slight
pain in my lower back. I thought I'd lose control. I got nervous and pan-
icky. I thought "I have to get out of here." I did some deep breathing,
talked to myself—the pain went away. I'd do well for a few days then I
could feel myself going downhill—that sinking feeling in my chest,
thoughts of death. I saw a lady at the store with her grandchild and
thought, Will I ever have that experience? I talked to my immune system.
Sometimes my coping mechanisms would work quickly, sometimes it
would take awhile. I've always been very open with everyone about hav-
ing breast cancer. I learned who I couldn't be honest with—I was bitter at
first because a few friends avoided me. They couldn't handle negative
reports, but I have so much support that I didn't need them. But we
remain friends—superficially, unfortunately.

As Pat struggled with one recurrence after another, she also felt a sense of estrangement, and anger at others.

Hearing I had breast cancer was one thing—hearing I had mets was
another. I mentioned my labile mood (with depression often present). I'd
get very angry—the old "why me." At times I didn't want to be with any-
one but my immediate family—I felt and sometimes still feel different.
Chris and I attended an anniversary brunch about two months after my
diagnosis with mets, and I sat there thinking how different I was from
everyone else there—I was sick, I wasn't sure of a future, I had to endure
suffering—and I hated everyone else for the "good life" they had.

I've become very impatient over the years with other people and their complaints. "How dare they complain to me?" I usually get over it and become my old supportive self. I want to be the one to be there for my family and friends—I hate always being on the receiving end. Sometimes I feel so inadequate—and yet I know how much I'm loved and how lucky I am.

Like many other women, Pat also worried constantly about the ways in which her illness affected the people she loved most:

It is illogical, I know, but I often feel my family would be better off without me, that it would be better for me to die quickly so they don't have to suffer. I'm glad to be alive but when I don't feel well, my thinking always focuses on this. I've even thought of suicide—overdose—but I couldn't do that to my family and I don't have the courage. I definitely ride the roller coaster. My mood was getting so labile that I recently started an antidepressant. It has helped. I have scans on January 22, and hope for a report that at least says no new mets and the old ones haven't grown.

Pam Hiebert, when her cancer came back after a three-year remission, also came to the point of recognizing she needed some help.

In desperation, having spent almost an entire weekend in misery and condemning my partner, the very person who is such a stable, positive force in my life, I called Ralph to obtain antidepressants. The new drug (Paxil) worked within a few days and vastly improved my mental state and quality of life. I don't like adding another drug to my daily medication routine but the physiological changes occurring by my use of this hormonal drug are something I must consider as another part of working with this disease. As my dear friend Gilda said to me, "Give thanks you have something that actually works. You'd be much worse off without it."

It's common for people in this situation to long for normalcy and resist treatments that make them feel "medicalized" or dependent. PJ Hagler commiserated with Kathy Stone about not wanting to take medication for depression.

I understand how you feel about meds. I have tried to just feel "normal" or free from all medical sensations myself. I hate meds. I have fought them for so long and have to admit I finally agreed to take Zoloft. I hate to admit it because I want to do this on my own but I do feel better. I like to think that I can do this by myself sometimes. I hate to admit any weakness in myself and part of that to me is giving into meds. I am trying to fight this stupidity. I can't do this on my own. That's what the meds are for. I have had this dumb morphine drip for over a month now and I really know my limits with pain management. I know I need it and I was getting so depressed and low on energy that I trusted the oncologist who has not misled me yet and agreed to the Soloist. I like to think that I at least made the choice on my own as to take it or not. If it helps I will give it a try.

Kim Banks recalled her own struggles with depression, and offered some of her strategies for coping:

When I was sick from the chemo and all alone at home, I wrestled with the demons of depression and hopelessness, daily. I took an antidepressant during those times which helped me from dropping into one of those deep depressions. That had happened the first time I was on chemo and it really scared me. At that time I didn't want to get out of bed and didn't want to experience the daily pain and haunting worries anymore. I had lots to live for, but at that moment it was hard to remember those things.

The times when I was very depressed, I would force myself to get dressed and go for a walk, no matter how sick I was or how miserable it was outside. I wouldn't be skipping back home, but the walk usually broke my chain of thought and lifted me out of that dark hole I felt I was in. I would remind myself that if I could just get through this minute and then the next, I would ultimately feel better. So I'd concentrate on the minutes and pretty soon an hour had gone by and slowly, I realized that I felt a little better.

There were times when I felt especially vulnerable and learned that I had to avoid people and situations that I thought would pull me down. I decided that if I was going to beat this, I had to make myself number one for a while and focus on what was going to make me better. It's hard for women to be selfish, but we've got to be in order to get better. We won't be able to take care of anyone, if we don't take care of ourselves first.

Lisann Charland also found that paying attention to her own needs was crucial, and sought the help of a therapist to do so:

I had to find a way to conquer the fears and loneliness I felt, due to the seriousness of this metastasis, as well as learn ways to improve my life. In parallel, I sought a psychologist who helped me deal with my fears and pain. I learned to put Lisann first, deal with my fear of death and dying and the loneliness I felt with my family so far away.

No matter how much progress I feel I have made in accepting death and dying, the fragile state of my mind becomes evident when I lose members of my support group, or friends to cancer. However, the nightmares are not as bad as they used to be. I have also learned to choose my words carefully when relaying test results to my husband, who suffers from depression at times, and to my family. When they are in pain, I feel the pain, and then have to work hard to get rid of the guilty feelings of being a burden to them.

Some days, I feel like I am "untouchable." Other times, I really feel the loss and pain of living with cancer. I react differently than I used to, and recognize that everything happens for a reason, and I always look for the good side of things. My personality is such that you make the best of a situation, and don't waste time—and move on.

I am fortunate that the low days are very rare. I get mild anxiety pains after routine checkups, which are easily handled by a good cry or a good talking to myself that I will handle what comes my way accordingly, and by taking a pro-active role in obtaining the results.

I have accepted losing the body parts and the scars and the limitations set on me physically, but I will not lose my sanity. I am more determined now to survive than I have ever been before.

Though inclined to approach life in a controlled, rational, problem-solving manner, Sharon Multhauf felt she had finally learned the value of getting in touch with her emotions, despite the sadness she found inside, as she shared in this poem:

My Heart Knows

Inside my head, I talk of life's march onward.
Inside my heart, I sob and mourn my youth.

Inside my head, I analyze and measure.
Inside my heart, I cling to hidden truth.

Inside my head, the options stand before me.
Inside my heart, the choice dissolves in strife.

Inside my head, I grasp my heart's awareness:
I've lost the open-endedness of life.

Offsetting the emotional traumas she experienced as she dealt with her escalating illness, Mary D'Angelo discovered an increasing intimacy with her husband:

I've had numerous times of overwhelming grief, usually when I get
bad news. This is characteristic—it always seems like I'm alone—that's
why I don't like to call for counts, because I know if they're not good,
they're going to depress me. So sometimes, I have Charlie call, or I just
wait for the next month.

When Charlie comes home, I'll just become hysterical, and we'll hug
each other. I'll just break down and let it all out, but only with him. He
hugs me, and then it's okay, because he accepts what I'm feeling: "Yes, this
is happening to you, and I'm here and I'll be with you. We will get through
it together." And then, there's no anxiety. There's still sadness, but it seems
to go away almost magically with his love, because whenever I'm really
upset about being ill, or the news is bad, that's when he comes, well—
crashing in, almost—with this bear hug of love that you can never
weaken or not get in touch with. So it's always at the saddest moments
that you get these great rushes of love. This intensity that you know is
there, but you don't actually viscerally feel at other times.

With wry good humor, Jenilu Schoolman expressed some of the frustration she experienced, as a psychotherapist, preparing her patients for her loss:

On occasion, I felt angry and put upon. "It is bad enough," I would
mutter to myself, "that I have to deal with my own death. Now I have to
help others deal with it too." But since I've never allowed my patients to
indulge in long periods of self-pity, I kept my own fairly short as well.

However, the pain would come unbidden and overwhelm me, and I
would cry. I soon realized that twenty minutes of crying at one time is suf-
ficient, and I learned never to let myself go on crying; enough is enough.
After a while, pain turns to self-pity and all that gets you is a headache.

In the same boat: Support and self-help groups

For the past two decades, self-help groups have proliferated in the United States, from 12-Step programs in church basements to the myriad support communities now on the Internet. Sociologist Frank Riessman referred to the phenomenon that makes this possible as the "helper-therapy principle." When people with a common affliction reach out to one another, and work together to transform personal tragedy into something meaningful, this enhances the self-esteem of people whose sense of themselves has been compromised by illness or other misfortune.

While some self-help groups are actively "anti-professional," rejecting the group facilitation skills of mental-health professionals in favor of the hard-won knowledge of those who have "been there," other groups, especially hospital-based support groups for patients, tend to have professionally trained leaders.

The online breast cancer support group that made this book possible has been discussed at length elsewhere, so it won't be dwelt on here, except to point out that this, too, clearly represents a complementary self-help treatment.

There are some good reasons why a face-to-face group for people with metastatic cancer needs an experienced mental health professional as a facilitator. Here is how Sharon Multhauf described the support group she attends:

> *Because I am by nature an optimistic person who seldom spends much time in tears, I needed to be taught that sometimes the best thing for a person in crisis is to cry and feel sad, and that this does not equate with giving up or lacking hope. During the two years that I have attended a weekly support group for women with metastatic breast cancer, I have heard over and over again the gentle words of our skilled and compassionate facilitator, "How does that make you feel?" She seldom lets us stop with reporting the facts about our pain, our treatment, our test results, our life circumstances. We are invited to look closely at the effects these more tangible things are having on our less tangible emotional state. Time and again, we see someone move from anxiety or despair into more peace and optimism through the process of acknowledging her fears and sadness.*

It is very hard for a person who has always been "in control" of herself to deal with the inevitable emotional pain and fear that cancer brings, if she is not allowed (by herself or others) to reveal the cracks in her armor.

Disturbing and painful issues are bound to come up in such a group as its members frequently encounter medical crises, treatment failures and are unable to attend for health reasons. Over time, some members will die. If the group is to remain vital, the feelings raised by these events must be explored and expressed openly. This confrontation with common issues of mortality and loss will often will lead to further growth for the members, but it is never an easy process, and always fraught with deep emotions. Sometimes the grief is too overwhelming for some of its members. Pat Leach left her longtime support group after her third recurrence because, as she said, "all the oldies were dying."

Here is Nancy Gilpatrick's experience with a support group as she wrestled with her decision about high-dose chemotherapy:

*I just began attending a support group for breast cancer survivors with mets. I had heard of this group around town and just found it in May. Last night was my first time. It was great. There are five women who have had high-dose chemotherapy with stem cell transplants, which is where I'm headed next. Two were there and talked about their experiences. They told of their experiences and talked about the process of making the decision and being comfortable with it being more important than whether it's right or wrong. One woman said she just realized that she makes decisions every day without expecting a known outcome and yet once with breast cancer and making such serious decisions as we do, we expect more certainty in the outcome. That helped me a lot. They also talked about the area of my greatest fear: going through this treatment and coming out with active disease. The two women who were there still had active disease after the transplant. They are doing well, a year for one, and one and a half years for the other after the transplant **and** with active disease.*

For most of those I interviewed, the only support group they've "attended" has been on the Internet. This support has helped enormously with the sense of isolation and stigma PJ Hagler had felt in her life before:

*One thing that is taught in any counseling class is that the most important thing to do is encourage the person who is needing help to **talk** about everything and especially what is bothering them. It is how one gets well. If we keep our feelings in we don't ever get the support we need. How is a person going to help if they don't know our feelings? I know if I'm depressed, sick, excited, happy or even unsure of my feelings that I can come here and you all will help me. You're all better than one therapist. I have hundreds of you to listen to me and help me. I try to explain to my friend and my sister why you all mean so much to me and they both say that when I'm cured they hope I will quit. Little do they realize I will never be cured unless there is a miracle in my future.*

For Glenn Clabo, a great deal of help and comfort came from participating in the Breast Cancer Discussion List, after he made the discovery that it was easier for him to write about what he felt than to attend a group or see a therapist. Although his wife, Barb, chose not to participate directly, it helped her as well.

Barb didn't like to post (write messages) but she loved to read mine. It allowed her to see what I was feeling without the cover of toughness that I sometimes put over myself. I've also made some very understanding and helpful friends, All this without ever meeting anyone eye to eye. It still amazes me. I kept a running daily account of her progress during her first Taxol treatment and it sure helped me deal with it. The response was wonderful and helped me get through each day.

Barb Pender found a compatible group, although she was uneasy about upsetting the newly diagnosed women:

Initially, my sister dragged me to a support group for all cancers—I was in my own world during that time and really wanted to talk to women with breast cancer. I found a support group at the hospital across the freeway but found it to be a much older group. They were wonderful and wanted to take me under their wing but I needed current information and younger "hope." I finally went to a weekly support group in a neighboring town. It was wonderful—a mixture of ages but all seemed to be able to relate. I went faithfully for the first year but when the metastasis hit I felt as though I was scaring the new people away. I went more and more infrequently.

It seemed that I knew in my heart when I needed to go back and each time that I did I was greeted by lovely old friends. It's a place that I feel comfortable—they are probably the only people who know exactly what I am feeling. I have strong support at home but there are times that the only one who really knows how I am feeling is one who has walked in my shoes.

Sometimes, though, a group does not turn out to be very supportive. As a man with breast cancer, Bob Stafford had a more difficult time finding a support group that would accept him:

I did attend a support group and didn't feel welcome there. One woman that I had known for several years told me that she found it difficult to talk to me about breast cancer even though she had a bilateral mastectomy some twenty years previous. Breasts are too sexual an issue in our country. I did find a group that now has about 25 women who consider me an adopted "son" in a way.

Bob has since gone on to set up a number of resources for men with breast cancer. Pam Hiebert also felt different than other group members:

During one of my initial visits to the local breast cancer support group it seemed to me most women were grossly concerned with their appearance rather than their actual health. I sat on the floor refusing to conform to these fluffy topics of conversation. They wore wigs while I just pulled my old baseball cap down over my shaved head. I felt very alone. Everyone there talked of earlier stage treatments. It was a shock not to have any others around who were also battling mets.

Although face-to-face professionally led group resources for metastatic patients are still hard to find outside of major population centers, they are well worth investigating as part of your treatment plan. Online resources, while they cannot provide professional guidance, can also be surprisingly effective in gathering information and support and combating isolation, even when "real life" groups don't meet this need.

One reason people shy away from support groups—as well as from psychotherapy in general—is that they fear becoming more depressed and frightened by their illness than they already are. They are afraid that the expression of grief and fear in such a group will lead to an increased negative focus in their lives, which seem limited enough already by the disease.

Won't it just make me feel worse? they wonder. Isn't it better to "try to look on the bright side" or to "keep a positive outlook?"

In fact, just the opposite appears to be true. Sharing feelings in a supportive setting actually helps people to feel calmer and more able to think rationally about what needs to be done. Whether cancer patients are any more likely than other people to suppress emotions, as some studies have suggested, there is ample evidence from well-controlled studies that expressing strong feelings in a group setting, to quote Dr. David Spiegel, "has a powerful and positive therapeutic effect."

> In our psychosocial treatment laboratory, we have obtained recent evidence that attempts to suppress emotion are counterproductive. Metastatic breast cancer patients who rated themselves as high in emotional suppression on the Courtauld Emotional Control Scale (5) turned out to have higher total mood disturbance scores on the Profile of Mood States (6) than those who were low in affect suppression. In other words, suppression of adverse affect [emotion] does not work. It seems to increase, rather than reduce, dysphoria [abnormal generalized feelings of ill-being]. The patient who suffers constant intrusion of her fear of death may be relieved by the opportunity to discuss that fear with others in a similar situation. As one support group member commented, "The world hasn't changed, but I feel less alone with my feelings about it."[17]

The Psychosocial Treatment Laboratory at Stanford University School of Medicine has pioneered group work with metastatic breast cancer patients. In their *Treatment Manual for Brief Supportive-Expressive Group Therapy*, the staff make clear the vital importance of the kind of group support they offer:

> There is strong evidence to suggest that a social structure, such as a support group, provides meaningful support, encouragement for the expression of relevant emotions, and buffering of patients from stress. It has the potential to impact positively on both adjustment to illness and, ultimately, the course of the disease. Many studies have shown positive effects of group therapy interventions for cancer patients on such psychological variables as mood, adjustment and pain.... It is clear from this research that the expression of relevant emotions and direct discussions of difficult subject matters enhances rather than hinders quality of life, and may actually increase the life expectancy of women with breast cancer.

The group experience offers to these patients a place to belong and to express feelings.

There is an intense bonding among the members and a sense of acceptance through sharing a common dilemma. This serves to counter the social alienation that often divides cancer patients from their well-meaning but anxious family and friends. Involvement in a group also allows patients to better mobilize their existing resources as well as to develop new coping strategies and sources of support.

....Being with others who have the same illness and who share similar experiences mitigates the anxiety of facing the illness on one's own and normalizes disease-related feelings and experiences.[18]

Whether or not your life will be extended by reaching out to others, by expressing your emotions, by seeking new meanings in your experience with illness in the company of other people struggling with cancer, many people have found these pursuits to be worthwhile in and of themselves, for the sense of connection and clarity they can provide.

Support groups may not be for everyone, however. For some people, privacy is a crucial issue. A one-to-one relationship with a therapist, a close friend, or a spouse may feel far more supportive. One or two contacts with other patients may be all that you want—or perhaps none at all. For some women, the prospect of witnessing fellow group members experience progression of their illness and die is simply too disturbing and disheartening to even contemplate. They find it impossible to believe that any benefit could offset these upsetting realities. If you feel this way, but find that the stories in this book have been helpful, you owe it to yourself to give a support group a try and to see if your fears are founded. Still, while a direct confrontation with mortality can indeed be life-affirming and meaningful, it is wrong and insensitive to force that which is unwanted on anyone, in the name of its being "the right way."

You must find your own way. Seeking that delicate balance between honoring your own inclinations and challenging your preconceptions is something no one else can do for you.

Curing, healing and being whole

In summary, while a cure for metastatic breast cancer may be elusive, the healing of body, mind and spirit can be a worthwhile and achievable goal. It is toward this goal of healing—through information, commonality of experience and inspiration—that this book is directed. In this very broad definition of healing falls much that gives our lives meaning. The importance of this vital pursuit will be addressed in the final chapters of this book.

Michael Lerner puts it all in context for us:

> *Understanding choices in healing begins with understanding the difference between healing and curing. A curative medical treatment is something your doctor ardently hopes to provide. Healing, by contrast, starts within your own mind and body. The capacity to heal is what you bring to an encounter with illness.*[19]

What are you bringing to this encounter? Take a close look at yourself in your current circumstances. What are you doing to take care of yourself? Are you getting the best medical care? Are you seeking and finding support, encouragement and love from those around you? Whatever pain and discomfort you are feeling, do you have a sense that there is still meaning and purpose in your life? And is there something more, from among the many possibilities open to you, that might enhance and enrich the time you have, however long it may be?

Simple questions, yes—but the answers are always complex. And the story continues to unfold.

> *Discovery is a journey*
> *An attitude*
> *A way to teach yourself to say*
> *"So. And where does this new thing*
> *that I have learned take me?"*

> —Pam Hiebert

CHAPTER 8

Living with Side Effects and Symptoms

BY AND LARGE, it was not specific coping strategies for dealing with treatment side effects or disease symptoms that really mattered to the people interviewed for this book. Surprisingly, in what they had to say, there were no lists of helpful hints, no special diets, no recommended reading.

Instead, what concerned people most was how they were going to be able to cope emotionally, to keep their spirits up, to continue their roles with their families, to work as long as possible and to prevent their lives from being consumed over long periods by their disease and its treatments. This chapter speaks to the small but relentless daily struggles that wear down metastatic breast cancer patients. Having to live with uncertainty and waiting for test results. Feeling their lives become increasingly medicalized as their disease progresses. Fearing the isolation of long hospital stays. Dreading the prospect of intolerable, unrelieved pain. Asking for help or accepting help from others. Being forced to relinquish the meaningful roles they had played in their own lives before illness forced a change. Losing control of their bodies and of physical functioning. Becoming burdensome to those they love.

And yet, the people I interviewed have without exception managed to cope and adapt, surprising themselves with their strength. While there are no simple remedies for any of these difficult issues, what follows in this chapter is testimony both to their resilience and their candor in "telling it like it is."

Testing, testing...playing the waiting game

Living with a life-threatening illness that is likely to return or worsen at any time is a waiting game anyway—but it is testing that often forms the focal point for anxiety. Medical testing is an integral and unavoidable part of the landscape of metastatic breast cancer. Tests monitor the progression or remission of the disease, and the success or failure of treatment. Oncologists use the information gleaned from tests to guide their recommendations. Some tests are painless and non-invasive, involving drawing blood from a port or taking an x-ray or scan; others, like liver and bone marrow biopsies, are quite invasive and can cause considerable pain.

But every test, difficult or not, evokes anxiety while waiting for the results. What is a routine aspect of daily life in any medical laboratory or doctor's office is far from routine for you, since the results can alter the course of your life. Some providers are sensitive to this, while others seem largely oblivious what it's like for cancer patients to undergo tests and wait for their results. Sometimes, you can make a difference by making your needs known. You can arrange to get the test results before the weekend, for example, or arrange a time in advance when you can contact the doctor.

Cindy Wirth was 34 years old and had just given birth to her second child when her breast cancer was diagnosed at Stage IIIB in 1991. Despite aggressive treatments, including Cytoxan, Adriamycin and 5-FU, the cancer soon spread to her supraclavicular nodes and lung. Two years after her original diagnosis, Cindy underwent high-dose chemotherapy, but again the cancer recurred within a few months. She qualified to participate in a Her2-neu study and traveled from Illinois, where they lived, to San Francisco for ten consecutive weeks to participate in it. Her husband, Gerry, reported that while he certainly did have to spend more time running interference with the children during parts of her treatment cycles, they actually managed to maintain a semblance of ordinary life during almost all of this time—except for one particular point in the treatment cycle.

> It all became normal...except for the every-cycle chest x-ray. That is how we knew the treatment was working. She would get it done on Saturday so the oncologist would have the report on Monday, chemo day. The weekends were such hell that the oncologist showed Cindy how to get a recorded report on Sunday. Every time you always wondered if the spell was broken.

Sometimes it seems as if the procedural bureaucracy of hospitals and clinics must be designed to make things difficult. Nearly every woman in this situation can recall some story of tests results lost, delayed or otherwise mishandled, and of the emotional cost to her.

As outspoken and unafraid to advocate for herself as anyone I interviewed, Lucie Bergmann-Shuster has put her finger on what it is that makes the process of testing so excruciating:

> I wish I knew the answer for a fix on this kind of emotional pain. I go through it every time I have a battery of tests done. The waiting and the uncertainty is just so devastating. I have told my doctors that this kind of pain is worse than any physical pain I have ever experienced.
>
> All I can say, that once you get the reports back, the gnawing, mind twisting suspense will be over. Even if the results are not in your favor, at least you will be able to go on to chart a new course of action. It is the infernal wait that kills us. Let's hope that there will be some positives in the results, but at least the waiting and the suspense will cease.

In and of themselves, of course, almost all tests, including biopsies, are minor procedures, and are frequently treated offhandedly by medical personnel. But because these tests are intimately tied to revelations about the course of a life-threatening disease, the entire process can take on enormous emotional weight. This discrepancy between your subjective experience of the testing process, and the routine, often depersonalizing way the process is handled is a source of much unnecessary distress.

As a high-risk patient two years following intensive chemotherapy, Ellen Scheiner has found that one way to minimize anxiety is to have blood drawn a week before her quarterly checkups, so that the results are available by the time she visits her oncologist. Despite the inconvenience, she finds that this simple act of foresight permits this visit to be both definitive, and reassuring.

And it's not only the patient who worries, of course. It can affect the whole family. Sylvan Rainwater, Pam Hiebert's partner, reflected on the role that testing played in their lives since Pam's diagnosis at Stage IV, three years earlier, and the ways in which both of them had changed in attitude over time:

> Pam goes in for another bone scan today. She's had two more, one each year, since that first one. Each one she has faced differently. That first one was new and terrifying, in a time of crisis and facing the unknown. The second one she faced with anger, cursing the machine as she lay down. Last year she approached it with dread, having lived with health again and fearful of going back into medical crisis. This year she's

getting the scan a few weeks earlier than the previous two years. She's had increasing body pain again, in spite of exercise and generally improving health in most ways.

After two weeks of the pain not clearing up, she made another appointment to get it checked on, and found that her tumor markers were up. The oncologist drew blood again and said that if they continued to rise she would need a bone scan. So here we are, with markers rising and body pain, facing another bone scan.

We've gotten used to relative health and well-being again. Pam's remission has been a gift that at first we didn't know how to accept, but have learned to be grateful for. We know now that her markers have risen before and fallen again for no apparent reason, and that body pain is something she has lived with for a long time, with flare-ups certainly not unheard of. We know this could all be nothing, a false alarm like other false alarms in the past.

When you live with metastasized breast cancer everything sounds an alarm. We also know that it could be the recurrence we've been told will most likely happen sometime (no one can say when) and we want to be timely and responsible about treatment options if that turns out to be needed. We've learned that you don't have to respond to a test result the same day. We've decided that when we get the results, no matter what they are, we will continue with our plans to go to the family reunion in Kansas and defer decisions about treatment until after that. There's a measure of calm acceptance that wasn't there before, just because we know so more now than we did then.

I find that I fear losing that calm acceptance and being thrown back into medical crisis. That was such a horrifying time. I tell myself that we've changed and grown and learned and that the experience will be different, which is certainly true, but still...the what-ifs lie in wait, trying to shred my self-control, threatening my ability to concentrate on my work once again. I breathe deeply, trying to meditate, and find the monkey mind jumping crazily from one thing to another. I re-center again and again.

As Pam and I talk about our anxieties, we recognize that this test is only a procedure, which will give us another piece of information. It will *not give us The Answer, but it does have the power to lead to procedures that will alter our lives. For me, the fear and lack of control is centered in the fact that it is not even my own body, but that of my beloved. For her, similar feelings surround the fact that it is her own body. For neither of us is it easy.*

Every woman with metastatic breast cancer becomes expert in the anxious art of waiting. Two years after high-dose chemotherapy for inflammatory breast cancer, Bonnie Gelbwasser tells her own experience.

I have not found an easy way to cope with the waiting, whether it is for test results or waiting until you can have the test (sometimes tests or procedures are scheduled days or weeks in advance). I try to maintain my normal daily routine—I get to work and get involved in that, or stay as busy as possible on weekends. I do not eat well during these times, have trouble sleeping and am often distracted and edgy. Fear and anxiety appear to have taken up permanent residence in my psyche. I admire and envy anyone who can stay relaxed and focused in the face of a disease that seems to always be threatening to return.

Still, Bonnie is actually one of the lucky ones, whose providers, sensitive to the stress she is under, arrange for her to get tested and obtain results in a timely way.

To my great relief and comfort, my doctors have consistently given me results as quickly as possible. Three examples: I have had three bone scans so far. Each time, the M.D. who reads these scans has come to me before I left the room to tell me that everything looked okay (twice) and to reassure me that although it was possible that a more thorough examination of the results might indicate a problem, it was unlikely. The last time, when a shadow did show up, he walked with me to the Hematology/ Oncology Clinic and he then met with my oncologist, who talked to me shortly thereafter.

I had a biopsy that was totally unexpected—the oncologist found something she wanted biopsied immediately and sent me to the surgeon. My next appointment that morning happened to be with my therapist. My surgeon arranged to get the report very quickly and to interrupt (with my permission) my session with the therapist (less than one hour later) to tell me the results were benign. Had the cells been malignant, I would have been with the therapist when I got the news.

I had a lumpectomy on a Tuesday and was told not to expect the results before the following Monday. The surgeon's nurse said she'd call me if they came in earlier. That Friday I received a call from the surgeon himself, who said his nurse was not in the office that day and the pathology report indicated no cancer and he didn't want me to have to worry over the weekend.

To top it off, about half an hour later, the nurse called. She said she'd called the lab, gotten the results and wanted to let me know. I had a similar experience after my mastectomy, when the nurse called me late on Friday afternoon to tell me that she'd just learned that my lymph nodes were clear and thought I might like to celebrate over the weekend.

Many women are less fortunate, and the anxiety often becomes even worse when test results are not forthcoming. Pat Leach reported frequent frustration in obtaining this information:

I'm usually a basket case waiting for test results. And many times the docs keep me waiting. I bug them with calls, etc., but it doesn't always work. Then I usually take the "no news is good news" attitude and go on with my life. It works some, and as long as I feel reasonably well and can keep occupied I do okay.

I agree that frequent testing means increased nervousness and anxiety. I'm not sure what the answer is. Even if I have a "test break," I'm anxious over what might be going on. Receiving good news—and that can be anything from tumors are gone or decreased in size to tumor size is stable and especially, no new spots seen—is about the only thing that calms me down for awhile....

Barb Pender has discovered a strategy that works for her:

My health care providers have been very sensitive to my needs— emotionally and physically. My doctors have been very sensitive as well. With every scan, I remind my doctor's case manager, "Don't forget, Sarah, I'm waiting on pins and needles. The weekend is coming and I would like to know something." If the official results are not in, my doctor calls the radiologist and gets some sort of a preliminary idea of what is

going on. So, I think expressing your needs is the most important sugges-
tion I would give to someone battling the waiting game.

While many of the tests used in following breast cancer patients are not in themselves physically painful, there are a few that are. PJ Hagler, who has endured many of these tests, speaks as a veteran:

> I will admit that over the past six years especially I have had every
> test known to man and then some. I have an oncologist who believes in
> being 100 percent sure of what he is dealing with and doesn't want to sec-
> ond guess why I feel the way I do. He wants to be sure of chemo and also
> he knows because of the expense of the Taxol, that the insurance com-
> pany would not agree to treatment unless he could justify the need. He
> will fight any insurance agency for full payment if he has to fight end-
> lessly.
>
> The worst time was the beginning in 1990-1991 when he was trying
> to find the mets to the lung. He was so sure there was cancer and he
> couldn't see it anywhere. It finally took opening my back and looking at
> my lung to be sure. I prayed very hard for the strength to endure the pain.
> The hardest tests, while they helped slightly, were not worth the pain in
> my case. I had a bronchoscopy, two thoracenteses and two liver biopsies.
> All but the last biopsy came back inconclusive.

Reading the harrowing description of one of PJ's liver biopsies, Pat Leach, a nurse herself, became angry.

> I think all of them should have to undergo these tests just to feel
> physically what it's like, especially the painful ones such as bone marrow
> biopsies and liver biopsies. I always ask for sedation and if the doc says
> no—I take my own. Ativan is a wonderful drug to keep around. A couple
> work wonders on my anxiety, pain level tolerance, etc. And I wish I could
> let every woman know that sedation **can** be given for these biopsies. Duke
> did it and I tolerated the procedures much better than those done here in
> Connecticut where the doc said, "No sedation, I need you to be alert."
> Bullshit—I get so mad that they make us suffer—PJ should not have had
> to endure what she did. I try to be as honest now as possible with my docs
> and am at the point where if they won't do it the way I want it done, I'll
> refuse.

Whether you tolerate the waiting with equanimity or insomnia, whether you endure painful tests stoically or insist on pharmaceutical help, it helps to know that you are far from alone in your tribulations. It makes sense to have a support person with you, if you find that comforting. And it makes sense to assert yourself to arrange to get your test results as soon as possible. For the woman with metastatic breast cancer, these routine events are anything but routine.

Getting through chemotherapy

This is a Day

This is a day of rest
lying in bed in a pillow nest
today the light hurts my eyes.

This is not many things.

This is not the flu—an interruption.
This is not my period and cramps
—a regular rhythm that is now stopped as a side effect of drugs.
This is not a hangover, but I feel the deep, deep poison and nausea.
This is not a mental health day to play hooky from work

This is not many things.
This is cancer.
This is in my very bones, now moth-eaten and fragile.

This is what dictates my activity.
And permission comes
yes or no
depending on my blood counts.

This is a day when my red blood
cells are low and I am short of breath.

This is a day when I cannot go
out because my white cells
are too few to protect me.

This is a day of very low energy.
This is not comfortable.
This is cancer.

This is still a day I cherish.
This is a day that is mine.
I am not the cancer.
I am in my pillow nest
secure and fortified
looking ahead to tomorrow.

—JB Boggs

There is no denying that chemotherapy treatments for metastatic breast cancer can be toxic and debilitating at times. Many of the same cytotoxic drugs are given as with primary breast cancer. These, of course, temporarily damage normal rapidly-dividing cells and cause side effects. Many of these side effects, however, can and should be effectively treated, and some can even be prevented.

Cytotoxic chemotherapy is myelosuppressive, meaning that it affects the bone marrow that produces the white blood cells that control our ability to fight off infection, the red blood cells that carry oxygen to the rest of the body, and the platelets that form clots and control bleeding. When white cells are low, you are more susceptible to fever and infection, and may be placed on antibiotics or even hospitalized if you run a fever. When red blood cells are low, you may become anemic and feel very short of breath and fatigued. When platelets are very low, you must be careful to avoid any activity that could prompt bleeding.

Growth factors are often used to stimulate the bone marrow and avoid fevers, infections, bleeding and low white blood counts. This new and rapidly progressing field of medical research has made chemotherapy much safer. Neupogen (the brand name for G-CSF, granulocyte-colony stimulating factor), which stimulates white cell production, has enabled doctors to safely give much larger amounts of chemotherapy in the past several years. Growth factors that stimulate red blood cell production (erythropoietin) are now in wide use, and a new growth factor that stimulates platelet production still in clinical trials, may soon be commonly used, greatly reducing the risks of intensive chemotherapy. Red blood cell and platelet transfusions, as well as the bone-marrow or stem-cell reinfusion (also called transplant or rescue) given with high-dose chemotherapy, are also ways to deal with the myelosuppressive effects of chemotherapy. Your doctor will monitor your blood counts, and give you specific instructions for the precautions you should take during the times in the treatment cycle when your counts may be lowest. This period of time, sometimes referred to as the nadir, usually occurs ten to fourteen days after treatment. It is important that you understand the side effects of each medication you are taking and how they interact, so that you can be alert for any problems and report them immediately to your oncologist. Often you will be asked to take your temperature daily, and report any significant elevation to your doctor.

Among the most troublesome and debilitating effects of chemotherapy are nausea, vomiting, diarrhea, mouth sores, thrush infections and other symptoms caused by the chemotherapy's effect on the rapidly dividing cells in the gastrointestinal tract. Generally, GI side effects diminish after the first few days following treatment, although onset of nausea and vomiting may be delayed until the better-working intravenous drugs wear off. Everyone experiences these side effects differently, too. Some women have very little nausea and no vomiting, while others are plagued with it, and may feel sick for days on end. No one knows why there's such individual variability.

The good news is that nausea and vomiting can usually be controlled. Effective anti-nausea drugs are widely used now, with the newer, more expensive but far more effective Zofran and Kytril augmenting older drugs like Compazine. Make sure you insist on adequate relief from nausea and vomiting—most of the time, even if you are very sensitive, this will be possible. Have your doctor or a nutritionist skilled in dealing with cancer treatments discuss non-pharmaceutical ways you can control these symptoms, like having frequent, small, bland meals, nibbling on crackers upon awakening, learning self-hypnosis and changing the timing or administration of treatments.

Many women find that it is the persistent fatigue and malaise that most affects their state of mind, especially if it is constant. Usually these symptoms are cyclical in nature, allowing people at least a few days of fairly normal life before the next treatment. But when treatments go on and on, with little respite from side effects, it's not at all unusual to become worn down emotionally as well as physically, and experience symptoms of depression and anxiety. Even though you may know, rationally, that the symptoms come from the treatment, not the disease, feeling "sick and tired" most days can make everything else about having metastatic breast cancer seem all the more real: the actual and emotional isolation you may feel from friends and family, the hair loss and other physical changes, the overall loss of self-esteem that goes with being on leave or disability retirement from work, and the sheer medicalization of your life, with its rounds of doctors' appointments, treatments and tests.

Dr. Wendy S. Harpham, author of *After Cancer: A Guide to Your New Life* and three other books on coping with cancer, has undergone treatments for cancer recurrence since 1990 and has become an expert on the fatigue cancer patients often feel.

> *There are many things that can be done to counter cancer-related fatigue, starting with a search for treatable physical factors, like low thyroid or blood count, and learning to recognize and respect one's limits....* *Many patients try to keep life as normal as possible and in the process, they overdo it.* [1]

Fatigue can have a variety of causes, and at least some of them are treatable. While cancer treatments themselves are certainly one clear cause of fatigue, Harpham says, so is the depression and anxiety that is so common among cancer patients. Inactivity can play a part, as well. Regular exercise, attention to nutrition and plenty of rest can be helpful. Harpham recommends consulting a dietician for ideas on how to deal with poor appetite as a result of treatment. Avoiding unnecessary stress and saving limited energies for the things that matter can help with relieving fatigue. Asking for assistance with household chores, for example, can free a person to do the things she likes most. New habits, like taking naps during the day, and eating frequent small meals, can also help a great deal. When anemia is a side effect of treatment, it can often be treated with drugs to encourage the production of red blood cells. Sometimes, the fatigue is simply so profound, it must be yielded to and accepted as part of the process.

Most women find that they are able to cope, with adequate rest and getting the help they need, throughout the treatment process. Not all treatments are toxic; some hormonal and experimental treatments are not particularly disruptive of daily life. Whatever your side effects, however, it's important to speak up about them and ask for your oncologist's help in dealing with them effectively. Your quality of life ought to be the first concern of your treatment team.

At Stage IV, when Barb Clabo's initial Taxol infusions failed to produce any objective response in her tumors, she and Glenn were becoming desperate. Her doctor started her on intensive doses of FAC (5-FU, Adriamycin and Cytoxan) another standard treatment for metastatic disease, and her liver tumors disappeared. But she had problems tolerating the treatments. Each cycle of treatment seemed to land her in the hospital with fevers.

> *Took my temp at 6:00 p.m.—102. Panic and anger set in. I immediately started to cry and say I don't want to go to the hospital again—I don't want to go. Was acting pretty much like a small child, but I was really frightened. My last stay in the hospital was 8 days. Glenn called the doctor and again we were sent to the E.R. Spent 4 hours in E.R. before finally being admitted—WBC was .5. Here we go again.*

> *I had a very difficult time in the hospital emotionally this time. I cried a lot. I would look at Glenn and just start crying. Every time I looked at him, I thought to myself that I was not ready to leave him, but oh so afraid I might. I would think, How am I going to say good-bye? Every time this thought came to mind (and it came quite often, even when he was not around) I would try to suppress it because it was so painful to deal with. I would see myself on my deathbed having to tell him good-bye. I would try to tell him how much he has meant to me through the years and what a wonderful husband and father he has been. I cannot express in words how I feel about this man. Words don't seem to be enough. I didn't think I was near death with this treatment, it just made me wonder about the future. The doctor said he might have to change my treatment because I was not tolerating it very well. This, too, is very scary to me. We finally have a chemo that is reducing my cancer and we might not be able to use it? What if we switch and another one doesn't work. I was feeling very down about this.*

Barb's husband, Glenn, felt demoralized too, seeing his wife become so despairing during her treatments.

> *Beside the fact that Barb is just plain down and out...she continues to mention the fact that she thinks her mother's fight with cancer ended in her death from the treatments. It is always on her mind and, in fact, she almost broke my heart when she asked me on the way to the hospital, "I'm going to be all right aren't I? Please tell me I'm going to be all right!" I thought she was thinking of her mom.*

> *Barb keeps saying, "I want me back! This isn't me. I'm not the person in the mirror. I'm not the person watching someone else working in*

the garden. I'm not the person who acts like this stupid crybaby!" I sit there unable to say anything. What can I say without being stupid?

Such setbacks, upsetting as they are, are almost always temporary. Depression during chemotherapy is not at all uncommon, as partially suppressed feelings of fear and sadness tend to emerge during these vulnerable times. Transient times of despair, hopelessness and grief as you and your family make the necessary but painful adaptation to your changing circumstances should not be confused with crippling major depression, under-recognized and under-treated in many people with cancer. The cancer itself, or the treatments may help cause depression. As mentioned in the previous chapter, a study of depression among hospitalized cancer patients found that fully 42 percent met the psychiatric criteria for major depression.[2] Many cancer patients, and health care providers, for that matter, fail to recognize the symptoms. If you are suffering from extended disruptions in sleeping or eating, extreme fatigue and loss of motivation, long bouts of tearfulness and despair, or are plagued with thoughts of suicide, it's crucial to bring this to your doctor's attention. Skillful psychiatric intervention can make a world of difference.

From this point in her induction chemotherapy, Barb went on to have high-dose chemotherapy and a stem-cell reinfusion. She recovered and was back at work, full time, three months later. During the months before her relapse, Barb was able to get her "Me" back, and so was Glenn.

However temporary, these feelings of loss of control and loss of function are difficult for everyone to cope with. Jenilu Schoolman described her feelings as she moved through her chemotherapy:

> *While cancer certainly seemed to control a good deal of my body, chemotherapy controlled much of my life. As I moved through the treatment cycle each month, my white blood counts dropped and I became very susceptible to infection. Because of this, I carefully avoided concerts, plays and other events since someone in the audience undoubtedly had a cold. This was truly painful because I enjoy these activities, but the effort was worth it.*
>
> *Of course, the control issue is much broader. I had so little control over my own body it would have been easy to feel helpless and abandon the efforts required to maintain control of my life. When my body didn't*

do my bidding, all I had left was my mind, and even then I had to make a conscious effort to give up control over people and events.

Ellen Scheiner found that her training and expertise as a physician worked both for and against her as she underwent her chemotherapy. Two years after completing rigorous treatment for high-risk breast cancer, she organized a symposium about health care professionals with cancer at an international psychooncology conference. She expressed the difficulty physicians face as patients, their need to maintain facades of professionalism and objectivity and their often ambiguous relationship to their treating physicians.

> *In this self-perpetuating situation, the physician who becomes ill finds him or herself struggling to replicate what was taught: to maintain control, to resist becoming vulnerable and not to be weak. Being ill means being weak in this context.[3]*

At 61, Ellen had been considered too old to undergo HDC. She described her choice to join a clinical trial at the hospital she'd once practiced at as an internist:

> *I knew the odds: less than a ten percent chance of five-year survival with conventional chemotherapy. It was then that I saw an oncologist and learned that I would have to devote the next months entirely to the ATC protocol. I would have to close my practice and make arrangements in less than three weeks. The recommended regimen was a Phase II study involving Adriamycin, Taxol and Cytoxan, given at high doses, three doses of each drug at two week intervals. I would be hospitalized at least six times. There were, in fact, three additional hospitalizations for neutropenia and fever. Before consenting, I read the actual research protocol, in addition to the one usually given to patients. I thought I knew what the words nausea, fatigue, fever, chills, low blood counts, shortness of breath, bone pain and trouble swallowing meant. When I experienced them myself, I saw how very little I had really comprehended.*

As a single woman, Ellen didn't have a spouse or partner to get her through the rigorous treatments.

> *Since I live alone, I had to be responsible for the carrying out of nine treatments, six in hospital, a series of scans, blood counts three times a week and all of the other usual needs of life: food, shopping, paying bills,*

dealing with insurance companies. I had closed my practice in psycho-
therapy and had arranged coverage. As the protocol proceeded, I got
sicker and sicker: my hands and feet swelled, I developed fevers, mouth
sores and shortness of breath—a hypersensitivity reaction to Taxol. I
hired people to be with me and take care of me.

One aspect of human resiliency in the face of difficult symptoms is the capacity to forget. When PJ Hagler was worried about having to endure the potential side effects of yet another treatment, Kathy Stone reminded her:

You know how it goes, while we are going through it, it seems so
unreal and terrible and then when it's over, it's a lot like pregnancy and
labor, you can't really remember all the details.

Still, one of the most difficult aspects of dealing with metastatic disease can be coping with the unrelenting side effects and medicalization of near constant treatments, tests and doctor's appointments. Even the presence of medical supplies can be upsetting. In the days following her HDC, Jacque Fisher lamented to the breast-cancer list,

I HATE TURNING MY HOUSE INTO A HOSPITAL!!!!! Getting all
of this stuff just makes me feel sicker! Does it effect anyone else this way?

Laurie Feldman, another metastatic patient who underwent high-dose chemotherapy, commiserated:

I had all those same things around before and after my stem-cell
transplant, then six months later had to have a total hip replacement and
added a high toilet seat, wheelchair, walker, crutches, lots of other
"invalid" supplies. Having two small children at home as well, it was a
toss up whether our house was more like an old folks home or a pre-
school—and sometimes like both at the same time. I'm sure my husband
thought we went from newlyweds to senior citizens in record time. I was
only 34 at the time.

And Sue Tokuyama recalled her own feelings as she recovered from her HDC:

My linen closet was turned into a pharmacy, and the first thing I did
when the ABMT and all was over was pile everything into a couple plas-
tic bags and give it to my oncologist for people who couldn't pay. Then I
put expensive, superfluous, fragrant soap where the stuff used to be. I

*can...almost...forget what it was like. The other thing was the Neupogen
in the fridge, and the Compazine suppositories. How about the big red
garbage bag with BIOHAZARD INFECTIOUS WASTE on the outside
that I had to leave on the porch for the home nursing service to pick up?*

For some women who elect HDC, the possibility of being able to avoid ongoing treatments for a year or two, or even some months, seems worth going through the much more intense short-term distress of this treatment, and the several months recovery. For them, a single treatment, even one that causes a severe "interruption" of normal life, seems easier to bear psychologically than the chronic treatments of chronic disease that signify "intrusion" or even "immersion" in illness, to use sociologist Kathy Charmaz' formulation of life disruption. For the majority of HDC patients, sadly, this goal does not turn out to be attainable, and treatments will eventually resume. To a greater or lesser extent, most people with metastatic breast cancer face ongoing treatments as their best strategy for keeping cancer at bay.

Many report that it is not so much the day-to-day trials, but the cumulative effects, the loss of normal functioning and the dependency on others that proves to be so difficult. And it is not so much the physical symptoms, as the emotional impact of the physical symptoms, as they drag on for day after day and week after week. Here is what Bob Crisp felt in retrospect about his wife Ginger's treatment following her relapse after HDC:

*We are approaching the one-year mark since recurrence. Treatment
of one type or the other has been near continuous for this year. While she
has tolerated the treatments well, the cumulative effects have taken a toll.
We are both emotionally exhausted from this year of treatments. Not
ready to give up, but certainly tired.*

*Long-term, continuous treatment is physically and emotionally very
difficult. I once used the analogy of someone giving you a 20 pound ball
that you had to drag around wherever you go. At first, no problem, you
yank that ball and go full speed ahead. After a while, you don't do as
much as the ball gets heavier and you get tired. At some point, you quit
and just stay with the ball.*

When Kathy Stone's oncologist discovered that the continuous infusion pump didn't seem to be working, he decided to give her a brief treatment holiday. Kathy was jubilant, and immediately planned a trip with her husband.

He took me off the 5-FU and off all chemo...in fact I don't have to go in and see him for three weeks. I can hardly believe it. It is only the second time in almost two years I have been off of chemo or radiation treatments for that long a period, and I have never in all that time gone three weeks without having to have some type of a doctor's appointment or blood draw.

I plan on having the time of my life in Hawaii...even if it is just to sit on the beach. I just love each new day and find they go far too fast anymore...maybe that's why I don't go to bed at night sometimes...too much to do...to feel...to live and time just keeps clicking away. Don't get me wrong, I don't feel pressured or panicked or "hurried"...just feel like there is SO much to enjoy and do and feel and I WANT IT ALL....

When I return I will be ready to "do" whatever it is I need to do for the next "phase"...anything other than stop chemo.... I'm not ready for that yet.... I still have visions of knocking the hell out of this stuff. I just have to find the right cocktail to do it...my job is to stay sick long enough for a cure to take place...so I'm going to stay sick and keep kicking...and stay on the go as much as possible so the Grim Reaper will get tired of trying to catch up with me and give up.

Not everyone becomes disheartened or stays that way, of course. A lot depends on the success of the treatments. Nothing is more difficult emotionally than treatments endured for little or no benefit, which was the case with Ginger Crisp. Knowing that the treatments she was given significantly prolonged her life, Caren Buffum felt positive about her treatments. Despite rigorous and continuous treatments for over five years, she made the observation:

I have been fortunate that I have not experienced the degree of side effects that some have. But I can't say how my experience compares with others in the same sense that we can rarely say one individual is experiencing more pain than another. We all have different thresholds and different capacities to deal with pain and discomfort—how much is objective and how much is in the mind? So I think I have had to cope with less to begin with, but I think I have had a lot to help me cope too, and I'm not sure where the line is.

To some extent, this also has to do with temperament. Barb Pender's attitude toward all of her treatment has been one of acceptance, and making the best of the situation. It was no different during a rigorous treatment that involved not one, but two HDC's.

> I didn't want to be a hero—I just wanted to get through the situation. I didn't have a problem taking the prescribed medicines for nausea. I didn't have mouth sores during either transplant. I also don't have a problem with just resting—like I said I didn't set out to be a hero. There were times when I would wonder will I ever be the same—but my answer to myself was always "yes" and I would rest enough to build myself up. I also placed a lot of faith in Neupogen. I know my body responds well to it and it just needed some time to kick in. I think the infections and fevers became a part of the game. I have allowed myself the privilege of allowing my body to recoup. I came to the realization that for me, I was not going to fight my body but rather work with it to heal. At the first sign of an infection, I call the doctor. At the first sign of a fever, I'm on the phone. It has helped me to work with and not against my body or rather the cancer. My periods of isolation for the two transplants were not bad. The 21 and 23 days went rather quickly. I became the talk show guru for the nurses during the day and had many soul-searching conversations with the night nurses. It wasn't bad. I used the time to reflect on my life, choices, paths—I cannot complain about the isolation or the experience for that fact.

Like Barb Pender, Ellen Scheiner lived alone and had to take charge of her own care:

> During the last hospitalization my gums were bleeding and I did not dare to ask my platelet count. When I returned from the hospital I could not walk around my apartment. What kept me going? Fierce determination, a lifetime of professional discipline and the ability to let go into the treatment, realizing that it was the treatment that was making me ill, not the cancer. I knew that this protocol, though horrendous, arduous and experimental, was my only chance for survival, and I wanted to live.

> It's not that I sat and said, "I want to live." But something carried me along—I call it life force and one doesn't have to will it, it wills itself.

I asked those whom I interviewed to share the ways they had coped with various side effects, the nausea, loss of appetite, peripheral neuropathy (loss of nerve sensation or pain in hands and feet, a side effect of Taxol), fatigue and a host of other symptoms, some annoying, some debilitating, some dangerous. As I indicated at the start of this chapter, few of their replies included specific coping strategies. So many had written at length about their emotional state in the face of these troublesome symptoms, that it has seemed a better choice to focus here on the process of adaptation and acceptance as the crucial issue. Appendix B, *Resources*, contains suggestions for readings on specific helpful coping strategies.

Lucie Bergmann-Shuster has given a great deal of thought to how she can preserve her own strength and optimism during difficult times of treatment:

> *While I actually agree that biologically some of us are endowed with more or less happiness capacity, I still maintain that our life experiences and coping strategies can significantly alter the quality of life we enjoy or lack. Simply stated it comes down to the old "glass half full/glass half empty" concept. Personally, I have had some horrid experiences and have had to deal with depression and anxiety in occasionally crippling forms. But I have made it my private goal to latch onto the good and the glorious potentials in whatever yucky situation I might find myself.*
>
> *A few months ago, I found myself in the "3M" stage—morose, moronic and meltdown—while doing chemo and recovering from abdominal surgery to remove my cancer. My three-week chemo cycles would be as follows. Week of chemo, meltdown, a human vegetable with zippo life force who couldn't care less if they were to have carted me off in a casket while still breathing and set me up for burial. Week 2, moronic, celebrating such events as having a bowel movement and standing up or walking about for more than an hour at a time. Week 3, rebound and happy to be alive again, forgetting totally what I had been like the 2 weeks preceding.*
>
> *Now I know that I am one of those overly endowed happy people else I would not have found myself bouncing back so well. At the same time, when I am in the pits, I do use several life strategies to help me distance myself from the morose or morbid aspects of my disease and treatment. I avoid all negative input, be it food, media or social contacts. When I am severely wiped out and vegetative, I request that I be left alone and ask to have zero stimuli except for the medications I need and the fluid/nutri-*

ents that I can put down. I tolerate those, but just barely. This gives me sufficient recovery time and allows me to conserve what little life energy I have. When I am ready for stimuli again, I make sure those are positive ones. To me this is just a simple strategy to manage my physical and mental resources. However, this coping strategy was not something that has come my way since cancer came into my life. The strategy has evolved over years of living and practicing it in less intense and threatening situations.

Caren Buffum also reported being able to manage her responses to the side effects of treatment somewhat through the compelling distractions that her life provided:

I love my work (teaching) and I have been able to express myself creatively through music and writing. Even through tiring chemo cycles, I have worked and created and continued to do a great deal—I fill my days with so much activity, I don't have time to feel ill. Well, of course, that isn't entirely true—being fatigued or queasy or in pain have not been in my control. But I cope well because I am so often distracted from my physical condition.

Attitude toward treatment can make a big difference in how you feel. With primary breast cancer, where surgery, radiation and chemotherapy are used to remove the primary tumor and prevent further recurrence, the treatment often causes more distress, both physical and psychological, at least initially, than the disease itself. The cancer itself, while terrifying, seems far away, not actual and immediate. With metastatic disease, it is a different matter. There is usually a measurable tumor that does or does not respond to treatment. There may be pain from the tumor itself, especially from metastases to bone, and the treatment, rather than conferring pain, may actually relieve it. If the treatment is successful, there is a measurable decrease in the disease, as shown in scans and tumor markers. Psychologically, this often leads to a real difference in attitude. However arduous, the treatment becomes associated with hope, and from that hope flows the strength to endure the treatments.

During the time I was gathering material for this chapter, Joleene Kolenburg was experiencing unusually severe side effects from the course of Taxol treatments she was undergoing. In response to a question on Taxol, she wrote:

I hesitate to go into all the problems I have had. I would not want to scare anyone into not having a treatment that will help them. As long as it works, I'll do it. But the fatigue is unbelievable. I literally did not do a thing for fifteen weeks. I could not read, watch TV, do crosswords. I mostly slept. I could not eat, food tasted blah. And the neuropathy, which does not affect every one, just completely disabled me. I have not shopped for groceries for five months, because I cannot walk. I have been unable to drive because I can't judge what the bottom of my feet are doing.

I don't like to keep mentioning my age, but I am three years older than I was when I had Adriamycin, and the body does seem to wear down at 66, even though I am what the doctors say "in very good health." But for the record, I had it all, the low blood counts, low hemoglobin, both requiring transfusions, the racing heart beat (monitored for forty-eight hours and put on lanoxin and Rhythmol) the buckling knees, dizziness.... But as I said, the tumors shrunk, so I would do it again.

Some months later, in remission for the time being and once again able to walk and drive, Joleene had obviously found ways to accommodate the persistent side effects.

I feel great.... I feel like I could run the marathon, but my feet and hands won't work. The peripheral neuropathy is still there. I walk kinda flat footed and use a cane. Sometimes I lose my balance. I can't turn pages, button a button, unscrew a jar, open a Coke (that's terrible, but I have one of those little do-jiggers that pulls the tab back) and oh so many other things. But I do lunch real well (can drive now) so I meet people everywhere, Pizza Hut, Wendy's, specialty restaurants in town. I am becoming known as the lunch girl. "If you want to go to lunch, call Joleene."

Hospitalization

Most people with metastatic breast cancer will face several hospital stays, to deal with the effects of treatment or with the symptoms of the disease itself. A hospital is a unique environment, nurturing and frightening by turns, a dangerous place and a place of refuge. It is often a setting where patients easily feel intimidated, as Scott Kitterman observes:

The problem is that when you are the one that is sick, there are a lot of psychological pressures to shut up and believe what they tell you. This is why we have a policy in my family of not leaving anyone alone in the hospital during the day when they are most likely to be mucking about with you. If the individual is really sick, then we go 24 hours. Adult or child, makes no difference. If you're really sick, you need someone there sticking up for you.

Pat Leach, as a nurse, describes the insights she has from both a patient and a health care professional's perspective.

I've been in the hospital three times in the last two years. I brought along loads of photos, CD's (I love 50's rock and roll, and I jitterbug and twist in my room), I walk the halls if possible, read lots of good books. My daughter has stayed with me all night and my husband is with me as much as possible. I talk a lot with staff, question everything but tell them why I am questioning. I try to get to know them by expressing an interest in their life and I've been lucky in that my hospitalizations have gone smoothly—I've had no real complaints—being a nurse I know how busy a unit can get. I also know they're all human and can make mistakes so I try to discreetly stay alert to what's being done, given to me, etc. I've tried to talk to my family and educate them to be on the alert, to question and to please advocate for me if I am unable to do so myself. It's scary, what could happen—what did happen at Dana Farber (a medication error where two patients were given four times their HDC dosages). Staying as well educated as possible about treatment can only help.

Kim Banks echoes her thoughts:

While in the hospital, I feel comfortable with acting as my own advocate and am more assertive in that environment than I am in everyday life. Although I'm assertive about asking for things when I need them and asking questions about what I'm being given, I do treat the staff with respect and thank them for their care. I also try to be understanding when they are busy. I know that many hospitals are cutting costs by cutting back on nursing staff and that they are all taking on more tasks. As in most situations, I've found using honey gets quicker results than vinegar.

Many women find ways to resist the depersonalization of hospital life. PJ Hagler, a veteran of many hospital stays, felt easier knowing her oncologist was willing to go to bat for her if need be:

When I went to the hospital in the beginning of all this the only thing I would bring was my personal toiletries and pj's. I have been in and out so many times over the last six years that I now take my pillow, quilt, my mascot (a stuffed giraffe), tapes, tape player, etc. I find that if it is going to be a long stay these things help a lot. I'm always in the middle of a book so that always goes. All this helped me to be able to tolerate my stay better. I get homesick and unless I'm in isolation I get visitors and that helps unless I'm very ill. When I was in isolation for low white cells and an infection, I had an awful time and the only one allowed to see me was Mike.

I was in a room once where the nurses were awful—they didn't give me pain meds when I was supposed to have them. My oncologist is the head of oncology and a board member and trustee at the hospital, so within one day I was on the other floor. He's always made arrangements for a private room on the second floor where the nurses are who he knows will take care of his patients the best. We live very close to the hospital and Mike works only two miles from the hospital so I insist he gets some sleep at home and I also want him to work to keep his mind busy, especially the last time when I was getting so many tests. Otherwise, he would have to just sit and wait for me to have x-rays and whatever for days at a time.

Jenilu Schoolman brought a small part of her work as a weaver into the hospital:

Even in a medical crisis, it is important to me that I retain my sense of identity. One thing I do to insure this is to put on regular clothes in the hospital and wear pajamas only at night. My little spinning wheel comes as well. Besides being a novel conversation piece, anxious hours move more quickly to the rhythm of the wheel.

During her lengthy transplant stay, Barb Pender found comfort in reminders of life outside:

My transplant stays were very special to me. I took many pictures of my children and grandchildren, precious reminders of why I was there. I took my computer, my CD player with my favorite go-to-bed music. I also took books I didn't read—no concentration—and I took some crafts to work on that are still unfinished in my closet! Before my second transplant I went to the river with my friends—they made a video of the wonderful weekend we had—I watched that over and over just to remind me of the life I had waiting on the outside of those walls. I didn't care for visitors during that time—I spent most of the time resting and recouping from the high-dose chemo and I didn't want to expend my energy entertaining guests—they didn't require entertaining but I felt as though I needed to be "up" and perky. UCSD hospital staff was the best.

Like many other women, Bonnie Gelbwasser was impressed at the quality of care she received during her lengthy stay for HDC:

My only long stay in the hospital was the 25 days I spent in the BMT unit. I never wore the nightshirts I brought because it was easier for the medical staff to access my catheters if I wore the johnny. I brought a computer but didn't have the concentration to do anything with it. I did bring books, puzzles, note cards and notes and photos from friends and family to put on the bulletin board in my room. I also brought a cassette player with me—that was the best thing because I could listen to music that calmed me.

I have always felt comfortable discussing my concerns with my doctors or nurses. There has been no need for an advocate. I have a strong voice and on the rare occasions when I feel I have not been well-served I have no problem articulating my views. My experience with hospital staff has been almost entirely positive. I think it's most important to be polite when you have a request or a complaint, and to be sure that what you are asking for is not unreasonable. I have found the medical professionals who worked with me to be dedicated to providing the best care they can to each patient. They try, within the limits of their knowledge, ability and time, to understand each patient's specific needs and personality and to adjust that care to take those needs and that personality into consideration.

Since Bonnie preferred not to have visitors, even family members, during the most difficult times, she devised an ingenious way that she could still feel their support:

I had cards made before my transplant. They were yellow postcards with a chicken coop on the front. The flip side said, "I'll be cooped up for a while having an autologous bone marrow transplant" and provided dates and my hospital address and encouraging people to call and write. They worked like a charm. People saw that my sense of humor was still intact and came through for me.

Like Bonnie, Jacque Fisher prepared for the loneliness she knew she would feel in a most creative way:

I took as much of home with me as possible. My favorite green and white-striped throw, pillow shams, stuffed animal to hug during the long nights, lots of tapes, a tape player, EASY crossword books (your brain goes on vacation), my own comfy pj's that buttoned up the front, sweats to roam the hall in. I had several knitted hats (like skull caps that my mom knit me). My bald head got VERY cold sometimes and the turbans, etc., were too lumpy. Since I wasn't able to take or have live flowers, I made an "angel" basket of pretend flowers. I made a template shaped like an angel about 3 to 4 inches and traced that shape onto all of the cards that I had received before entering the hospital. I then hot glued a pipe cleaner to the back of each and stuck them in a paper straw-covered oasis that had been arranged in a basket. Each evening and morning I would take an angel out and say a prayer and remember the sender of that particular card (I forgot to mention that I had written each sender's name on the back of her/his angel). Then I poked a hole in the opposite end from the glued pipe cleaner and made a chain of them to hang from the window in my room. This really helped me take my mind off myself...very important during this procedure.

JB Boggs, a former aerobics instructor and rock climber, managed to get around, with some difficulty, using a walker, and wore a morphine pump for her extensive bone metastases. In a writing workshop, JB reflected on a process that had become a part of her life in a prose-poem she entitled "My Hospital Bag":

The bag is there now packed with my comforts. The radio, the earphones. A book on tape. A paperback. My own lotion and toiletries. The bag is all ready to go if I am pulled into the hospital again. The contents have grown with experience. I have learned to take along my own special sleeping pillow. In the thirteen months just past I have been in the hospital nine different times, most stays at least a week, often longer. The bag is always ready.

Who knew it would become an easy routine to pack to go to the emergency room? How can it be a regular part of my life to rush to the hospital in response to some crisis or to thwart some developing problem? I see the bag on the floor of the closet, ready and waiting. Also, now it is full of paperwork. My duplicates of power of attorney. My will. My specific wishes about not allowing the "heroic" measures or anything to keep me here when it is time for me to go—to go where my traveling bag cannot. I'll leave it behind then.

I won't need the contents anymore. I will be light and free and traveling to a new place with no baggage, no tubes, no cane, no CADD pump, no pain. I do not fear the process or the journey.

Pain relief: On myths, undertreatment and persistence

In any discussion of pain relief, there is no better place to start than by dispelling a common and tragic misunderstanding. Despite what you may have heard, the effective relief of cancer pain does *not* create addiction. The misconception that a patient will become addicted to pain medication is what so often interferes with cancer patients getting the pain relief they need, whether that misconception is held by the doctor who underprescribes or by the patient who is afraid to ask, or both. Dr. Ronald Melzack, of McGill University, debunks this popular misconception.

Two widely held myths often prevent physicians from prescribing adequate doses of narcotic drugs to patients in severe pain, especially those not terminally ill: the belief that narcotics inevitably produce addiction, and the notion that repeated doses produce rapid tolerance so that escalating amounts of the drugs are needed. We now know that both of these concerns are based on observation of street addicts and do not apply to people in severe pain who do not have a history of substance abuse.[4]

Several large, persuasive studies, each involving more than 10,000 chronic-pain patients, including patients on burn units injected with opiates for months on end, have consistently revealed that only former drug abusers are likely to display addictive behavior. Despite prior fears, when post-surgical patients are given pumps to self-administer morphine, they utilize only reasonable amounts, and decrease the medication as their pain decreases.

It is the patient herself who can most accurately assess her own needs, as Lucie Bergmann-Shuster points out:

> The way I look at it, nobody knows my body as well as I do. My doctors know through training what the dose ranges are on average and how they may be stretched. I trust them to follow their guidelines on the chemotoxic agents, but I always make sure that I get the right meds and research each one in the same literature they use. In some ways it gives me a sense of personal control over this disease that is eating away at my life. I never mess with the chemo, but I do take charge of the palliative aspect of treatment, like pain or nausea meds, antihistamines, antacids, stool softeners and, of course, steroids.

Studies have also found that once an effective level has been found, while patients do develop a physical tolerance for opiates, they do not become psychologically addicted, as had been previously feared. Increased needs usually signify a change in physical status, Melzack says, and pain patients do not generally experience symptoms of withdrawal and are able to decrease and discontinue pain medications when and if they no longer need them. If there is an ongoing need, if pain medication is taken regularly, around the clock, no signs of addiction occur. Yet patients who experience even severe pain are widely undertreated for it. It is the confusion in minds of doctors and patients alike about the nature of addictive behavior that is in part to blame, Melzack believes:

> The patient uses drugs to relieve pain and maintain a normal relationship with the real world; the addict takes narcotics to escape from reality. Society's failure to distinguish between the emotionally impaired addict and the psychologically healthy pain sufferer affects every segment of the population.

But what of cancer pain, specifically? A widely read guide to pain control on the Oncolink website, available on the Internet, written by an interdisciplinary pain treatment team, confirms the important distinction of legitimate physical need from addiction:

> Addiction is a psychological or emotional dependence on feeling "high." People with cancer do not take drugs to get "high" but to relieve their pain. When the proper dosage of medication is taken around the clock, addiction does not occur. People with cancer can take pain medica-

tions indefinitely, if properly used, without concern that they will become addicted. People also worry that if they take their medications continuously, they will become "immune" to that dosage and need higher dosages until no dosage will work. There is no such thing as "running out" of pain medicine.[5]

If you're like most people with metastatic cancer, one of the things you fear most is being in intolerable pain. Along with loss of dignity and loss of control, this is the most common fear—and it is one that, if not addressed, can even lead some cancer patients into suicide. But studies show that almost all cancer pain, by most estimates 85 to 90 percent, can be effectively relieved, yielding a quality of life that is acceptable.

In a review article on pain relief in the medical journal *CA*, Doctors Nathan Cherny and Russell Portenoy state that overall, about two-thirds of patients with advanced cancer experience some pain with their disease. Because unrelieved pain can be incapacitating, impair day-to-day functioning, interfere with normal life and lead to heightened psychological distress, it is imperative that it be effectively addressed, the authors write. Yet, despite the existence of effective strategies for management of cancer pain, numerous surveys consistently show that 40 to 50 percent of patients in "routine practice settings" fail to get proper relief.[6] Physicians frequently do not believe patients' reports about their pain, fail to assess pain properly and have the most rudimentary understanding of up-to-date techniques. A large survey of over a thousand cancer specialists found that only 51 percent felt that their patients obtained adequate pain relief. Despite increasing efforts, comprehensive cancer centers still have a long way to go in allocating resources to palliative care and pain relief. Issues of emotional suffering from physical impairment and other psychosocial causes are often intertwined with physical pain, and require multidisciplinary, comprehensive treatment. The authors conclude:

> *The relief of pain must be emphasized as a cardinal goal of cancer therapy, and patients need reassurance that efforts to secure comfort will not be at the expense of efforts to control the underlying cancer. The individual practitioner can effectively treat most pain problems by attending to careful pain assessment and implementing analgesic therapy. Successful long-term management requires continuity of care that provides an appropriate level of monitoring and responds quickly, flexibly, and*

*expertly to the changing needs of the patient. Patients with pain or suffer-
ing related to other losses or distressing symptoms that persist despite the
best efforts of the treating oncologist should have access to specialists in
pain management, palliative medicine, and psychooncology, who can provide expert assistance in the management of these complex problems.*

Compounding the fact that some physicians may not yet be knowledgeable
about the constantly evolving science of pain relief, you yourself may have
been concerned about not becoming dependent upon or addicted to strong
drugs, or that you will need ever-increasing doses to be effective. You may
also feel a subtle pressure to be stoic and strong about your disease, to be a
"good patient." Pain is invisible, and not easily measurable. Like many subjective experiences, your pain may not be taken seriously enough by your
doctor. You may also be worried about being perceived as a complainer or as
weak, and so you may be hesitant to ask for the help that you need. This can
lead to needless suffering.

Physical pain is like a black hole: it absorbs energy and attention. If you are
living with pain now, you're already familiar with the way that pain can
diminish your world and limit your experience. It can prevent you from participating in activities you'd otherwise be part of. Because a person in pain is
often irritable and self-involved, relationships can suffer as well. All of these
problems are compelling reasons to seek help.

It can be of great help to address the suffering on a mental and behavioral
level as well as a pharmacological level. Stanford psychiatrist David Spiegel
writes that "Pain consists of both a physical signal and a mental message:
Something is wrong with my body and I cannot think of anything else."[7] He
finds that the experience of pain can be complicated by an inability to put it
in its place.

Self-hypnosis and other techniques that go a long way to help control pain
can be learned by anyone. These generally involve two activities: some form
of voluntary muscle relaxation and some process for directing or focusing
attention. "Absorption in work or play is a natural analgesic," Spiegel
explains, adding that most people who deal with chronic pain are already
aware that their pain decreases in certain situations, for example, when a
compelling other concern intervenes, or when they are distracted in some
other way. Conversely, when they focus on the pain, with little other distraction, the painful sensations often become more intense.

There are two simple lessons to learn with regard to controlling pain, Spiegel says: first, that muscle tension actually causes pain, and second, that you have to pay attention to pain for it to hurt. This is not to say that the pain is any less real, but only that there are strategies that you can learn to control its domination. Anxiety and depression are known pain-enhancers, and the meaning pain has for the individual, for example, that the cancer is progressing, plays a crucial role as well. The chapter on controlling pain in Spiegel's excellent book, *Living Beyond Limits*, offers a clear and helpful explanation of these techniques. Appendix B contains suggestions for some other sources for learning these techniques.

To get help with pain, you must first find ways to communicate how you are feeling. An important first step is to keep a diary or record of your pain, using as complete descriptive terms as you can, indicating where it hurts, the circumstances, the specific nature of the pain and its duration. This will help the doctor know how to help you. If your doctor can't or won't help, ask for a referral to a pain specialist. Pain specialists have had advanced training in this field, and should also be knowledgeable about non-pharmacological means of controlling pain. If your doctor won't refer you to one, call the Cancer Information Service (1-800-4-CANCER) for a referral in your area. Hospice staff are generally expert in pain relief as well, and are generally available for outpatient consultation to cancer patients even though they may not be in a terminal stage of their illness. Kim Banks wrote in some detail about the ways in which she sought relief from her pain.

> When I learned that my breast cancer had recurred two years after I was first diagnosed and treated, I was most frightened by the thought that I may die soon. I was willing to do anything that would prolong my life. A surgeon's knife cut away the new tumor and chemotherapy dripped into my veins. Several months later, a bone scan showed two new tumors on two vertebrae. How could the cancer grow so quickly when I was taking such strong chemotherapy? I switched to a different chemotherapy and alternated that with radiation. I took vitamins and shark cartilage, changed my diet and started meditation and visualization. Throughout this I endured a lot of pain, but I knew that it was only temporary. It was like the aches I endured after a long workout, a good pain that signaled a breakdown and rebuilding of a stronger, healthier body. I would constantly remind myself that the discomfort from chemotherapy was short-term and would help me to live long-term.

The chemotherapy didn't shrink the tumors as the doctors had hoped, but it did slow the cancer down. I've had only a very slight increase in the size of one of the tumors and no new tumors in a year and a half. But what I wasn't prepared for was the pain that started up months after the tumor in my lower back had been discovered. The tumor hadn't changed, so why was there such intense pain now? My doctor explained there was often no correlation between the growth of the tumor and the occurrence of pain. I soon learned that we have a long way to go in understanding chronic pain—what causes it and, more importantly, how to stop it. I no longer worried about dying; after all, I believed I would be going to a better place, a place without pain. I was now far more worried about living with chronic debilitating pain.

Radiation stopped the pain completely. I was ecstatic. But, the effects were short-lived; the pain returned two months later. Next I tried cortisone epidurals. The shots helped some initially, but the relief lessened after several shots. My doctor then started prescribing more powerful pain killers. I had a long history of migraine headaches and knew that all medicines that contained codeine or a synthetic version of codeine would trigger migraines. So, I tried hydromorphone (Dilaudid)and Duragesic patches, both narcotic drugs similar to morphine. These worked reasonably well for a number of months. But then, as I had to increase the dosage, I started to get migraines again.

I want to make it clear that most people will not have the difficulties in tolerating the pain killers like I have had and will get along fine with one or more of the many pain killers available. Also, doctors are now realizing that they've been under-medicating patients for pain and are changing their mindset about prescribing narcotics. They used to worry about addiction, but studies have shown that the risk is very small. They realized that there's a much greater risk of patients giving up on life if they are in constant pain.

I'm sharing this because I want others in pain to know that there are other ways of dealing with chronic pain. I use a TENS unit for sharp pain that works by emitting small electrical charges from electrodes placed around the painful area. The electrical charges send a sensation that competes with the pain sensation, which reduces the pain I feel while I have it on.

Swimming seems to help loosen the muscles and produces endorphins that lessen the pain for several hours after leaving the pool. I'm excited about an aqua-exercise class that I'm to start next week at a local therapy pool where the water temp is kept at a balmy 90 degrees.

This week I've called to make appointments with a therapist to learn self-hypnosis. Many patients have had very good luck in reducing their pain through hypnosis. My pain lessens when I'm relaxed, so I hope that I can take it a step further with the hypnosis. I've also set up an appointment with an orthopedic surgeon to review my MRI's and x-rays to see if surgery would help. My oncologist says that he doesn't recommend surgery for pain alone, but I've learned to get second opinions. My oncologist may not be aware of a new surgical procedure that could work for me.

I've also found that when I get depressed, the pain worsens. Antidepressants not only help me deal with the pain, they actually seem to reduce the pain. I read later that this has been proven in studies as well. Researchers think the anti-depressants may cause an increased production of endorphins, those natural pain killers our bodies produce.

Lastly, I researched the drug Aredia, which was recently given the OK by the FDA to treat bone mets. The preliminary studies show that the drug helps some patients with pain and may lessen bone loss in metastatic areas, with very few side effects. It's the best news I've heard in a long time. The point I want to make is that there are a number of ways to deal with pain and there are new treatments being developed all the time. You may not find a miracle drug that completely eliminates the pain, but you may develop a combination of treatments that allows you to live a more normal life and makes you feel you are more in control of your life.

Because of the location of her tumor, its resistance to chemotherapy and her allergies to opiates, Kim's situation has been unusually difficult. And yet with persistent effort, she has been able to get the help she needs.

Nancy Gilpatrick, suffering bone pain from metastases and fractures in her pelvis, reports on her experience:

What I've learned from my doctors is that with a good combination for pain relief you should be able to have little to no drowsiness. My goal was and is to not be drowsy on pain meds. I think this has kept them from recommending anything any higher on the scale. If the drowsiness remains, you may actually be on too high a dose. They said when you get the pain relief of the meds, then you would feel little or no side effects such as drowsiness and being drugged out. I am rarely drowsy from the meds. I am still struggling to get a good amount. The oncologist today said to try changing the dose upwards every 3 to 4 days until I get relief (I'm to call the office to let them know I am increasing a dose). I've tried to be a "good girl" and not bother them too much, thus I've suffered with too much pain.

Scott Kitterman, whose wife, Mary, suffered with one of the most painful of all cancers, a metastatic spread of breast cancer to the central nervous system, known as carcinomatous meningitis, was able to secure good pain control for her. He wanted to pass along what he has learned in the process of caring for his wife after she came home in hospice care:

Don't be shy about raising the doses. For the last four or five days, when Mary was at home, we ended up increasing her morphine dose roughly 50 percent per day. Over time, people will develop a tolerance to opiates like morphine. You can keep going on the dose, so if you need it for pain control, don't be shy. Use it.

There's no reason to be in pain. And if the doctors you are dealing with are not managing your pain, you need to be persistent about that, and not accept it. All major hospitals have a pain management service. So don't get to some point where you feel, "this is just pain I have to live with." That is not generally the case.

For Pam Hiebert, coping with chronic pain that preceded her diagnosis with metastatic disease, the real help didn't come from conventional Western medicine:

My experience with pain started very early on, even before my diagnosis. I was in the emergency room weeks before my cancer diagnosis because I was in such excruciating pain with my lower back. It was a sudden attack of rippling muscles up and down my lower back that put me flat in bed for five days. The emergency room doc did little more than give me a prescription for pain medication. A follow-up visit with my osteopathic doctor offered more help. I was puzzled when the doctor told me that the E.R. doc had not written a high enough dosage for pain meds— seems it's an emergency room trick for some people to try to get more drugs—I frankly had never considered this fact and had trusted the doctor to provide what I needed to get better.

I've had to do a lot of growing since then and it's not a pretty sight when it comes to pain. This is the worst area of my treatment where I feel I have gotten inadequate support. I am, in fact, not able to break the code of communication needed to find adequate care. I have chronic and recurrent pain that I wish I had better techniques in coping with. Time has been my greatest healer. My doctors have failed miserably in this dimension. They have failed to communicate an acceptable method of treatment and I have failed to be persuaded that pharmacological treatment affords the quality of life I need.

My pain is primarily neurological or musculoskeletal. I have experienced ongoing pain for the last three and a half years and have found a few things I would like to share: In my search for ways to communicate the pain I was experiencing, I found a Guideline For Pain rating chart, numbered from 0 to 10 and designed to distinguish all the way from no pain to moderate to distressing and intense and finally immobilizing pain. I developed a journal that used this verbiage along with a graphical segmented illustration of the human body (front and back) and mapped out different areas of my body giving each area a number that would indicate the location of my pain. Combining these two elements, pain rating and location, gave me a method to track and scale what I was experiencing.

I further developed a daily diary that was formatted to reflect diet, medications and supplements, exercise, sleep, stress and doctor activity. I tracked this information for one month and then showed this to each of my doctors. This action alone did, in fact, get me to a point where change happened.

At the advice of one doctor I quit exercise to give the large muscles a chance to relax. During this time I came to realize that this pain was chronic and that I really wanted to get on with the life I had to live, and actually told the doctors that I understood now, they could not help. I would accept where I was and live with it. It is fascinating to me that the veil lifted with this recognition (this coming over) and soon after that I found something that worked for me and added greatly to the quality of my life.

I found a form of exercise that practiced gentle stretching and length-ening of the torso (Pilates) and I began to get better. My chiropractor said it was my persistence and my willingness to work at finding a solution that was the key. I saw how my final willingness to let go precipitated the change.

I believe pain is a mind thing and different states of intensity of the same pain can be felt at any one time, depending on the holistic state of the person. Maybe this is where mind-body rests. I have much to learn about this area and am searching for ways to understand and use these principles. Motivation is not a problem. I'm plenty motivated—it's just that I tie myself in knots at times when help from professional caregivers could guide me through so much faster.

Pam's partner, Sylvan, comments on the sobering meaning that physical pain has taken on for both of them since Pam's recurrence.

One thing different about pain now than before diagnosis is that now we always wonder if the pain means recurrence. It has to be taken seri-ously and monitored. Pam has done a lot of work trying to figure out how to work with pain in responsible ways, and has finally resigned herself to the fact that she will always experience some pain. We found some forms of exercise that she can do, and these help her a great deal.

Before a recent course of Navelbine reduced his pain, Bob Stafford was beginning to feel desperate and incapacitated by the pain he was feeling. Still, he also expressed the ambivalence about the pain medications he was forced to take:

I've come to realize that pain consumes your thoughts when it reaches a certain threshold. When great enough, all you want to do is alleviate your pain. I guess I understand some people going to Dr. Kevorkian because of pain. Nothing else matters except getting rid of the pain. My recent battle confirmed that. First it was extreme bone pain and then pain in the kidney area. No great spiritual thoughts, no thoughts about others, no thoughts about family or friends...just get rid of that pain. The unfortunate part is that there are several of the myriad of peo-ple in the medical community who don't take pain relief seriously. Some are still afraid that we'll get addicted to pain medications. But, as a hos-pice nurse told me, there is a difference between want and need. My body, because of its condition, needs pain medication. I really don't want them.

Living the patient role: "I just hate to ask"

Going through an extended period of physical pain, malaise, fatigue or outright disability that interferes with normal day-to-day functioning takes an emotional toll as well as a physical one. As a result of treatment side effects, or disease progression, you may no longer be able to work, at least temporarily, or find that your other everyday roles are compromised. Maybe you aren't able cook or shop for your family, or chauffeur your children to their lessons or games. Maybe you have difficulty with walking or just getting around. Maybe you worry about how your husband will cope with a lengthy period of caring for you if your illness progresses. Other people must take over doing accustomed tasks, and it's hard for you not to feel badly about burdening them. For an independent woman who has always taken care of others, it can be extremely stressful to become dependent upon others, to feel a loss of control over activities you've always taken for granted. However much the people in your life understand and accommodate themselves to your needs, all these changes represent a blow to your self-esteem. It can be particularly hard to ask for the help you need.

When Kathy Stone was told she'd need three weeks of radiation for a tumor that had appeared in her chest wall, she spoke of her difficulty asking for and accepting help. "I am very fortunate," she said, "that I do have a lot of friends who still do care and offer help and I know it won't be a problem getting my ride schedule filled.... I just hate to ask."

Laurie Feldman responded:

> I feel the same way. My friends keep telling me that doing something for me makes them feel that they are not completely helpless in the battle against this disease. It makes them feel that they are doing something that will really help. I know how hard it is to ask for more help when you have done it so many times before and you probably feel like I do, that there is no way you will ever be able to pay back these wonderful caring friends for all that they have done for you...but just let them help. I know from my experience with my sister and my dear friend who succumbed to this beast, that I cherished the memory of the times when I was "allowed" to do some small thing to help them, even if it was a ride to the hospital, a meal for their family, some fragrant smelling body lotion as a hospital present that they loved, whatever.

Remembering her own problems with neuropathy, Joleene Kolenburg commiserated with Kathy as well:

> I am so glad that you have friends there that can drive you. It was hard for me to ask my friends to drive me, too. (I could not drive because of my feet). If I ever have the opportunity to help someone, I am going to be the transportation chairman and line up drivers for chemo. People are so willing, but it is so hard for the patient to ask.

Kim Banks felt the same way about having to ask:

> I've always been a very independent person. Recently I've had to rely upon friends and family to take me to appointments, which really isn't that big a deal, but I hate it all the same. I'll put off asking, and when I do, I apologize repeatedly for being such an inconvenience. Actually, I've learned that it's at least **something** they can do for me, and probably makes them feel better. I still hate it!

Loss of function, however, bothered her still more, though Kim still felt hopeful that one day she could become active again:

> I've also been a very active person and was diagnosed with cancer at the age of 32, when I felt like I was in my prime. My husband and I had just moved to Colorado to hike, bike, ski and generally enjoy all that the mountains had to offer when I was first diagnosed. In the past 10 months I've had to dramatically limit my activities because of my back. I cried last week when I looked through our photo album—was that me powering up the side of a hill on my mountain bike? It made me feel even more like an invalid. We went home for Memorial Day and I just couldn't play the crazy games with my nieces and nephews like I used to. I so wanted to scoop up little Nathan in my arms, but knew my back wouldn't take it. I'm used to being in the center of things and now must stand at the sidelines. Guess I'm going to have to learn to be a better cheerleader, but I haven't given up the idea of being on team again!

Nancy Gilpatrick, whose pelvis had fractured soon after her diagnosis with Stage IV breast cancer, shared Kim's concerns:

> I have been physically disabled by the cancer. I started first with a cane, then graduated to a walker. I use a wheelchair if I'm going out for what would be a long walk or a crowd of people or I would have to stand

for a long time or my boyfriend thinks it would really be easiest for me. The doctors never recommended any of these except the wheelchair when my hip fractured; however, they've all supported the equipment when I showed up with it.

I do know other women with bc and mets and I'm in a bc support group. I continue to be the only one who is disabled and feel really alone and like I stand out everywhere I go. It is one of my frustrations in that I am never able to get away from the cancer. I use humor and jokes, make up names, etc., to deal with it.

PJ Hagler also mourned the loss of normalcy:

I miss getting to walk like I used to. Mike and I used to go for long walks and this is tough for me now. On Taxol, I have an awful time getting up in the morning with my sore legs and swollen hands. I soak my hands to help the swelling. I can't exert much energy in doing much. My job is working at a computer most of the time and general secretarial duties. I don't walk around much in my job. I'm learning to cope with my limits. However, I still wish I could get some of the energy back that has been taken from me. I even get resentful when I see everyone else doing or going wherever they want without a second thought. I have to know if there is a long walk required or are there stairs to climb, etc. I miss not having the energy level I used to. I hate being so tired so early in the evening or even needing a nap. I'm now just 46 a few weeks ago and I mentally am still young, but physically I'm getting old.

Ellen Scheiner, who had lived with disability her whole life, found that in some ways, breast cancer helped her to deal with her feelings about being disabled.

There was another unexpected fallout from my cancer experience. I had never made peace with my paralyzed right arm. I still felt like a victim because scoliosis had forced me to give up my work as a physician. I felt sad, depressed, angry, and pushed away many opportunities and people, out of rage. I was forced to work half time, give up running, could not stand for more than 10 minutes and was limited in traveling and in many other usual activities. I had learned new skills and pleasures that were within my abilities, but I still felt bitter. Knowing that many other people suffered (my support group helped here), forced me to put my life in perspective. I finally saw that I had had a full and productive life despite my prior disabilities. In a sense, breast cancer and mastectomy were less limiting than my previous, chronic orthopedic problems. On the other hand, they were not life-threatening. Somehow the realization of the uncertainty of "all that is" has crystallized something in me. I found a new way of seeing that enabled me to realize the richness of what is now and to give up victimhood.

For many other women dealing with metastatic disease or at high risk for recurrence, it was the more subtle issues of control and dependency that plagued them. Bonnie Gelbwasser described her own emotional responses going through HDC treatment and recovery:

The possibility of being dependent on others was the worst part of learning I had breast cancer. I am a control freak who is very independent and not one to be particularly demonstrative—or to enjoy being hugged by strangers. With the help of my therapist and the example of my caregivers and friends, I have learned to loosen up a bit. Seems like everyone wants to embrace a cancer patient. People would envelop me in their arms to comfort me (or perhaps to see if I would break!). I learned to accept it, even to welcome it, as just a warm gesture from someone who cared—and to be soothed by the expression of their caring. I now find it easier to hug other people. Strange world, isn't it?

The people involved in my care at the hospital accepted my need to maintain my independence. They quickly learned that I would always take my medicine and show up for appointments and would not do anything to compromise my care, but they also learned that I knew who I was and what I needed to keep up the illusion of living a normal life, so they gave me leeway whenever possible (one example: they let me drive to my chemo after the third session because I convinced them that I felt strong enough to get there and home without my husband). For my part, I have worked very hard at accepting the intrusions and the restrictions that come with being a cancer patient.

Jenilu Schoolman found it difficult to deal with her loss of control regarding the farm she helped run:

During this time, I think I had the most difficulty with the issue of control and how to give it up. When I was still very ill, I could not do much for myself, let alone carry my weight with chores. I had to give up complete control then, but now that I was better, I wanted to take control again.

Late that first summer one of my partners told me with much pride that she had ordered the hay for the animals' winter feeding. When chores are shared, a division of labor evolves and ordering the hay was one task I had always done. She was pleased with herself and expected me to be comforted by the knowledge that she could take over. But I felt horrible. "I'm still alive," I cried. "Why didn't you talk it over with me?"

Many people found that their relationships with family members were altered, sometimes in unexpected ways. Sue Tokuyama felt a new connection with her mother, who nursed her through her recovery from HDC:

I am a very independent person, oldest of four girls, always carrying the weight of the world on my shoulders. In fact, one of my favorite bits of T-shirt wisdom (since diagnosis) is, "For peace of mind, resign as master of the universe." I am trying to resign.

My mother once told me that I was a "bottomless pit of need," and this was pre-BC. After my diagnosis, for the first time in my life, I was her first priority, and I will never forget how much she's helped me, and been there for me in the last year and a half. But now, when I am not hurting, and the beast seems further away, she is also further away. And I have to fight to not feel hurt when she tells me that she wants me to delay the reconstruction until July, because she's going to Europe. The unreasonable child in me says, "I am the most important thing, and I didn't give you permission to go to Europe!" The grownup in me says, "this woman is entitled to her own life, ENJOY the relationship you have with her."

Mary D'Angelo, the oldest daughter in her family as well, also cherished her mother's caretaking and attention as she went through her induction chemotherapy, and felt it softening old feelings of resentment for the disruption and loss of mothering caused by a younger brother's severe disability. She also reported feeling touched by the feisty way her elder daughter took care of her after surgery in the hospital:

Danielle got in an argument with the nurse. I remember hearing this, because I kept drifting in and out. They were giving me injections. I was feeling so happy that Danielle was there, because I knew I was safe. But I could not believe her tenacity. She just dared them to try to remove her. I remember her saying, "I work in public relations, and I'll have your name on the front page! Get a nurse if you want me to leave!" I was just in awe. I had thought of her like a child, so that was a very important experience for me to realize the bond that we had, that she was there. I'll never forget that. Then, by the next morning I was fine, I had makeup on and the fear was gone. It was such a strong bonding experience between us.

Pam Hiebert also experienced a similar reversal with her daughter, Amber, who helped her mother through a financial crisis of her illness:

Amber and I have always had a special bond. I have grown in wisdom at her side as she rises to her authentic self. She has been my great teacher and I have mirrored my older years for her. I began to see her in different eyes when I became ill with the disease, for she took the role of an adult when I could not walk without help. She came and offered her strengths—unselfish, young in energy and as steadfast as I could ever have imagined.

The cradle was reversed and she worked long hard hours to help me get through the financial crisis that was before me. On her first visit, she sat with me in council and offered her resources to me. I felt such pride in her willing commitment to deal with a frightening situation head on. She shared her wisdom and we plotted the course together. It was such a noble gesture. It was such an act of compassion and love. She comforted me and the money that she sent became my safe haven. She never wavered from her commitment, but continued to send money each month until I was able to work more hours and again grasp hold of the yoke.

Lucie Bergmann-Shuster, who had cared for her mother at home during her dying process, offered the other perspective on the reversal of parenting roles:

My mother felt very badly that she was such a burden to me. I had to constantly assure her that I was okay and that I, too, was getting massage treatments to make me feel better. Then when the hospice volunteers came to stay with her, I would tell her that this is my time to get away and to please allow them into her room. She didn't necessarily like all of the volunteers that came but we worked around that.

I think some of us feel pained to be so burdensome when we, as women, in particular feel the calling to be nurturing. Likewise, I think that some of the men on this list with breast cancer feel compromised to be demanding of their supports in times of need. At best it is very awkward and quite uncomfortable to be so compromised.

Like others, PJ Hagler has found a way to graciously accept the help offered to her, and explains how this understanding came to her:

Years ago I was helping care for girls in a group home and we had a psychologist who was there for the staff. I tried to do it all myself and not rely on anyone else to help me. I was taught a powerful lesson. This observant man said, "You know how much you like to help others, well there are others like you out there who want to help and you are doing them a favor by asking and then letting them help where they can." There are people out there who have talents that they want to use and we need to let people use those talents. I still have a hard time but it's mainly because I want to be able to do these things. I now let a friend take me to chemo treatments, and when I came home from the hospital, people from church brought meals for a week, and at work another secretary does all the copying, which is down at the other end of the hall. I appreciate and thank people now for their assistance. But I still wish I could have my life back and do for myself.

Mary D'Angelo articulated what many women with metastatic breast cancer feel about what lies ahead, as she discussed her fears about becoming a burden to her husband and children:

If I would have a long, lingering end, I'm concerned that I would disturb all their lives. This is ridiculous, I know. But I worried that they would have to be taking days off from work, and that I would cause them a lot of pain. So if I feel sad about anything, that's what I feel sad about. And that's silly, too, because that may not happen at all. I know they won't feel that way. I know they'll all rally together.

CHAPTER 9

Families and Friends Speak

"It's happening to us, too."

IF DEALING WITH METASTATIC BREAST CANCER takes patients on a roller coaster ride, this ride is no less difficult for those who love them. This chapter will focus first on the experiences of spouses and partners, then on children, extended family and friends. It will examine the emotional highs and lows, the typical conflicts that arise about needs and priorities within the family, issues of caregiving and changes in family roles, and problems with sex and intimacy, communication and closeness. It will detail the stigma of cancer and the awkwardness often felt by friends and associates, as well as the extraordinary caring and generosity that sometimes graces the lives of cancer patients.

Most of the people I interviewed for this book were currently married or in committed relationships. If you are not, please consider that most of the issues between couples—the stress of the cycles of the disease, the need for clear communication, the difficulties of asking for help and the possible deepening of relationships—also come up with family, friends and other caregivers. Being single does not have to mean being alone. Single people are often able to develop their own rich network of significant others, who are able to respond with great caring and concern when the need arises.

As you read these stories, think of your own life and that of the family and friends who surround you. Ask yourself some questions. How can your family find the support they need? How can you keep the lines of communication flowing freely? Consider the many ways you can open yourself up to the love and practical support of family, friends and community. Think of the ways you can make it easier for them to cope with your illness. You are not alone with your disease.

Scenes from a marriage: Cycles of remission and illness

Any crisis in the life of someone in a long-term relationship tends to highlight both the strengths and problems of the bond between the two partners. The ongoing medical ups and downs of advanced breast cancer are no exception. Typically, the cycles of illness consist of periods of suspicion, waiting for test results, diagnosis, mobilization of resources, treatment and remission, followed by periods of relative normalcy before the next cycle begins. Sometimes these cycles are widely separated, but at other times, it can feel like one long crisis, with no recovery time.

Even during times of remission, the awareness of cancer haunts everyone in the family, as Leo Charland notes:

> Since Lisann's treatment ended last July, I have been trying to close that book. I think about her all the time and hope that she doesn't have a recurrence. I remember my personal pain of watching Lisann being tortured by the poisons injected into her body. I could dwell on this for the rest of my life, but this isn't helping me or her. I am trying to forget.
>
> I think about the future and pray that we will never have to go through another recurrence. Deep in my soul I know how insidious cancer is. You can not let your guard down. And you subconsciously await for the next occurrence, hoping it will never come.

Lloyd Multhauf wrote about the adaptation he and Sharon have made to the disease, so far, and the changes cancer have made necessary:

> After Sharon had her first bout with breast cancer, we were able to put it behind us and go on with life, regarding cancer as one of life's memories. Metastatic cancer is different. Sharon can't escape the reality of cancer, and as a spouse, neither can I. But I don't live with it as she does. I read books that take my mind in different directions. But there is seldom a day that we don't talk about cancer, and I have to accept the very understandable fact that Sharon does not engage as deeply as she once did in my intellectual interests. We really must understand each other's needs. Perhaps we are even sometimes using coping mechanisms, though I lack the skills at penetrating the subconscious to know.

I believe cancer has the potential to cause great stress in a marriage. It's easy for either spouse to feel pangs of guilt—Sharon, because so much of her time is focused on cancer-related things (much of it on the Internet) that other things get neglected, and me because I feel I don't do enough to help, or I shouldn't get tired or grumpy, but I do. Fortunately, neither of us regards feelings of guilt as being very productive. I think we're handling this okay. But when I look at other couples, I realize how different the patterns are. Sometimes it's the spouse who's heavily involved in the cancer network. Sometimes, as with a friend of mine, the spouse seems to want to deny that the cancer is happening, or at least to believe that it will be possible to get past it. Successful patterns for living with cancer seem to be quite varied because the emotional needs of people are so different. I would be quick to recommend professional counseling if a relationship became very stressful.

A number of partners and spouses remarked on the emotional fluctuations that the disease provokes. Bob Crisp described what he and Ginger went through this way:

We both go through highs and lows, not always in synch. This makes things more difficult particularly when one is high and the other low. We try hard to maintain some balance but this is difficult. Cancer is like a cloud that hangs over your head and never goes away. Sometimes you can forget it for a while.

Glenn Clabo, in the time following his wife Barb's HDC, noted a certain perverse consistency in his own emotional responses.

I'm finding a pattern to all this. When Barb is going through hell, my instincts and dedication take over. I just focus and get with the program. Of course I don't think about me much during this so when she feels better I fall off a cliff. Both emotionally and physically drained to the point of wanting to crawl into bed with a blanket over my head when it's "over." It lasts a couple of days, then poof! it's gone. The first couple of times it was tough for us both. We seemed to cross paths, with Barb going up and me going down. Now we know the whats and whys and just deal with it. Just another new adventure in the highs and lows of the roller coaster ride from hell.

Leo Charland found the same sort of pattern in himself:

> I think that the caregiver gets so locked up into doing everything and
> our minds don't have time to think about anything more than the one we
> care so much about. All else is done by rote, until our loved one is feeling
> better. Your mind is lost and you really don't know what happened. You
> have been focused on only one thing. Now every other thing comes to
> mind. You are overwhelmed with inane things. You find that you have
> neglected your everyday chores and have been living for only one cause.
> Now it's time to get back to the normalcy of life. You have a lot to do but
> just don't know where to start. You say, I've got to do this or that, but all
> you really want to do is rest, not so much physically, but mentally.

> I was going through this from November '94 through December '95.
> I'd had it and began to feel depressed. I told Lisann that I had to get away
> and be by myself, and do absolutely nothing. I went to Palm Springs and
> lay in the sun for two weeks. I did not think of anything. When I came
> back I felt human, my brain was mush but I felt good. This was my way
> of getting back to a normal life.

Partners and spouses also often feel powerless in the face of their loved one's
reactions to treatment or disease. Glenn Clabo recalls his own feelings when
Barb was newly diagnosed:

> The surgeon's eyes were not able to hide what he knew. How could I
> keep giving Barb hope, knowing it wasn't going to be good news? I wasn't
> ready for this. I knew that it was very probable that the cancer was some-
> where else. I was supposed to die first.

Bonnie Gelbwasser remembers her husband's pain following her high-dose
chemotherapy:

> My husband said the worst thing for him was talking to me on the
> phone in the days after the chemo hit. I would cry about how sorry I was
> I'd chosen to have the transplant. Obviously there was no turning back at
> that point and he felt pretty helpless.

Patients also worry a lot about how their partners are coping. PJ Hagler's
concern for her husband, Mike, was evident in this message to the husband
of another woman with metastatic disease:

It's getting so hard on Mike, I know it must be hard on you as well. If there was just some magic you guys could perform that would give you something to do to feel you were able to achieve something. I keep telling Mike that his being there and holding my hand when I need it is the greatest gift. We don't need much. Just having you in our lives is what keeps us fighting in the first place.

Kim Banks believed that for her husband, Richard, doing work around the house that she couldn't do anymore was one thing that helped both of them to cope with the feelings of helplessness:

Richard has taken up some of the housework and errands that are difficult for me because of the mets to my back. He rarely complains about the additional work he's taken on, and I think it's made him more aware of how much work is involved in keeping up our household. Of course I praise and thank him repeatedly, which he soaks up. Remarkably, I think this has helped both of us. He sometimes feels powerless in our battle against my cancer. By helping me with the house, he feels that he's at least making things easier for me so that I can focus on fighting this disease. My guilt over relinquishing my duties to him is lessened because I know he feels better by helping out.

Helpless though they may feel, partners help immeasurably just by being present, providing physical contact and listening, allowing for and participating in the process of dealing with the strong emotions that cancer forces, as Barb Clabo wrote:

As always, after the initial shock, which could take a few hours— Glenn and I would start discussing it. This is one of the many ways in which Glenn helps me through this so much. He lets me get all my emotions out, whatever they are. He'll just hold me and let me scream, cry, rant or whatever. After I settle down, he'll let me tell him what I'm feeling and he'll give me his assessment of the situation. I just don't know what I would do without him.

Talking about it: Problems in communication

Before couples can make accommodations like this, however, they must be able to communicate openly about what is going on. This is often extremely difficult, as Joleene Kolenburg discovered during the time when the peripheral neuropathy from her Taxol treatments had left her bedridden over a several-months period.

When Jack and I left the oncologist's office on Monday, I could see that he was discouraged that the scan did not show better results. But as we talked, I said that I had a feeling that I would get many more reports such as that before I am through and we have to take the bad as well as the good (or something like that). When we got home after five hours, I was very tired, my feet were hurting and my emotions were shot. I cried quite a bit. He went to his regular Boy Scout meeting after supper, and when he came home he asked if I had called the girls. I told him I had not, but had sent them an e-mail. Like most families these days, I would only have talked to their machines anyway. I thought if I e-mailed them, they could call back at their timing.

Tuesday was uneventful, we had some company and I got up to visit with them, but my feet were still hurting. Wednesday morning Jack got up early and came in to see if I was okay. I told him I felt pretty good, but would stay in bed for awhile because a friend was coming to make my breakfast at 9:00. Just before she came, my daughter from Ohio called and was crying, and asked how I was. I said okay except for my feet, and she asked if I had talked to my doctor. I said there is nothing he can do for my feet. And then she told me that Jack had tried to call her and she wasn't home, and he had called our daughter in Illinois, and told her that I had given up, that I had come home to die and would not even call them to tell them. He indicated to them that there was nothing more to be done. He also told them they should come home as soon as possible. My Illinois daughter was, at that very moment, trying to get the oncologist on the phone. So daughter #1 called her and then daughter # 2 called me and said, "Who am I to believe, Pollyanna (me) or the Grim Reaper (Jack)?" I could not convince her that I did not have the comforter over my head ready to give it all up. My friend had arrived by this time and took the phone and told her that I was smiling and hungry, etc., and I was not turning myself in yet.

When Jack returned from his nursing home ministry (he was a hospital chaplain before retirement—how ironic!), we talked about his calling the girls. I tried again to explain what I was talking about Monday when I said there would be more bad news. I also told him there were all sorts of other things that could be tried before I would give up. I just think he was scared and when I even mentioned my death just might come before his, he heard nothing else. I hope and pray that we will be able to discuss this more openly from now on, say what we mean and listen to what the other is saying. After 45 years, you'd think we could do that.

I am ready to die and not afraid of death, but I am not ready to leave yet. And I believe that the will to live is an instinct in all of us. I have thought constantly since diagnosis of how hard it would be to leave Jack alone. Since I have been in bed almost 16 weeks, I have thought of how hard the illness must be on him. However, I know how I would feel if it were the other way around.

Caren Buffum felt that her husband, Dave, who hadn't been much involved in her treatment decisions, seemed unaware of the seriousness of her situation:

I sensed that he was really in denial, couldn't deal with thinking about my having cancer—everything was going to turn out just fine in his mind, so why go out of his way to fix what didn't seem broken? What helped was coaxing him to a meeting at the doctor's office where I let the doctor speak to the issues, so he wasn't getting it all from me. The doctor was able to say enough about my situation to scare my husband (in my case, my scans had worsened) and my husband had a very strong reaction, after which, for a while, he was most cooperative. Recently, I got three bad scan reports in a row, and it was the first time Dave was willing to talk about my possible death and what it would mean for the rest of the family. Since then he has volunteered to do some of my nutritional preparation for me and is more sympathetic to my feelings and needs. Little by little, he is beginning to understand what it means to be a team in this fight.

In response to a woman who asked what she should do to improve her relationship with her husband who didn't want to talk with her about her cancer, Caren advised:

Be sure you are actively communicating with him and not just expecting him to reach out and guess what you need, as obvious as it seems to you. Try to ask as many questions of him that will encourage him to share his feelings and don't judge him or make him feel that there are right and wrong answers. He may be harboring concerns, but not know how to speak to them without feeling that he is encouraging you to dwell on the cancer even more.

Scott Kitterman had similar advice from the "receiving" end:

Mary has always been a very strong, independent person. It is difficult for her to ask for help. Our biggest problems have come from her reporting a problem and my misinterpreting the report. I typically think that she is providing information that she wants me to accept. Often what it means is I'm supposed to do something about it. The classic example is when she told me her back hurt three times in half an hour. What that meant was that I was supposed to give her a back rub to make her back feel better, but it was too hard to ask for help directly. We've gotten through that now. She asks for help when she needs it. If she doesn't, I'm more attuned to the chance that she might, so I ask her if I have any doubt.

Adding to problems in communication are temperamental differences. The "thinker" and "feeler" split, articulated here by Bob Crisp, is a disparity many couples will recognize:

She is much more emotionally expressive and much more in touch with emotions. This is probably one of the bigger differences between us and one that creates more problems. In a difficult situation, I want to think to a solution and she wants to feel to a solution. The two don't work well together. Yet, understanding this helps some. She appreciates my objectivity and rational approach to things—sometimes. And I admire her ability to be in touch with the emotional side.

Along with his rational, problem-solving approach, Bob also shares with many husbands a certain stoicism:

I am not an emotionally expressive person. Sometimes, but rarely, when alone, I may cry. Venting anger is a problem as it often wants a target. It's hard to target a disease, to target anger at cells that have bad DNA. Racquetball helps dissipate some of the adrenaline.

Kathy Stone's husband, Chuck, had similar stoic tendencies. Her discussion of this with him led to a crucial and satisfying change in their relationship.

Chuck was very quiet as he sat and drank his coffee and told me everything was going to be okay no matter what the diagnosis was... and it dawned on me that although we truly loved each other and he had always been there for me through lots of adversity, I could not and would not go through having cancer without talking about it and talking to **him** *about it and* **him** *talking about it...the good, the bad and the ugly...* **all** *of it. It was going to be a* **must***, a high priority and I might as well confront him then and there about how I felt...and so I did.*

He acted very surprised and made some noises about always under-standing, never trying to keep me from talking, etc., (which was all very true)...but I just kept insisting he understand that he was going to have to **speak** *words, not just actions...I needed to hear from his mouth what he was thinking, how he felt, if and when he was scared...I needed to hear him speak of it openly to others, not be quiet about what was happening to us. It was one of the best things I have ever done. After reminding him of some examples of things he had always "stuffed" ...he agreed that he would try. It was hard for him at first because it is against his nature to discuss "bad" things...his family is very private...but he did it for me right from the beginning and as he did, it got easier for him.... He now sees the benefit of opening up to each other. He still is quiet and private, but will talk to others about breast cancer, about me, how I'm doing, how he is doing...but more important, he talks over feelings with* **me** *and lets me talk over everything with him...over and over and over I'm afraid.*

When one partner is more expressive, even in the best of times, keeping communication flowing often takes continued conscious effort, as Caren Buffum found:

My husband and two boys are probably typical in that they are there for me, but don't always know how best to interact with me regarding the cancer. I wish, at times, that my husband was more aggressive in this fight with me—he does not initiate a lot of the "fighting activities" and rarely volunteers to join me for doctor visits, treatments, etc. But he clearly cares deeply and is willing to do pretty much whatever I ask. I think he has had a relatively high level of denial through most of this, and the faith that has been a source of great hope and comfort has probably also made him at times "too optimistic." I don't mean he has had too much hope for me—I don't think one can have too much hope. But his "everything will be all right" attitude sometimes interferes with his realizing that this is a very serious and difficult battle, and that we cannot become passive in our response to it. One of my biggest struggles regarding his involvement is wanting him to notice when I don't have the strength to carry the ball myself, and to jump in and pick it up for me. I am understanding more and more that I am expecting too much and that I must simply ask for what I need, because he is more than willing. But I struggle with feelings of guilt for asking too much, imposing myself.

Answering a wife who wrote that she hesitated to ask her husband for his true feelings about her illness, Glenn Clabo articulated some of the problems and rewards of the process:

I don't know your husband but I do know what it's like being a man dealing with this. My experience with Barb says you really don't want to know how he's dealing with this but you really should try to find out for all the right reasons.

The process was horrendous for us. When I finally got to the point of wanting to say what I felt...it made her cry. Even though it was a "good" cry.... I am a man and crying means hurt. That in turn made me want to stop. I'd clam up and make statements like "You ask.... I tell... you cry. Don't ask!" It took quite a few of these moments to get through it all. Actually, I don't think we'll ever get totally through it.

As you may know, Barb's situation is pretty bad. It's really not if, it's when. That's not something anyone should stuff. I've gone from not believing depression existed to...not being depressed was fantasy.

*I guess what I'm saying is... If you really want to know, ask. However, make sure you **really** are ready to know. Be prepared for some difficult moments. Don't think that everything he says at first is really everything he feels. He may be much better at all this because of his education and training...but I still believe that unless he's worked his way through some man things...it will be tough for you both. However...it really is a great feeling when you finally get working on it and see how it is beginning to change how you look and feel about each other. We had a very good and strong marriage before all this. I believe it couldn't get much better than it is now.*

In response to another woman's lament about her husband's lack of involvement, Scott Kitterman expressed his perception of what might be going on, and his belief that however grim the prognosis, being there as an advocate is an important role for family members to play.

> *I think what your husband lacks is a sense that anything he does will matter. If he can't affect the outcome, why bother to try? I think caregivers can affect the outcome. As I'm sure you know, the person being treated is not generally in an optimal frame of mind to defend her own interests. In my family, we have long had a policy that if someone is in the hospital, adult or child, you don't leave that person by him or herself (an adult does get to spend the night alone in most cases). This is because experience has shown us that the patient needs an advocate and no one in the medical community fills that role. Maybe what he needs is to know that what he learns and does will make a difference to your prognosis?*

Attending a monthly group for couples dealing with cancer sponsored by the local Wellness Community led Caren and Dave Buffum to some new discoveries:

> *The group was very interesting. We got to talking about communication between spouses and it got rather intense at times. I feel this is especially good for Dave and me to hear how other couples are dealing with cancer, and boy, did we have some discussion afterwards. In fact, it was a pretty intense week as we brought all sorts of things to the surface. It felt very negative at first, because we were being more honest than we have been in the past, and sometimes honesty can hurt. But it gave us a place to move on from and I feel like we are now headed in a positive direction.*

Despite the intimacy and openness of their relationship, Glenn and Barb Clabo found themselves constantly challenged by the fears they both felt:

> *I didn't realize how important the art of listening was. Barb always told me that I helped her by doing all the research. I helped her by taking on all the responsibilities of day-to-day life. But the biggest help I gave her was when I sat and just listened. Believe me it wasn't easy. I was programmed to help. I had to continually remind myself to not try to help...just listen.*

> *Even though Barb and I were together for thirty-two years and took pride in how well we communicated, this fight led us to find new ways to talk. The tears and the anger took on brand new meanings. The hugs and touches went far beyond words. The fear was real. I can't tell you how*

many times that Barb indicated to me, in many ways, that she was just plain scared. Scared of the next chemo... scared of it not working, scared of it working so she could go on to the next torture... and, of course, scared of death. It started to come up more and more. Is there anything more difficult to face? It's never a good time to talk about it. It was always there and always on our minds.

"Love doesn't worry about looks"

The physical changes wrought by metastatic breast cancer and its treatments often have a profound impact on how women feel about themselves and their attractiveness to their partners. Though they may have experienced it before, the repeated hair loss of chemotherapy may still be deeply disturbing to women, even though it is temporary. Glenn Clabo wrote about his wife Barb's reaction:

> *She kept saying, "I'm gone. I don't see me when I look in the mirror." Her normally low self-image was compounded by orders of magnitude. Because she always felt overweight and not pretty she clung to her very thick and beautiful hair. It was the thing that everyone commented on. It was the only physical thing that she had pride in. I always told her that I and all the people who ever got to know her loved her because of her basic being. Her love of life and compassion for others. No one to my knowledge ever disliked Barb the person. She really had a problem with this. "I don't get it" was a statement she made many times a day.*

PJ Hagler also found losing her hair one of the more difficult, ego-bruising parts of the cancer experience.

> *I combed my hair. Then, not realizing what was happening, I got the comb stuck in my hair (which was very long, blond and pretty) and didn't know why it was stuck. I looked at the comb when I got it out and saw the amount of hair in the comb. It was almost like the shock all over again. I ran to the phone and called Mike at work. He asked if I wanted him to come home. I said no and just cried into the phone, "please love me, it's so awful." He came home as fast as he could.*

Menopausal changes are difficult for most women. For cancer patients who endure a premature abrupt menopause from the effects of chemotherapy, these changes can be particularly devastating. Gerry Wirth related the impact these drugs had on his marriage:

> I hesitate to write this next paragraph but I guess I should. The HDC made intimacy impossible for Cindy to enjoy. She underwent menopause and lost elasticity and lubrication. We tried many things but none of them really worked. What was frustrating was that I enjoyed giving her pleasure. It was a gift that we reserved for each other. While my love for her was deepening, I was no longer able to give her that special gift. She, on the other hand, wanted to please me and tried very hard. But I was never satisfied because I could no longer give her pleasure. While now it seems simple, it took us a while to realize what was going on and to communicate it to each other. In the end the issue ceased to be important as her condition worsened.

Pat Leach and her husband also experienced this common problem:

> With all the anti-estrogen medications over the years, and then chemo, my vagina is like sand paper, no lubrication no matter the amount of passion and on the whole I'm really not interested in intercourse although I want to cuddle with my husband. Lots of foreplay is fine but I dread actual intercourse despite KY, vitamin E, etc. Thank goodness for my loving, caring and sensitive husband. We are doing fine but we miss vaginal intercourse.

For Lisann Charland, the visible physical signs of her treatment were particularly troubling:

> I broke down continuously, especially during our lovemaking and as I looked at my physical state. My poor husband had to reassure me that it was okay, he loved me for what I was, not for what I looked like today during this difficult time. I felt less and less like a wife and the girl I used to be. The physical scars kept reminding that I could not be the same again—something very difficult to cope with mentally. I refused to let anyone see me without a scarf around my head. I would not even look at myself in the mirror. I was losing myself to this disease slowly and he kept encouraging me to hold on. I was embarrassed to talk about the side effects of chemo with the gynecologist. This fatherly-type man slipped a tube of lubricating gel in my purse as he asked me questions about sex

during my visit, and I could not look at him and answer him. This is still
a subject I cannot talk openly about due to my Catholic upbringing.

Kim Banks and her husband, Richard, found ways to adapt to the situation.

> *Oddly, while we have sex much less often, we are far more intimate*
> *in other ways. I've gone into early menopause from the chemotherapy, so*
> *my libido is much lower than it was. My back problems have also added*
> *to the decrease in sex. So we hold hands, give each other back rubs and*
> *snuggle a lot. We talk and are open about it and have decided that enjoy-*
> *ing this level of intimacy is right for us now. Still, I miss our former sex*
> *life very much and hope that our sexual activity returns more to normal*
> *as we adjust to all of these changes.*

Only 27 when she was first diagnosed, Sandra Yandell, newly divorced and living in Portland, Oregon, began a new relationship with the man who had been her first boyfriend. She was rediscovering and savoring that first love just at the time her breast cancer spread, three years later. Metastases in the bones of her spine, pelvis and leg left her with difficulty walking and with expressing the passion she felt for her boyfriend despite all the treatments and changes:

> *All I want to do is walk. I took it for granted for 32 years, and now I*
> *have dreams about the simple act of putting one foot in front of the next.*
> *Is it so much to ask in the great scheme of things? To stroll around the*
> *block and see the flowers blooming, to walk into a restaurant and have*
> *people look at me because I'm beautiful, not with pity in their eyes*
> *because of the crutches. And I want to be able to make love with this*
> *incredible guy of mine and not end up crying because the slightest wrong*
> *move and I'm in agony. All this awful stuff that's happened to me, yet*
> *somebody still finds me beautiful and desirable. And one of the few things*
> *I have left to give him gets more and more difficult and painful, and he's*
> *almost afraid to touch me.*

Like Sandra, Nancy Gilpatrick suffered from widely metastasized bone disease. The breaks in her hip and pelvis have left her in a wheelchair. And like Sandra, Nancy had begun a new relationship with a man at the time her cancer was diagnosed at Stage IV.

> *Terry moved in around January 1, 1996, to be with me, care for me*
> *while going through treatment and to love me. My life has been filled with*

a wonderful, passionate, mature love. We respect one another. We laugh together, share similar values and work on living in the present with one another. Our lovemaking has been over the top, before and after diagnosis. We've needed to be creative and since we were already creative it continues. I've gotten the relationship, the joy, I've always wanted. And here I am living with Stage IV breast cancer, a disease with no known cure.

Kathy Stone expressed the profound gratitude—and sense of mystification—many of these women feel about the tenderness, care, affection and even passion their mates express for them.

I have no idea what I would do or how I would get through this without my husband...you partners who stand by us are wonderful. I looked in the mirror the other night as I was getting ready for bed and I didn't know if I should laugh or cry...there I was—fat, bald, one boob off and a fanny pack hanging around my waist. I told my husband it was bad enough before I started wearing the fanny pack of 5-FU hanging off my stomach, then it just looked like he was going to bed with Buddha, now it looked like he was going to bed with a Sumo wrestler. He just hugged me and laughed and said LOVE didn't worry about looks. How is it that at my ugliest he can make me feel beautiful. I guess that really is what love is all about and therefore you husbands/wives/partners hurt with every pain we have and agonize over every test with us...and we can never thank you enough for being there.

Deepening of love

Those fortunate enough to have partners who stay with them throughout this ordeal often experience a deepening of their love. Just as individuals come to feel as if they themselves are challenged and enlarged by the experience of dealing with cancer, so the same can be true of loving relationships, which can also grow in meaning and depth and mutual respect, with the shared experience of the two partners. Bonnie Gelbwasser's love and admiration for her husband grew in the course of her illness:

My husband and I met when I was 15 and he was 18; we were friends for four years, then dated for two more before we married. This is a long and loving relationship that has grown deeper since my breast cancer diagnosis. Cancer took away my breast and, for fourteen months, my hair, and there were times I feared it would rob me of my sanity. I did not have a strong self-image before cancer; the disease did nothing to enhance that image. But my husband did. His gentleness, concern and commitment to my emotional well-being and his total acceptance of my new body (I also lost 40 pounds these last two years), have enabled me to focus on the challenges of living—rather than the pain and the disfigurement. He honors me with his love. I could not be more blessed. The bone marrow transplant was just part of the protocol. Cancer is the reality that each of us has had to integrate into our marriage and into our individual lives. And integrating cancer into our lives has been, and continues to be, our greatest challenge.

When asked how her husband had coped with her having cancer, Bonnie replied:

My husband is an uncomplicated, patient, practical and focused man. He has always believed that one does not choose how or when one dies and so he has never feared death. He has coped with my cancer the way he copes with the other parts of his life: he gives thoughtful consideration to the issues, evaluates the alternatives and determines his course of action. That is not to say he doesn't cry (he's actually someone who cries a lot, usually because of something one of the kids is going through), but just that he finds the strength he needs to keep himself and the rest of us moving along. He told me years ago, when we were still teens and I could not see myself spending the rest of my life with him, that I could be certain of one thing—that he would always be there for me. There was no decision for him when we learned I had breast cancer. He would do whatever needed to be done to make this easy for me and for himself and for our family. And he has done just that—with grace and courage and love.

Kim Banks also felt that the cancer had drawn her and her husband closer:

I'd heard that cancer could break a marriage or make it better. Ours has definitely followed the latter course. We're best friends and I feel that we don't take each other for granted anymore. We share and make plans together more often now. While we plan more, we're much more "in the moment" than ever before. There's an intense intimacy in staying in the moment, really enjoying each other. We don't put off the things we really enjoy doing (like sleeping in and snuggling on a Saturday morning) and we're much better at prioritizing our lives. We love to camp and have spent every other weekend this summer up in the Rocky Mountains.

When camping I try to put the cancer behind me and I feel healthier hiking in the woods and breathing in that wonderful, clean air.

For Mary D'Angelo, as for many of those I interviewed, the reality that time was short was what served to enrich and deepen an already good marriage:

When you think you have the rest of your life, you love each other but you keep putting things off. You think there will be time. But we went through a period when we thought I didn't have much time, of traveling every place, and that was great because when we were traveling, I thought—well, I had read in books that you shouldn't go on vacation while you're on chemotherapy, because you'll get depressed—but when we were traveling, everything was just so intense. We felt that maybe it would be the last time we were in Paris, or the last time in Italy. I was able to let go and enjoy every moment more than I ever had. We realized that these trips are so much better, and we're taking a lot of them. We never would have allowed ourselves to do that. My life is so much fuller now, because I'm ill.

This year, the trips have calmed down, because we ran out of money. But I also feel that the traveling was like an immediate reaction. The trips are not even that important to me now. It's just being with him. I notice this—well, I'm really glad there are no children at home now, because they're distractions from being with him. I like simple things now. He comes home and I want to have dinner for him. I always want candles and flowers, a bottle of wine and conversation. Not because I think it will be the last, but because we spent so many years with meals with three children, and high chairs at the table, struggling.

Charlie feels sad about that. We put off a lot, struggling to raise a family and thinking that we'd have all this time, and he feels cheated. I don't feel that way. I feel grateful that I was able to raise my children and that they're all well-launched. In a sense, the major part of my work, with them, is done. So I'm grateful about that. I just want the remaining time to be as good as it can be.

PJ Hagler and her husband, Mike, wrestled with feeling their lives had not taken the direction they hoped for:

Mike and I have been together since we were kids and truthfully we always thought of our wedding vows in the positive: for better, not worse, in richer, not in poorer, in health, not in sickness, and that death would be in our very old age. So at 34, being told I had cancer and that it was very bad and that statistically (in 1984) I had 5 years at the most, our entire lives were changed. So for the next 12 years and counting I have dealt with cancer every day of my life. I am limited in what I can do, where I can go. My entire life has been different than we planned.

Stories from partners: "Things are back to normal"

Three of the partners of women with metastatic breast cancer wrote about their sense of what life was like for them, with all its fears and changes. It is not only their devotion, but also their sense of the pleasures and problems of ordinary domestic life that form an eloquent testimony for human coping and adaptability. For Lloyd Multhauf, a metaphor best expressed his experience of what it was like to live with his wife's metastatic disease.

> I have at times thought of the experience of Sharon's cancer as floating down a river in a boat with no means of control, while hearing the ominous sound of a waterfall ahead. When we were first told of her metastasis, we felt we had heard a death sentence. We would not have acknowledged it then, even to ourselves, but I believe we both felt it. We right then were in the churning river, knowing we were approaching the waterfall without any hope of avoiding it. You might ask why I say "we" were threatened. For me it was because the thought of approaching Sharon's death, and of living in an emotionally depleted beyond, was frightening.

> Fortunately, for both Sharon and me, our reaction to crises is to focus on what we can do, rather than to dwell on what has happened or how it might have been different. Neither of us is inclined toward self-pity or a sense that life, or even God, is unfair. So, we read extensively, talked to doctors, and in general, tried, as quickly as possible, to get information so that we could make the best decisions possible to gain a sense of control and avoid feeling victimized. The immediate treatment decisions were made, and after a time, we began to feel reasonably well informed.

> Several months later, after we had taken a Caribbean cruise, we found that it didn't feel like our last vacation. We went through the trials

of a rebelling teenager and were emerging from what seemed like a tun-
nel. The tamoxifen seemed to be working, and we were leading fairly normal lives. It was as though we kept drifting down the river, all the while
hearing the waterfall but never reaching it. In fact, the sound seemed less
intense. And at times, I even fleetingly wondered if I was hearing a waterfall at all. Maybe it's just wind in the trees. Doctors don't really "see" cancer in bones, they just see, on bone scans and MRI films, light and dark
areas that they don't really understand but, through experience, have
come to interpret as cancer. Maybe they are wrong in this case. Being a
scientist, I find these thoughts don't persist. But I do entertain thoughts
that perhaps the waterfall is a long way off. And I begin to think that
there may be an opportunity to get to the shore. Maybe if I try hard to
find a way. Maybe we'll be lucky. Maybe there will be a bend in the river
and we'll be caught in an eddy where we can grab a branch. These, of
course, are those hoped-for cures, or new ways of achieving long-lasting
control.

But even time itself is a gift. After all, mortality is a fact of life for all
of us, and my fears are mostly associated with the effect of my own death
on the lives of those I love, or of Sharon's death on the family and me.
Those fears have already diminished as our children have gotten older,
although as long as there are cherished relationships, they will always be
there.

For Terry Houlahan, life with Nancy Gilpatrick was difficult to describe to
the outside world, marked as it was by subtle realizations and "ordinary"
moments—and a new sense of what normal had come to mean.

Well-meaning friends and acquaintances approach me at work or on
the street, in shops and stores and say, "How is Nancy?" They pause and
search me for any clue I'm giving a perfunctory answer or putting up a
brave face, stoically holding back my pain.

Living with someone who has cancer means I'm enmeshed in the routine of our lives. I don't begrudge anyone inquiring into Nan's health but
questioners want to know the highlights. Once in a while there are big
events—these are what the people who ask usually want to hear. The
"Nancy has metastatic disease in her bones and her hip fractured and
now she has to use a walker to get around and a wheelchair if we are
going any distance at all," or "Nancy is going into the hospital for super

high-dose chemo and a stem cell transplant," or "Nancy got the tests back and it looks like the chemo has stopped working." That kind of stuff. Unfortunately, cancer is a chronic disease and chronic is mostly boring. For us down here in the midst of things, highlights type stuff is most always yesterday's news. Nancy and I live in today and lean towards an uncertain tomorrow. So when people ask, "How is Nancy?" I have to pause and think to see if some big deal has happened lately.

A friend at work asked the other day, "How's your girl doing?" It was about 45 days since the stem cell transplant and I stopped to think if anything had happened lately. Nothing. So after a moment I said, "She's doing good. I think everything is kinda getting back to normal."

Then I got to thinking, what is normal?

Next morning I read an article in the local paper. A staff writer had written a series of articles about hiking to the highest point in every county in Utah. Some high points were easy, some were real alpine summits. I was jealous. Washing the breakfast dishes, I was thinking about the article and about how much we love to hike. I thought, "I'd love to do that some day. I'd like to do it with Nancy."

Right about then my reverie was interrupted. "Honey, would you let Harriet out?" The dog needed to go out for her morning constitutional. Sitting at the table, Nancy was closer to the door but her hip pain had flared in the night and she was too sore. Considering how her hip felt, the task of rising out of her chair and walking seven steps to the door was more than she felt up to.

"Sure, honey." I said. I stopped washing the dishes, dried my hands and walked over to the door to let the spaniel out.

Things are back to normal.

Embracing his wife one morning following her recovery from HDC, Glenn Clabo struggled to express the complexity of fear, tenderness and joy that he felt in that fleeting moment:

Since the sudden death of my sister, when I was young, I've always wondered what would happen if I was placed into a situation like the one I've been in for over a year now. A situation where someone I let myself fall in love with again...faced death. Now I know...I wish I didn't. The *fantasy was many times easier than this reality. Something happened this morning that made me face the reality.*

During our morning hug I noticed something. When Barb settled her head against my neck I felt her hair. To the uninitiated that's no big deal.... To this man it somehow made me snap to attention and feel something down deep. At that moment, I couldn't understand what that something was. It was there and gone in an instant. Coffee and the plans for the day took over...until we headed off to work.

I couldn't get it straight and I couldn't get it out of my mind. That feeling of Barb's hair on my neck. What does it mean? Why was it so important?

It's the waiting that has crawled inside my head. I know that the long and torturous road has led us to this rest stop...but we can't rest. We can't forget where we've been, or who we were...nor do we want to. We have gone far beyond change and moved into something so different it doesn't resemble our past. It never will.

I now believe this rest stop was placed here to renew our energy to move on...to find what is ahead. It wasn't put here to just wallow in our own worry pit. It's here to focus our life...to help understand our meaning. Make us realize that we are different and will never be the same. Last year at this time we were both looking into each others' eyes wondering if we would see another Christmas together. Barb was so worn out from treatments that all she did was sleep and worry. Barb's hair is completely different than it was in the other life...but it's here! But **she is** *here!*

In a few hours, I'm going to leave work, grab my love by her hand and steal her away from her job. We are going to get ready for Christmas. Start with lunch, walk the stores, spend some money, take in a movie and spend a quiet evening at home. Tomorrow the tree that's been sitting on the deck will be put up and filled with years of collected decorations. The house will be filled with Christmas cheer and a realization that we have too much to be waiting for...too much to be thankful for.

Conflicting needs and priorities

In a crisis, most families are able set aside other members' needs to focus on a very sick person and doing what is right for them. But as weeks stretch on into months, and then years, conflicting needs and priorities are bound to arise. The drama of treatment and remission recede into day-to-day life, and become part of a new normalcy, of a kind. And life goes on. Other family members have problems, too. After a family crisis reminded her of this simple reality, Bonnie Gelbwasser wrote:

> I have come to believe that the lesson of this is that cancer patients are not protected from the day-to-day challenges of living. The flat tires still come, the kids do dumb things, the dog throws up on the rug just when your guests drive up, and the power goes out before you can shower!

When Sylvan Rainwater became seriously ill herself, her life-partner, Pam Hiebert, was suddenly thrust into the unfamiliar role of caregiver. Sylvan's analysis of this time is a classic report on the kinds of problems couples face in situations like this:

> The role reversal has been one source of stress, I suppose. We've learned how to have me be the caregiver and her be the one needing care (or, as we recently named the roles, "mother" and "queen"). I suppose at first glance she thought she already understood the mother role and would find it easier. In my hospital room after the surgery she announced to everyone that she would much rather be mother than queen. We all got a lot of laughs out of that.

> But there were two problems with the role reversal. One was that I expected her to do the mother role as I had, to give me the kind of emotional support I wanted, to be unfailingly there and patient and listen to my problems and give me lots of strokes for how well I was doing. For her part, I think she took on the support role as she would have wanted it to happen—the supreme organizer, the one clearing the forest to make it safe for me. Our different expectations eventually clashed in a variety of ways.

> The other problem with the role reversal was that she was still dealing with illness herself. It was difficult for her to process the recurrence she was going through once we discovered that I had health problems as well. She was being pulled too many ways. And her Amazon role came out in full—she wanted to do it all, and ended up taking on too much, even though we both knew the risks involved in that. I had learned, painfully, that I couldn't do it all, couldn't always fix things, couldn't, in fact,

save her life. Pam knew this all theoretically, but still bumped up against it herself by taking on too much and then crashing with fatigue. Inevitably, it came out as resentment of me. And of course, it was difficult for me to give her the amount of support and space she needed to deal with all her issues because I was involved in my own fears and issues.

During her illness, the loss of Sylvan's income had placed even more pressure on Pam. Already juggling medical appointments and a full-time job, Pam felt some resentment despite herself at the added financial responsibility. Sylvan was painfully aware of Pam's feelings. "Really not fair, and I hated it, but didn't know what else to do," Sylvan acknowledged, and reported a crucial moment that served as a turning point for them:

When Pam finally asked me what I wanted from her, I had to think awhile, but finally said I needed her to appreciate what a tough spot I was in. She thought that over and replied that she could call a bunch of people to come in and do that (what an organizer!). I could just picture it, and had to laugh, but said, no, I needed **her** *to appreciate me. Later that day she brought me flowers and told me how much she appreciated all the work I do. Exactly what I needed to hear. A good example of her sensitivity. Sometimes you just have to ask. And I suppose that's the crux of the matter. It's easy to fall into the trap of wanting the other person to "just know" what you need and provide it without being told.*

Pam was also candid about her own responses to Sylvan's illness—and to Sylvan's full recovery as well, an experience that was poignant for them both.

Many of the feelings I experienced once Sylvan came back from the hospital and began her eight weeks of recovery are difficult for me to fully admit about myself. I think ultimately I was projecting my own feelings of vulnerability on Sylvan. I think I was trying to get in touch with the likely possibility of my living with less quality of health and I was frightened. Maybe it was the dark side of me that saw her able to recover and this just reinforced the fact that my disease is a one-way road. Such a mixed bag!

When I heard her doctor say she would be feeling much better after recovery and that the worst was over, it brought home something I had forgotten: it was possible actually to have a disease that could be cured.

The optimism in her doctor's voice was far different than the pessimistic voice of my doctors. It seemed to drive a still larger wedge in my mental separation of wellness and illness.

Sometimes, differences in temperament and personality can lead to conflict. Although he loved her deeply, for Bob Crisp, taking care of his wife, Ginger, didn't come easily, something he attributes in large part to his personality, being by inclination a loner and thinker, the "prototypical college professor" type, a man who loves ideas but is often uneasy with people:

Being thrust into caregiving for me is like being a fish out of water. It requires special effort and directed thinking to do what needs to be done. I'm better at the physical stuff, like getting laundry done and taking Ginger to appointments, and not so good at emotional support. I have to make conscious efforts to give her a hug or kiss, to listen to her fears and concerns, and to be present for her. These things are not so natural to me and they take more energy than they would for others—particularly those where this comes naturally.

At other times, it is the patient's concerns about being dependent upon others that interfere with this process, as Scott Kitterman experienced with his wife, Mary:

One thing I have repeatedly told my wife is that it is not her place to judge the limits of commitment that others have to her. If she is too much of a "burden" people will bail out. No one has yet. If those of us around someone fighting breast cancer are willing to be there and help out, those who are fighting breast cancer should trust us to have our own reasons and not second-guess our decision to help.

There are also inevitable conflicts in priorities. A person with metastatic cancer may understandably be living more in the moment than in the distant future, pursuing short-term interests and goals, while other family members' interests may be different. Bob Crisp raised a few of the emotionally charged questions many couples face and yet find so hard to discuss.

Do people with cancer get license to do all the things they've wanted to do, even if it causes financial difficulty? Or does the person live life as normally as possible? Fighting the beast dominates the lives of people who have the disease, but how much should it dominate the lives of those around them? Should their children change behavior and patterns or go

on with the softball or band and live as if there was no cancer? Should the
spouse continue to play golf, or go fishing, or play poker, or other things
like they used to do, or give these up so as to have as much time and help
for the spouse with cancer? If the child wants to stay in band given the
time it takes, or the spouse wants to continue his regular Saturday golf
game, should the person with cancer ask them to quit to have more time
together?

Personalizing these dilemmas, Bob risked disclosing the sort of universal perceptions that are always so difficult to talk about—his sense that whatever his love and loyalty to Ginger, her road, in fact, diverged from his.

In some ways we are closer, but in others we are not. It's a weird
thing when I'm healthy and doing everything I would normally do while
she has become increasingly limited in what she can do. She now has oxy-
gen. Walking up one flight of stairs will put her heart rate to 145 and her
blood oxygen levels fall like crazy. I still want to do some of the things I
love to do: go to basketball games, play racquetball, go fishing, but she
became increasingly limited in what she could do. This continues to get
worse.

Cindy Wirth was six months pregnant when her breast cancer was first diagnosed. Their son Matthew was three years old. Gerry is candid in describing his feelings at the time.

When Cindy was first diagnosed I wasn't very understanding. The
way the adjunctive treatment changed our lives was hard for me to
accept. It got in the way of some personal goals. Lots of people had can-
cer and survived. Why did this treatment have to be so disruptive? Car-
ing for the new baby was very difficult for me. I resented not having all
the help and support that I had with Matthew.

His attitude changed, however, on her diagnosis with metastatic disease less than a year later.

I focused on getting her well. I really felt guilty about my earlier atti-
tude. So I just focused on Cindy's treatment and supporting her.

The time of her high-dose chemotherapy was particularly difficult for Gerry.

I found it hard to prioritize my time. Work was not an issue. My
supervisor told me to show up in the morning so he could take head

count. After that he didn't care where I was. My coworker kept up with the load so I had time. The right way to spend that time was a problem. When I was with Cindy I worried about the kids. Cindy was "sleeping" a lot so I had plenty of time to worry. When I was at home with the kids I worried about Cindy: was she okay, was she lonely? It didn't seem like there was a possible answer that was correct and felt right.

Gerry speaks for many couples who have been through this emotionally troubling time.

This experience had very positive and negative effects on our marriage. We cherished each other and our children more then ever. We were not as wasteful of time. When you are well there is always tomorrow. We were starting to realize that we might not have as many tomorrows as we thought.

This experience also added tension to our relationship. Each of us feared what would happen if the HDC did not work. Each of us did not know how much to tell the other of our feelings, in fear of hurting/worrying the other. Cindy wanted to live with more gusto, engage in long-term projects, like remodeling the house, etc. I was very hesitant to do that because I was unsure what the future held for us. Cindy had several side effects to the preparatory chemos that required hospitalization. That experience plus the pressure it put upon me led me not to want to disrupt our lives and routines because I never knew when I would need to go into hospital mode.

It's safe to say that there are no right or wrong answers to any of the questions posed directly by Bob Crisp and implied in the words of so many others. Each couple, each family, tends to arrive at an understanding about conflicting needs and priorities that makes sense to them. The important thing is for all the people involved to keep on talking and sharing their thoughts and feelings.

Who cares for the caregivers?

The subtitle of this chapter is, "It's happening to us, too." In a very real way, family members are also deeply affected by the ravages of this disease. Research supports this. In fact, psychologist Douglas Rait and psychiatrist

Marguerite Lederberg, of Memorial Sloan-Kettering Cancer Center, are concerned enough about the impact of cancer on the entire family that they identify the families of cancer patients as "second order patients." Yet the family's needs are frequently overlooked. The crux of the dilemma is this:

> Although family members themselves may be shattered by the diagnosis of cancer in a loved one, they are expected by others—medical staff especially—and by themselves to be able to contain their feelings and function supportively toward the patient.[1]

In addition to providing emotional support, shared responsibility for decision-making is also a crucial role that family members play, according to Rait and Lederberg:

> A diagnosis of cancer makes immediate complex decision-making demands on the patient at a time when he or she is perhaps least able to meet them. Family members routinely step into this breach, providing tireless involvement and often performing the lion's share of the work needed to explore, learn, and evaluate a sea of new and difficult information.... It has been repeatedly observed that family members are not just willing but have a deep need to receive information and share in the decision-making.[2]

Added to shared decision-making, concrete caretaking as well as financial and social costs are among the expenditures of emotional and practical energies for families. Finally, Rait and Lederberg point out, family members must work hard to maintain the integrity of the family. In addition to providing patient care, families must also cope with the emotional needs of all family members, and find ways to perform all of the roles and functions the sick person was once responsible for. Patients often worry more about the burden their illness places on their families than they do about themselves.

The support of the extended family and a community of friends is often greatest in the midst of an acute crisis, and then tends to fade away during chronic periods of remission or lengthy treatment, leaving family members feeling isolated and depleted, at a time when they most need help. Surprisingly, studies show that only about a third of families make use of the supports available to them at these times, even though they know about them.

Families, particularly those with young children, need to create extended networks of support to cope with a member who has advanced cancer. Improving communications within the family—between spouses, among siblings and between parents and children—is an important first step, involving frank discussions with all parties.

> *All children experience guilt about their possible causative role, grief and yearning for lost parenting from both parents, fear for themselves, and anger and resentment about being abandoned or shunted aside. This latter reaction can be quite realistic, as young children are often sent away and are almost always bypassed in the illness communication network. Therefore, fantasies replace fact, and, as child therapists have long known, these are more tormenting than even a grim reality.[3]*

Most families need some help in dealing with a seriously ill member. Getting the necessary outside supports, whether this means from extended family, from church or social organizations and from friends, or getting help from agencies and organizations to fill specific needs, like homemaking or counseling, can make all the difference. Later, in the sections on the final phases of illness, we'll hear more about how some of the people interviewed for this book manage to handle these needs, particularly in dealing with their young children.

Every family is profoundly affected. When I asked Bonnie Gelbwasser how much of a return to normal family life there had been following her high-dose chemotherapy for inflammatory breast cancer, she placed her response in the context of change.

> *A total return. But we are no longer a "normal" family. Three of the five of us have worked with therapists, and cancer colors almost every decision and seems to lurk in the background of every family encounter or event. Still, we can laugh and enjoy each other again without crying or hugging like we could never let go (as we did in the months after my diagnosis) and we're moving on. Our youngest daughter is relocating to Phoenix in June, our older daughter has created a satisfying life in Connecticut and our son is happy in his job in Boston. The constant phone calls have ended and we touch base whenever we can—not because we feel we have to.*

As Joleene Kolenburg found after four months spent in bed with the side effects of treatment, sometimes families do manage to find out things about themselves they never knew:

I can see a little of what God has taught me through this. I could be real honest and tell you how I always thought my family would fall apart if I weren't totally in charge of everything. But over the past few months, I have found that they can get a meal on the table, they can get the checks written, the groceries purchased and a million other things that only I could do before.

Friends and extended family: Needs, kindness and fears

Not everyone dealing with metastatic disease is fortunate enough to have a loving partner close at hand to see what is needed and to provide "built in" help. Some people with metastatic breast cancer live alone, and must make special efforts to deal with loneliness and isolation, on top of all the other physical and emotional stresses of the disease. For these people, having a support network becomes crucial, whether this takes the form of a loving group of friends, extended family members nearby, or the services of a tight-knit community at church or temple.

While Ellen Scheiner found it possible to hire the help she needed to care for her physical needs during the intensive chemotherapy treatment she underwent, her emotional needs were more complex:

At the time of diagnosis and surgery, I was dating someone who was available some of the time, but was also very occupied with taking care of her mother. She comforted me at mastectomy time and the night before surgery we tearfully and solemnly said good-bye to my right breast, thanking her for the sexual pleasure she had given to me and my lovers. This relationship ended in April, when my lover developed serious health problems of her own. We had worn each other out and each had nothing left to give to the other. That left me without a significant other—no one to hold, touch or physically comfort me. I had wonderful friends, who did all kinds of things, but the element of pure bodily comfort was missing. A friend, who has been quite ill, recently told me that one of her criteria for potential friends is: will they hold me if I'm sick?

Barb Pender, divorced for ten years and taking care of her aging mother, recalls being devastated by the loss of her breast and pushing people away when she was first diagnosed:

I needed time to deal with my own issues before I could let someone else in. I truly tried to alienate everyone around at first—my children, my mother, my sister, my friends. I didn't want to be the cause of their pain in watching me go through everything. But then I found that I needed their support and their love—it ended up being the very thing that got me through those tough moments.

A woman alone, without a partner's reassurance of her attractiveness or desirability, can often feel woefully inadequate. In the company of the men she knew, Barb felt particularly self-conscious and negative about losing a breast.

During the period of my mastectomy and initial chemo I chose to keep the men at a distance because of my own insecurities. I could not believe that they would feel the same or treat me the same without my 44DD breasts. It was easier for me to distance myself from them rather than to deal with those issues while I was dealing with what was going on with me as well. It never occurred to me that I was loved and respected by them for who I am and not what I look like. I didn't find that until many months later when I finally "let them in" so to speak.

There was an article in the newspaper August of '94 that told of a young man with leukemia at one of our local high schools. All of the males in his class shaved their heads in support of his baldness. My friends are all married couples and we were talking about this article when I had to ask jokingly, as I sat there bald, where was their loyalty? As the afternoon went on, I had to go to the store. When I returned, there in the garage were the husbands shaving their heads—we were the three bald buddies. I never felt so loved.

Unmarried or unpartnered does not mean that one must confront illness alone. Barb Pender feels as if she is part of a "village" that includes her grown children and grandchildren, her mother and sister, and many others, including her former employer, her doctors and nurses and even a particularly supportive HMO:

As we get closer to the center of my village we reach my circle of friends. I can't begin to tell you about the love, kindness and support that I receive from them. They go to appointments with me, sit with me during chemo treatments, keep my spirits up, take me away from it all every

once in awhile. They allow me to talk of death and any fears that might
be laying around in the darkness—we laugh together and cry together. I
am truly blessed with their unconditional love and understanding.

Not everyone is as fortunate, of course. As their cancer progresses, some people with metastatic disease find that extended family and friends start avoiding them, and stop coming for visits or even calling. They may begin to isolate themselves still more in response to this real or perceived pulling away. PJ Hagler felt as if people around her were beginning to withdraw from her.

> *I have been noticing that those around me are pulling away. People*
> *are saying "good-bye" before I'm ready to go. It's as if I have been given a*
> *death sentence that no one wants to deal with. I still have plans for a long*
> *life, yet others seem to have given up on me. Some at church are young*
> *and I think they are scared at the idea that someone even close to their*
> *age is dying before their eyes. My son is dealing with this by pretending*
> *nothing is different. He won't come around much because he cried the last*
> *time I saw him and he's embarrassed and afraid he might do it again. My*
> *sister has stopped calling since she left here. She visited in February and I*
> *think for the first time in her life she realized this could kill me. She used*
> *to call almost weekly with a new cure, now she is running away. Mike*
> *and I used to go out on weekends with close friends to dinner or the mov-*
> *ies. I don't even hear from them. Friends at church who I have always*
> *been very close to just say, "You look fine, you'll be fine, get well soon,"*
> *and then they exit. My very good friend and her husband, who Mike and*
> *I used to go out with almost every other weekend to dinner, or movie, or*
> *wherever, has disappeared. She was in church a week ago and told Mike*
> *to give me a hug and tell me to get well soon. Get well soon! It's very*
> *weird. Even my family is having a difficult time talking to me. I know*
> *they're scared, so am I.*
>
> *But I'm not dead yet.*

Joleene Kolenburg reflected upon the work she had done before cancer forced her retirement, which had made her sensitive to issues cancer patients often face in social and work situations.

> *In my work as benefits manager, it was my "job" to visit the ones who*
> *were seriously ill. How many times I saw them go for days without a visit*

except mine. And these were all people that had a wonderful, caring church family. One fellow asked me once, "Are people afraid of me?" I told him that some people just can't handle this. And we have to understand.

I think the hardest thing for me after I was diagnosed with mets to the lungs was going to church and facing those who loved me so much. I could not bear to see their faces. But I knew that it would be harder as time went on. So I marched in with a big smile on my face and greeted people (even those that were trying to avoid me). Once we got through the initial meeting, it was okay. Of course the tears did come, but it got easier each time. It just takes time.

I guess the problem is that people do not know what we want. There are two ladies at my church that I hate to talk to. Yesterday the one said, "How are you?" I started to explain that my feet were much better and that I was walking some without a cane. But then in that sad voice, she said, "Are you in any pain? Can you breathe all right?" I told her that I have no pain, no trouble breathing, and I just want to enjoy life. Someone walked in just then who had gone to lunch with me last week. I told her I was trying to convince this other lady that I was okay. She said, "She's all right," and the lady said "But...but...." I said, "Yes, I do have cancer, and it is not going away, but I feel fine, and let me enjoy these good days." So what do I want? Sometimes I want people to listen to me, sympathize, but I cannot bear the "crepe hangers" that are preparing for the dinner at the church after my funeral.

From her own negative reactions, Kim Banks developed a clear sense of what she wanted from friends:

I have been feeling lately—a disappointment that the majority of friends and relatives respond to my explanations of recent treatments with, "But, you sure look good." I know that they think they are paying me a compliment or are providing encouragement, but it feels to me as if they are discrediting my illness or assume I must not be that sick if I look this good.

Four months ago, a college roommate, Carla, was diagnosed with breast cancer. She has been having a particularly rough time with chemo and I mentioned that to another friend of ours, Tracy. Tracy replied that

Carla must be doing OK because her last letter had been so upbeat. This comment also made me think about what I would prefer hearing from friends and family. Here are a few things I would rather hear:

"I'm so sorry you're having to go through this. Is there anything I can do for you?"

"How is the radiation/chemo going?"

"How are you feeling?"

"If you need to talk, please don't hesitate to call."

"How is your family doing?"

"This must be a terrible thing to go through. I will pray for you."

Sometimes, while their intentions are good, people just don't know how to treat cancer patients—especially if the cancer is at an advanced stage. They may need some help and encouragement to approach you. People's own fears and fantasies often interfere with simple gestures of concern and caring. Part of this is simple human nature. Most of us fight an impulse to withdraw, to avoid confronting the painful evidence of mortality. As some of these quotes show, even when others don't physically withdraw, a common response is to minimize or deny the severity of the illness on the one hand, or to be prematurely "hanging crepe" on the other. Neither response is particularly welcome or helpful, however. What cancer patients hunger for is to be treated in a concerned, matter-of-fact, straightforward way. Even when your disease is no longer curable, encountering your friends' ill-concealed looks of pity, or their awkwardness as they struggle not to discuss the obvious, can be very difficult for all concerned.

No one is entirely immune to these responses, not even other cancer patients. One of the more striking examples of this kind of denial among the people I interviewed came from Caren Buffum, who recounted with sadness and regret her own response to a member of the Breast Cancer Discussion List who was dying. In her searching self-examination, Caren uncovered the essence of support:

I thought about Judith and my last exchange with her—and I realized that I must confess my own part in pushing her away. Ironic, because here I am, almost where she was at—but that "almost" makes a big difference. I had been corresponding with Judith for some time when she started writing me about her feeling that she was getting close to the end; she was out of treatment options and her symptoms were getting worse. And there's me, ever the optimist, telling her that it's probably just side effects to the chemo, blah, blah, blah—just trying to cheer her up.

She wrote back, insisting she knew the difference and she was sure it was symptomatic of the cancer. Looking back, I realize that I was refusing to allow her to express her deepest fears, and in all truth, I was not there for her. I should have acknowledged that her fears could be well-grounded and then just expressed my own loving concern. I should have told her I didn't want her to leave, but I had no say in the matter—and that all I could do was be there for her to share her feelings. That no matter how sad I might become by what she shared, I wanted to experience that with her, and that I preferred being sad with her to being without her. That I would not become unduly sentimental, but I would nurture her in any way I could and that I would listen, listen, listen—and I wouldn't feel like I had to say anything unless she wanted to hear my voice.

When I first realized how inappropriate my response had been to her, I felt guilty—I, of all people, how could I not understand what she needed? But I realized that I could not know—because even though we all know we ultimately face death, we are all not at the same distance from it. And more importantly, we all do not have the same perception of how far away we are from it. So Judith felt like she was staring it in the face, while I was holding it at bay with my arm stretched out as far as it would go. I still hold on to faith and hope and believe there is a miracle out there somewhere. I simply wanted Judith to do the same thing. But she was not in the same place as I, and she was at a point where she could no longer do that.

We cannot feel guilty for that divided response—don't leave me / you have my support as you leave—reaction. If even my own precarious situation did not sensitize me to Judith's need, I certainly understand how the people around me feel so inadequate in responding to my situation.

The visible evidence of cancer—the disability and hair loss—are often very difficult. Nancy Gilpatrick dreaded going out and having to deal with the reactions of former friends to the physical changes they saw. Her statement poignantly expresses the universal fears, avoidance and misunderstand-ings—and the acts of compassion—that cancer evokes in the "normal" world.

> *I also have difficulty going out; it feels almost like an agoraphobia. I fear people staring at me in my wheelchair or using the walker. I also fear them "not seeing" me. Tonight, for instance, I had an experience while at a wonderful outdoor concert where some people recognized me and some didn't "see" me. I used to have brilliantly red curly hair that was long and wild. No one missed seeing me. So I've wondered do they not recognize me? No, that's not it. I saw a woman I haven't seen since losing my hair and she came right up to me, hugged me and said what can I do? My response was call me, come visit me. I then realized if people are looking at the woman in the wheelchair or using the walker they would recognize me. It's painful experiencing their "cancer phobia." I do keep going to church and other events I enjoy and value. Some days I have to take a deep breath and give myself a good gentle and compassionate talk. So many prices to pay for this dreaded disease.*

The sense of estrangement from the normal, healthy world can seem acute, at times. When her hair had grown back, Nancy found that it was this that people seemed to focus on. "I'm not supposed to be offended by getting compliments," she wrote, but what she longed for was someone to relate to her inner reality, ask about her illness and what life was *really* like for her. Once again, she found that one authentic response left her feeling less alone.

> *People around me, like in my church community, seem to want to focus mainly on how great my hair looks, I have hair, or it's so curly, etc., etc. They tell me how great I look. Now, don't get me wrong, I love the compliments and love hearing that the outside looks so okay. My problem is that people don't seem to want to hear the real story, how my insides are doing or the latest development. They want me okay and getting on with life. Last Sunday this funk was just starting and I was just going under.... I needed people to connect with me and all my church women, who were there, stayed at arms length away from me telling me how won-derful my hair looked. One friend sat down with me and asked how I was doing, really doing...the tears flowed. Just what I had needed, someone wanting to connect with me. She happens to be a 20+ year breast cancer survivor so she knew exactly what I was talking about with my feelings. I felt so comforted.*

In every cancer patient's life, there are blessed exceptions, people who seem to know instinctively what is important. Kathy Stone wrote gratefully about her grand-daughter's precocious gift for candor:

> My granddaughter, who just had her thirteenth birthday, has already told me that she understands that the chances of me being here for her high school graduation are slim…but that she wanted me to know that no matter when I die, I'll always be right there with her…and she said she knew that I would be proud of her when she graduated and she would know that I was standing right there with her, hugging her when she gets her diploma and awards. She is already planning on getting her college through scholarships because there's no money for it otherwise and she wanted me to know that she was depending on my encouragement even after I died… especially if it was before she achieved her goal, she said. Let me tell you…when your grandkids can talk so openly and freely with you it not only fills your heart, but it makes everything so much easier.

Bob Stafford spoke of the qualities he prized most in friendship:

> The support of friends has been immensely important. To know that they care and I can call on them for help. They also treat me normally and allow me to talk openly about what is going on. I made some new friends last year. They are a neat couple, and very real. They know what is happening. She said to her husband one night, "We're going to get real close and love them, aren't we? Then he's going to die." They've decided to stick it through with us. Some others have, too. But some can't. Even my mom says that her next trip here will be the last one. My half-sister never stops by. We know who our real friends are nowadays. They're the ones who will let us say anything we want and know that it's part of what we're going through. And they still love us and don't try to impart guilt or judgment.

At the same time that former friends and some family members may withdraw, others are likely to step forward—particularly those who may have experienced something similar in their own lives, and feel a sense of empathy. Friendship and real help can come from surprising and unanticipated sources.

While everything I've written about social avoidance may be true, it's equally true that as cancer becomes a more familiar part of daily life, as people acknowledge its commonplace reality, more and more of them will reach out with help and support. The old taboos about talking honestly about terminal illness and the dying process are beginning to crumble.

For Gerry Wirth, it turned out to be the members of the scuba diving club he and Cindy had belonged to before her illness who rallied round, as well as members of their church group.

> At the end, when Cindy's death was near, we had two kinds of friends. First, there were phone friends. They would call once in a while, but that was it. Then there were doorbell friends. These people kept coming to the door even when the outcome was evident. What set these people apart was that they were always there, no matter how dark and desperate the situation was. I could live another 100 years and not be able to repay them for their kindness. I guess I will trust God to do that.

Not only did the doorbell friends provide emotional support, but they helped with a myriad of practical needs that Gerry himself was ill-equipped to handle at that time, dealing with two young children. With profound gratitude, Gerry recalls the help that Cindy's friend Mary Jacobs offered during her illness.

> Mary and Cindy were friends from church and our parish school. They were instrumental in continuing our Sunday Bible Stories for preschool children. I think Mary was Cindy's closest friend outside the family at the end. Mary helped make things nice for the kids when Cindy couldn't. Cindy and Mary carpooled to school and play-group activities. When Cindy was too sick to drive or go, Mary would make sure the kids were not left out. We visited their house two weeks before Cindy died. We went over on a Saturday night for pizza. I had to carry Cindy from the car because she was so weak. But once inside, it was like everything was normal, the kids played and the "girls talked." Cindy was starting to withdraw at that time, perhaps preparing to die, but for that one last night she was full of life.

Just as crucial during the course of Cindy's illness was the help provided by both sets of parents:

> My parents are elderly. My dad is currently 80, my mom is 79. Yet they were like marathon runners, always there in a slow, steady pace. When Cindy was in hospital, they watched the children so I could visit. When I needed to take Cindy to the emergency room at 3:00 am, they are

who I called. They made us Christmas dinner while Cindy was in San Francisco getting her treatment.

Her parents were forced into the role of sprinters. They live 300 miles away. Yet they are much younger than my parents so their support was more concentrated and focused. They would stay with Cindy when I had to travel for several days due to business. They were great to visit when the cabin walls closed in!

Filled with gratitude over the fine help from family and friends that they all received over the entire course of her illness, Gerry reflected on the advice he might offer other patients and their families faced with a similar situation:

There are two keys to support. First, you have to ask for it. Most people have good intentions, but do not know how to help. Asking for specific help is what is required. At first, asking can be hard. It is hard to admit that you can't handle it. No single person can deal with the illness and the family alone. You have to be humble enough to ask. Second, you need to allow them to say no. It is important that they never feel that they are obligated or trapped. This could lead to resentment and bitterness. You have to ask for help in a way that demonstrates that "no" is an okay answer.

Patients often have decidedly mixed feelings about involving some members of their families in their care, particularly when it comes to informing them about the progress of their disease. Sometimes it is the lack of family reaction that is hurtful, as Joleene Kolenburg found:

I have two brothers and two sisters who live in the same general area as me. None more than 300 miles away. However, I have one brother that lives in Alabama and another in Florida. My brother from Florida just spent three days in a local motel and we visited during this time. The brother from Alabama came two weeks ago for overnight. This was the first of my family that have come to see me. This has really been hard on me, because we have always been a close family. I have always been the one, however, who organized the get-togethers and the visits to the various members of the family. Finally, I wrote some of my brothers and said I really needed a sibling visit. That's the reason for the two from the distance coming. Yesterday, the one brother who was here two weeks ago called to see if anyone else had visited me. I was sure they had been on the phone talking about me. (I had told my first brother that I knew they would come to my funeral, but I would really like to have them visit me now.) This brother today told me that he had told the younger brothers who live in this general area of the country that they should not wait too long. Of course that made me cry, but that is just what I was thinking weeks ago, when I thought I might die from the treatment.

I wonder what would convince my family that I really do have cancer. No, I didn't have a stroke or a heart attack, but it is not "behind me now." We are a complex people and we do have to let others know how we want to be treated, I believe. It is easy to do with some. Impossible with others.

Bob Stafford reported almost the opposite problem, as he described his mother's reaction to learning about the spread of his cancer:

I didn't tell my parents right away. I told my brother so that he would know, but asked him not to tell my mother. She's had to watch many of her relatives, including a sister and her father, die from cancer and I knew the news would be rough on her. I also didn't know what she would do. When I told her and said how extensive it was, she didn't say much, but later she called and said that she and dad were going to buy a mobile home only five miles from my house. That caused a fight between us because I knew that I had longer to live than she thought. I did not want her camping out at my house waiting for me to die. I did not want her trying to take over my family. I love and respect her, but knew that being that close would not be good.

Kim Banks was also concerned about her family's reaction.

My parents, in-laws and sister worry about me a lot, so I find myself often downplaying my condition to alleviate their worrying. I know that I can't eliminate their worries and would feel bad if they weren't concerned about me. Again, the cancer has actually brought us all closer. I "talk" with my sister almost daily over e-mail. Before the cancer, we called each other around once a month.

As with my husband, my family often feels helpless in helping me fight this disease. They visit more often and pamper us while they're here. Mom and my sister, Julie, cook and clean while my Dad runs errands and plays handyman around the house. My sister-in-law, Laura, a fellow

*writer, visits and inspires me to keep on writing. My in-laws call fre-
quently to inquire about how I'm doing and send me articles and books.
At first I resisted a lot of the help, saying that it was unnecessary, and felt
out of place, not doing the tasks I've always been responsible for. Then I
realized how much better they felt doing those things for me and I relaxed
and enjoyed the pampering. It also gives Richard a break from some of the
extra work he's taken on. And best of all, a whole lot of love is exchanged
in the process.*

Whatever their fears, people are often glad to help. They feel happy to be
given a way to relieve their feelings of powerlessness, and will respond with
extraordinary generosity to a family's needs. Social and church friends
helped Gerry and Cindy Wirth to cover some of the costs of expensive transportation for treatments, as well as the treatments themselves:

*Last October Cindy mentioned that we were running out of insur-
ance benefits. In an instant, there was a fund-drive at the church. It
raised $4,000 in three weeks. Earlier, during her trips to San Francisco
for treatment, the scuba club had several fund raisers to help.*

Bob Stafford also found that people showed their concern about the months
of financial hardship his family faced.

*Most people wait too long to apply for disability benefits. We stress
our bodies out and that doesn't help in the battle against cancer. One of
the things we don't realize is that there is a six-month wait before benefits
begin. Most families have a very difficult time financially during this time
because no one seems prepared for this economic hardship. We've known
other families who didn't fare so well during this waiting period, so we feel
very blessed to have been watched over by others. But we were taken care
of by lots of people. The churches in the area took up collections for us
and brought lots of food for the family. My wife continued to work. And
God was good to us.*

Day by day, cancer patients and their families do manage to cope with the
isolation and stigma the disease evokes. If you are open, if you will only ask,
surprising acts of generosity, companionship and love will often come into
your life. From unanticipated sources, the help and support you need will
make itself known. But you must seek it out. You must take action. If these
stories speak to you, if you see yourself and the people you love here on

these pages, take some comfort in the strengths reflected here. In this nation of individualists, we somehow are led to believe in self-reliance and stoicism as the highest goal. These stories show something else: that we are interdependent rather than independent, that we discover our best selves in relationship with others. And when the need arises, we are pretty good at taking care of one another.

CHAPTER 10

Light and Shadow

Stories of Remission, Work and Identity

IN THE COURSE OF METASTATIC BREAST CANCER, there are often resting places, times when treatment and disease will not be playing a central role in your life. This chapter touches on the issues that belong to these sometimes extended periods, in particular the difficulties you may have with rejoining the "normal" world—the re-evaluation of priorities, the discovery of a balance between optimism and realism, the continued apprehension surrounding testing and new symptoms, and the awkward alterations in time sense as some sort of a future begins to seem possible again.

This can also be a time to reflect on what has happened. The story of Jenilu Schoolman is offered as an example of how one survivor did just that, writing the story of her own lengthy remission. Finally, the importance of work and career in your life are explored, as well as the impact of disability retirement, and other ways of seeking out sources of meaning.

"I am not busy dying"

The weeks, months and years spent in remission are often difficult for people with metastatic breast cancer and their families. Apprehension mingles with gratitude, and the sense of expectation and dread of a new recurrence of the disease both diminishes daily life and heightens its moments. There is a sense of return to daily life, but it is a return informed by a new sense of fragility and impermanence.

After a course of tamoxifen put Pam Hiebert into an extended period of remission, her partner, Sylvan Rainwater, felt that she could finally put their experience with cancer into words that took the form of a poem:

Now Maybe

Now maybe
Now maybe I can write
Now maybe I can write
the cancer poem
Now that the hair has grown back
Now that the daily threat
of separation forever
has receded
Now that uncertainty has replaced
certain doom
Now that the medical crisis has passed
Now that solid remission—
"no evidence of cancer"
has driven away
daily doctors, hospitals, clinics
Now that all the processing we've done
all those countless hours
of talking, crying, breathing together
has brought us to a balance
of acceptance and struggle and gratitude
for now

The terror of that time
still makes me shudder
memories vivid and painful
still make me cry
Then
we took no pictures
wrote no poems
just kept our heads down
into the wind

Now that we're both working
full-time
Now that we exercise regularly
at our own health club
Now that we eat at home more
low-fat meals
Now that our worries are
budgets, car repair, and buying a new computer

Now maybe I can write
the cancer poem.

In his book *Living Beyond Limits*, psychiatrist Dr. David Spiegel recounts some of the factors that make up the state of mind common to metastatic cancer patients once their treatment has been completed:

> *While life can pretty much get back to normal, it will never be the same. You have been diagnosed with a life-threatening illness. You have come face-to-face with a vulnerability we would all like to ignore. You cannot feel quite as insulated from danger as you did before. In part this is because the actual nature of your dying has taken shape. You can visualize the unthinkable because its form has become all too real.[1]*

Many patients struggle with priorities and choices during this time. Should they take a special dreamed-about journey now, while they are well enough to do so? Should a family's tight resources be used to fulfill lifelong wishes and construct treasured memories for later on, or should previous long-term goals be kept in mind?

The sense of regained normalcy is now forever coupled with a sense of imperative and a strangeness that places one outside the healthy world. Jenilu Schoolman was acutely aware of what separated her from others around her.

> *Frankly, remission is an awkward place because I am not busy dying. In fact, beyond the normal wear and tear of aging, I now look and feel as well as I did before I became ill. But I have not been able to go ahead with my life simply as though nothing had happened.*

Moments of panic

The uneasy truce of remission is punctuated by moments of panic, when any physical symptom raises the possibility that the cancer is active and growing again. Surprisingly, perhaps, this represents a commonality shared by high-risk and metastatic patients alike. Glenn Clabo recounts one such familiar moment:

> *One of those big old smelly boots came out of the sky and hit us in the head. The short version... She woke up to pee while I was getting ready for work. She almost fell over but made it back to the bed okay. When she*

lay down and closed her eyes the room began to spin. Panic! When she called for me she was pretty scared and so was I. It settled down after awhile and she was okay in a couple of hours.

OK, decision time... Should she talk to the doc or should she wait to see if it happened again? Being a man I said, let's see. She felt, because of the upcoming trip, she wanted to get checked out to be sure. Again to make a long story short.... We went to the doc and she was scheduled for an MRI of the brain the next day.

As you know, this is one of those things that flashes back all the memories from the past "it probably isn't anything" discussions we had with doctors. It was a tough couple of hours when we got home. It wasn't a bad couple hours...just tough. It was one of those moments when we let some stuff out about being afraid and not saying things that we want to because it always sounds like we are saying good-bye. It was a good moment....

What Glenn refers to as a boot from the sky is more commonly spoken of in terms of the proverbial Sword of Damocles hanging overhead. The sense of dread that permeates daily life for a metastatic cancer patient—and even for very high risk patients—is difficult to describe. While others may try, more or less successfully, to suppress thoughts of further recurrence and disease progression, or entertain optimistic beliefs about cure and remedies, the people interviewed for this book have chosen another way to "prepare" themselves. Armed with knowledge, involved with other survivors, they have chosen to live day by day—never feeling that they are very far from another skirmish with cancer and its treatments. This takes a certain toll in anxious moments.

Bonnie Gelbwasser wrote of the poignant awareness of this fragile time:

Since my ABMT, I have had a skin biopsy, a lumpectomy, a rib biopsy and an MRI to rule out recurrence, so my life isn't exactly a smooth ride, but I do okay and as I undergo more and more of these tests, I become less fearful of the future. I'm just going along for the ride—and what a ride it has been.

I am fine and celebrating my "promotion" to three-month appointments. It took me three years to get here. I am optimistic that I will remain medically stable for the foreseeable future; I appreciate the careful monitoring but still cope with the fears that these tests and office visits engender. However, the last few months have given me a welcome respite. Yesterday, my first three-monther, my oncologist felt my shoulder blades and said, "My God, you are so tense!" "What do you expect?" I responded. "I am terrified to be here."

This is a woman who is dedicated to her job, lost her mom to breast cancer and is very sensitive to all of us (I know many people in her care) but who apparently sometimes underestimates the stress of these office visits. I told her that I "do" cancer very well. I can talk and write about the disease and sound very wise and I can offer hope and encouragement and advice to breast cancer patients facing ABMT. What I do not do well is my cancer. When I am half naked on that examining table and this young physician is moving her fingers over my body with the intensity and concentration of a rocket scientist, I am not calm. I am watching her eyes and waiting for those fingers to stop and wondering what she will ask me about or make an appointment for.

And I understand it never gets better. As my mother says about her widowhood, "It doesn't get easier, you just get used to it."

For Ellen Scheiner, who had also undergone an intensive chemotherapy regimen, it was her awareness of her mortality and impermanence on an immediate emotional level—as opposed to an intellectual awareness—that affected her most.

Shortly after I finished chemotherapy, I had a kind of epiphany. I have been studying meditation with a Buddhist-trained teacher for some years and have been meditating for 17 years. One day I realized that I would die. Not necessarily of cancer, but of something—since we all will die. My experience as a physician and my meditation training have removed a great deal of fear about dying. When I had this experience I realized, in the most visceral sense, that there was nothing that I could count on and that nothing was permanent. For several weeks I was in a state of free fall. I knew, in the deepest sense, that all of our plans are tentative. Sometimes we make them to fill the future to assure ourselves that we will still be here then. Gradually I felt more and more freedom. I began to differentiate between made-up plans and real goals—those acts that truly are right for me. What a release that was.

Past-present-future: Changes in time sense

In remission, a sense of the future as possibility begins to re-emerge. In her book, *Good Days, Bad Days*, sociologist Kathy Charmaz believes that as patients move from immersion in symptoms and treatment into remission, their relation to time changes. Where in the past-present-future continuum do you locate yourself? And how does this change with the course of the disease?

Charmaz believes that for someone in the course of active treatment or disease progression, living in the present moment often becomes an important strategy for containing and controlling thoughts and feelings about the future and past.

> *Living one day at a time allows people to focus on illness, treatment and regimen without being overcome by dashed hopes and unmet expectations.... Living one day at a time mutes "negative" emotions—fear, guilt, anger, and self-pity—and even gives one a sense of control over them.... By exerting control over the day, people avoid feeling that managing illness is an unbearable life sentence.*[2]

Then, when a person emerges from illness and treatment, the immediate crisis ends and a greater or lesser period of remission begins, leading to a shift in perspective as the continuum of past-present-future expands to include past and future once again. What Charmaz refers to as "mapping a future" begins anew, as the patient starts entertaining plans and expectations that involve projection into the weeks, months and even years to come. At the same time, energy is devoted to "recapturing the past," as people make efforts to restore and regain lost aspects of self—activities, roles, functions— that had been a central part of life before the intensity of illness and treatment. "A desire to recapture the past reflects yearning for a lost self," Charmaz observes.

Sue Tokuyama, another of the high-risk patients I interviewed who underwent high-dose chemotherapy, mourns for that lost healthy self. Since her children are young, she's acutely aware of the possibility that her cancer may return and take her from them.

One of the things that breast cancer has taken away is the feminine phases of aging. I never expected to experience menopause at 33. I wanted to have a third child. Breast cancer has irrevocably prevented me from being beautiful. Before cancer, I could tell myself that I would be a goddess if I could just lose weight and shape up. Now, I will never be naturally beautiful, I will always be someone very different in my skin than who I was.

Recovering from a stroke, the writer May Sarton, who also had breast cancer, described this transition.

...to manage such a passive waiting life for so many months I have had to bury my real self—and now realize that bringing that real self back is going to be even more difficult than it was to bury it.[3]

Telling stories

Susan Sontag, along with many others, has observed how a serious illness transports people to alien territory. The strangeness of the medical world with its sterile universe of hospitals and clinics, its strange treatments and technologies, all catapult a cancer patient into another world.

Illness is the night-side of life, a more onerous citizenship. Everyone who is born holds dual citizenship, in the kingdom of the well and in the kingdom of the sick. Although we all prefer to use only the good passport, sooner or later each of us is obliged, at least for a spell, to identify ourselves as citizens of that other place.[4]

Often the means of reintegration into the flow of life comes in the form of a story or narrative, observing what Charmaz refers to as "time markers" and "turning points." People who have been very ill, who've returned for the moment from "that other place," often have the need to tell their stories, to construct a chronology of illness that integrates what has happened to them with the flow of ordinary life. Whatever form this may take, whether written in the pages of a journal, or told to a friend or a therapist, this storytelling is often a healing process. "Retelling the event becomes a means of sorting, defining, and clarifying old sentiments that constitute the self."[5] It is a way of rediscovering and reclaiming the person you were who has been immersed or temporarily obscured by illness. Remission inspires this sort of retrospective frame of mind.

Often, anniversaries spur such reflections. A year and some months after Barb's diagnosis with Stage IV breast cancer, Glenn Clabo paused, looking back at all they had been through:

> It was the most confusing, absolutely terrifying, and all-consuming time of my life. Every moment was interrupted by the thoughts of losing Barb.
>
> Now it's been more than a year and she's still here. Although we are still consumed by the thoughts, our lives have changed so much that we hardly recognize who we were before this monster came into our lives. We always feel that we could have done without this....However, it was the slap in the face that made us both realize what a real gift life is. No longer are things that make us feel good put off until tomorrow. Just breathing has become an absolute joy.

Pam Hiebert took the time to reflect on the time of remission she was enjoying, as well as what she would be likely to do with that time.

> I do not know why, but I am three years out and showing no evidence of cancer. Maybe the Chinese herbs, the adequate sleep I give myself, or the love I share with my partner and my family of origin. I find I spend my days going "to" something, rather than asking myself so many why questions. Oh yes, I think the cancer will be back. I think that this uncertainty of when could drive me bananas if I let it. But I am also determined to think of myself as "living with cancer" rather than having cancer.
>
> I have worked with writing in journals to help clarify what I desire, so I can have an idea of what it is I want to do with this sacred time I have now. From this writing I know that further chemo will be something I may choose as a way of extending the periods between recurrence. I shudder at the idea of choosing to do chemo once again, but I believe that I can adapt and manage to find some enjoyment in my life journey. And I do not dwell on trying to imagine the extent of pain and suffering that lies before me. For me there is no future (as I once knew) but only the "now."

Seeking the possible

Once people have had their innocent confidence in the future shattered and have come out on the wrong side of medical odds, often repeatedly, it is difficult for them to remain optimistic. Nevertheless, most regain this capacity. Psychologist Shelley Taylor suggests how this is possible:

> When a person experiences personal setbacks or tragedies, the mind responds with cognitively adaptive efforts. Just as the need for control, a positive sense of self, and an optimistic view of the future are essential for normal functioning and for meeting the small rebuffs of everyday life, they appear to be essential to the readjustment process following more devastating events. The themes around which these adjustments occur include an attempt to restore self-esteem, an effort to regain a sense of mastery, and a search for meaning in the experience.[6]

A "downward" comparison with "less fortunate others," as Taylor refers to it, is one common way in which people who are ill manage to feel better about their own circumstances. There seems to be a human tendency, Taylor and other researchers have found, for people in difficult circumstances to compare their plight with the real or imagined predicaments of those worse off than they are. If you are in remission, you're bound to be aware of other women whose disease is progressing. You may find this knowledge painful—yet the awareness of your own "fortunate by comparison" current reality also provides some comfort and hope. At times there can also be a sense of bittersweet remorse to the suspended, indefinite state of remission, almost a "survivor's guilt," as Pam Hiebert expresses in this poem addressed to a friend close to death from breast cancer:

> Who am I to have this emerging space to thus
> wait out the end that comes so near for you?
> To feel the surprising thaw in this gloomy winter's
> rock hard season. The suffering sounds
> I too have wailed too well.
> To see another's space swallowed while mine
> is neither in afterlife nor in full regress.

For Sharon Multhauf, a lengthy remission both prior to and following her first recurrence provides her with evidence of the long-term survivability of her disease.

> After nearly eight years, I had a recurrence at the site of the original tumor, accompanied by bone mets. Since the ER/PR results this time were strongly positive, I began tamoxifen, and that has been my only (conventional) therapy for more than two years.

*There are three of us in my face-to-face support group who recurred after seven, eight, and thirteen years, and we are all apparently hosting **very** lazy cancers that took a long time to reappear and are moving at a snail's pace, if at all, in the presence of tamoxifen. If you get a long remission under your belt, the chances are better that if a recurrence does show up, it will be indolent and more likely controllable. No promises—just my experience.*

Sharon is also determined to do whatever she can to control her disease, which she now sees as chronic.

*I bristle when I keep hearing that the goal of treatment is palliation. I'm sorry, but I have a much higher goal for my treatment. Sure, I want to get rid of symptoms and feel better, but my main goal is to be able to keep the cancer from spreading any farther in my body—and, if at all possible, to drive it into submission. I want to live to see my children become adults, to share my husband's retirement, maybe even to be a grandmother. If the cancer that is in my bones won't go away, then I will work to find a way to coexist with it for as long as possible. But I don't call this "palliation"—I call it **war**, and surveillance and strategizing are part of my battle plan.*

In the world of metastatic breast cancer, there is a very wide range of survival times. The doctors on my team know that I hope to be far, far to the right on the survival curve, and while they are honest with me about the bad things that enter into my case, they don't try to get me to settle for simply feeling better.

I don't have tumor marker tests done, but I do have blood chemistry tests about every six months, including liver enzymes and calcium levels. I have been having bone scans about every four to six months, with less frequent MRI of my lower spine. My lungs and liver are monitored with CT scans, about six to eight months apart. We want to be able to take action and change therapies when the disease shows progression. Obviously, I can't have a bone scan every month, but I'm not comfortable waiting more than six months either. So we compromise. And we keep our eyes set on the goal of longevity, not simply palliation.

Longevity, with breast cancer presenting as a chronic but controllable disease, does seem possible for some women. At 57, Joan Bengston, a glass artisan who lives in Rochester, Minnesota, has been living with breast cancer for over twenty-two years. First diagnosed in 1974, at age 35, and with multiple skin lesions for the last nine years, she's been told by her radiation oncologist that, while she has no metastases to distant organs or bone yet, recurrences are now inevitable.

> I do not speak "in past tense about events that happened a long time ago." Throughout all the years of my cancer experience I have never really been sick. I have never lost my hair. By all accounts, I have had it very easy. Yet the reality, according to my oncologist, is that even though I have **long** outlived their expectations, as I get older the tumors will become more aggressive, both in their numbers and in their rate of growth. I now know that mine was a serious cancer. I no longer consider myself cured, but in remission, knowing that I will probably have to deal with it again.

> Fear of recurrence or metastases never goes away. The sense of security I had for so many years before recurrence has been taken from me. Yet, the very fact that I have survived this long offers hope for the future.

Barbara Ragland also considers herself a long-term survivor, on her way once again to a state of remission:

> I have survived twenty-two years since my first Stage II breast cancer (in 1974), which had gone into the lymph nodes. Although I've had a recurrence, metastases and a new primary in the remaining breast, I am still a survivor, twenty-two years after the first cancer.

> The oncologist told me on Monday that it looks like we're getting the current problems under control and, if I continue the way I'm going now, he may soon be able to use the term "remission!"

A promotion in her company, which under other circumstances she might jump at, filled Sue Tokuyama with anxiety.

> The thing is, I am really scared to change anything, now that I'm reasonably crisis-free. The thought of managing any kind of transition like that is quite daunting. I really like getting up in the morning, getting the kids ready for preschool, picking up my paper and coffee at the train station, catching the 7:50 express and marching into the office at 8:35. I'm afraid that any kind of stress will invite the beast back (sort of like, "speak

of the devil..."). Part of me says, "Seize the moment!" and part of me says, "Keep things under control!" And what about the TRAM? And what about my renovations, and my garden and my daughter's plans to start kindergarten in September?

> Pre-breast cancer, I would have jumped at the opportunity. Post-breast cancer, I am conscious of myself as a fragile organism. I think I also project this fragility onto people around me, especially the kids. Now, in addition to the amorphous "mother-guilt," I have "cancer-guilt." What am I doing to my kids emotionally in dealing with this disease?

As remission extends and the intensity of active treatment recedes, the day-to-day sense of ordinary life expands and along with that, the surprise that some things haven't changed at all. It's also a time when other problems that may have been deferred during crises rush in to demand their due.

Jenilu's story

When Jenilu Schoolman decided to write about her experience with breast cancer, a memoir entitled *Within Measured Boundaries*,[7] she was eight years into a remission following a recurrence of the cancer to her liver. A psychotherapist and weaver, Jenilu was able to look back at this time of remission as a series of stages she passed through.

> To make even death a time to reflect, to learn and to grow, I watched myself and tried to extract meaning as I moved through this final experience. Since I feel the measure of people is not what happens to them but rather what they make of the things that happen to them, I decided to note my own progress through this frightening, though interesting, journey in the uncharted land I know as remission.

The early stages following Jenilu's diagnosis with metastatic disease and initial treatment will be familiar to you already: the panic and intensity of diagnosis, the "holding my breath" time when chemotherapy was beginning its work, the feelings of "profound sadness" at knowing the disease was not likely to be curable. "Wait and watch" were the words she used to describe her state of mind as she entered remission, and struggled with wanting to get on with life.

> There were fewer **intense** conversations during this period. The people around me seemed to calm down and my well-being was less fre-

quently questioned. I was looked at without that expression of focused concern as people inquired, "How are you?" I don't know if the reality of my illness was being denied, but the topic began to move out of the forefront of conversations. Thank goodness! It does get boring to be so self-involved.

With her doctor's permission, she eagerly planned for a long-awaited trip to Peru. Her old hiking boots were nearly worn out, but she couldn't bring herself to spend the money for expensive hiking boots she wasn't likely to wear again. It seemed like a waste of money. But the real challenge, coming home after the successful trip, was to decide how to go on living.

Somewhat reluctantly, Jenilu went back to work, and resumed as much of her normal life as she could. Sometimes, she wrote, she felt like an impostor.

> *The reality is I am going to die of cancer, but it certainly doesn't feel like it. It was confusing. I am grateful to be alive, and every day I wonder why I am still alive. I wonder what I should do or not do to keep this miracle going. I want to go on and act as if this were all a bad dream or like any other surgery that I've recovered from, but I can't. It is not the same. I can't act as if I were dying and withdraw from life. I am still well and who knows how long this will last. What if I live for years like this? I have to go on working, playing, loving.*

> *In those days, the rest of the world acted as if all were well, but it never felt that way to me. I felt I was balancing on the center of the teeter-totter. I had to plan ahead, but not too far. When you have terminal cancer, how much of your income do you set aside for retirement?*

> *Also, without prematurely welcoming it, how do I maintain an awareness and acceptance of the moment when the illness begins again? I don't want to give up even one hour of good time to the illness if I don't have to. Yet it is hard not to become preoccupied with worries over what will happen or when.*

Finally, Jenilu bought herself a new pair of hiking boots, as she entered the phase she described as a "Rebirth of Hope." Over the next few years, there were trips to Africa and then to Nepal and New Zealand. She bred the llamas she kept for their wool. She decided to build another barn and clear more pasture for the animals. "I still believe I'll die of cancer," she wrote, "but maybe I can postpone death a while longer. In the meantime, I've got barns to build, dreams to dream." In September, 1993 eight years into her remission, Jenilu wrote:

> *And so, with great gratitude, and the awareness of the sword still swinging over my head, I continue to try to live my life gracefully. If, as Joseph Campbell, the noted anthropologist, says, the point of life is to experience the ecstasy of being alive, remission daily gives me the opportunity to feel the passion of existence!*
>
> *This is as far as my journey has taken me, and this is all I know. I will continue, as I am able, to note my trail as it crosses this wild and seemingly uncharted terrain.*

Jenilu would have enjoyed this story that Pam Hiebert told.

> *One of my cancer friends, who happens to be a Tibetan Buddhist nun, has this way of greeting me. Gilda will put her arms around me (and I her) and she will say, "Aren't you dead yet?" Lately, I've begun to do the same. "Aren't you dead yet?" I will ask her while displaying a big grin. We both get a huge chuckle from this. I'm sure this greeting would sound very strange to most people. When we bring those great fears to the foreground, Gilda and I find a common ground to unite with one another. Something like a salute to the unknown or maybe a recognition that it ain't over till the fat lady sings. There's something about calling death by its name that releases me to life.*

Although they never met, Jenilu would also have found in Lucie Bergmann-Shuster a kindred spirit.

> *Personally, when I learned of my mets and in the months before, I was willing to let go and accepted my impending death with serenity. I was perfectly okay with dying about now, May or June given the seriousness of my illness. My first two chemo treatments did not work and caused continued tumor growth. In those two months, when I felt alert enough to do some serious thinking, I thought about how to deal with the finale. But I still had some spark left in me, so I alerted my docs that the chemo was not working and we switched to my present protocol. Within the first two weeks of treatment, I went from complacency with dying to an upbeat way of looking at my life and my future. Somehow, my brain learned that my cancer was heading into remission and it changed the way I felt. I doubt very much that this transformation was anything that I*

personally engineered or, for that matter, had any control over. Of course once the switch happened, I did do a lot of personal affirmations in terms of prayer and meditation and physical exercise.

Get this: six months ago, I thought I might be dead or close to it. Let me assure you, this past weekend when my husband and I sailed twenty-one miles across the sea to Catalina in gusty winds and a frothing sea on a small sailboat, we were anything but dead, and rather very much more alive than most people. It was a riveting physical and mental challenge, maybe even crazy to do the crossing. We survived and it was wondrous, albeit exhausting, to feel so intensely alive.

Work, identity and meaning

Many of the people I interviewed have been forced by their disease or by the treatments to take extended leaves of absence and even to resign from their work. Unquestionably, this can represent a great loss, not only financially, but in terms of a struggle for self-esteem and loss of purpose. If they are fortunate, work has become a source of pride and identity and meaning. It forms much of the substance of self-reliance and a feeling of contributing to others.

The problem is, the demands of illness often overwhelm people. In her study of people with chronic illnesses, sociologist Kathy Charmaz explains it this way:

*When life becomes founded on illness, illness is not simply intrusive. No longer can people add illness to the structure of their lives; instead, they must **reconstruct** their lives upon illness.... Most of these people don't work. They can't.*[8]

This throws many people into a crisis of identity.

Ill people wonder where illness will take them and ask who they can be during their odyssey—for self and for others. At this point, illness serves as both foundation and focal point of their experience. Ill people ask: Who will I be? How will this condition affect my future? How can I continue to be myself while having relentless illness? What will being dependent do to me? [9]

Having retired from her private practice as a therapist following her Stage IV diagnosis, and preparing for her high-dose chemotherapy, Nancy Gilpatrick reflected:

> Work is so often an important part of our identity, and while we are going through active cancer treatment being a "patient" becomes the primary identity (whether we want it to be or not). As treatment winds down and you enter a disease-free time, then comes the time of looking at the absence of work as part of the identity.

After her recovery from high-dose chemotherapy, further progression of her disease prevented any real thought of a return to her work. The long-awaited hip surgery that would permit her to walk again would have to be postponed indefinitely. Despondent at first, Nancy soon discovered that she had to look elsewhere for satisfaction and self-esteem:

> What I've found is that I'm pulling out other parts of myself that weren't as developed and that I can do now. I can't do my athletic ventures, which is where I put my energy another time I didn't work.... The point is looking inward to see what else is there to occupy and fill my time well; not just let time pass.

When work has served as a source of purpose and normalcy, it is often very difficult for cancer patients to let go of their jobs and careers, even when working may put their health in jeopardy. Barb Pender wrote about how difficult it had been for her to acknowledge when it was time to leave work.

> I have worked continuously throughout my cancer journey. In fact, to the point where I was not helping my situation any. The day after I got home from my transplant, I went to work for a couple of hours. I would have an infection that would land me in the hospital overnight—the doctor would tell me not to go to work for the rest of the week or the next week and I would ignore his instructions. Consequently, I was landing in the hospital more and more often.

> I think it was my need to be productive. I didn't want to go home and wait to die. I wanted to feel needed. Last November my doctor wanted me to talk to a psychologist. He helped me face the fact that I had not given 100 percent to getting healthy—that between work, children, grandchildren, play, home life, I was on overload.

I took the month of December off and my health was wonderful even though I was on weekly Navelbine. The first week in January I happened to be threatened at work by my boss—"write this speech for me or look for work" sort of thing. I immediately spiked a fever and was a wreck for the whole weekend. I made up my mind then that my doctor was right—I needed to concentrate on me. My last day of work was January 31, and I haven't looked back.

Bob Stafford wrote that it was his wife who had first expressed concern that he might not be able to keep up with the demands of his employment.

Finally, in January of 1993, the oncologist suggested starting chemotherapy again. I had been working as a bi-vocational pastor. I ministered in a small rural community and worked on the child unit at a psychiatric hospital. But I was burning the candle at both ends and couldn't keep up much longer. My wife knew work was important and was one of the things keeping me going. We discussed it one night and I confessed that I didn't think I could go on much longer doing all that I was doing. We decided that perhaps I should apply for disability. The next day I went to the Social Security office and applied for disability benefits. A couple days later I started chemotherapy again.

After Barb Clabo's several stays in the hospital with low blood counts, Glenn worried that his wife was pushing herself too hard during the difficult induction chemotherapy she was undergoing prior to high-dose chemotherapy.

The subject of work set her off again last night. She brought it up and all I said was.... You know how I feel. She just can't bear the thought of leaving. I know I'm being over-protective but I think her dedication and her feelings toward her friends there are not as helpful as she thinks. She went into work on Monday, one of her worst days, at 5 a.m. She went in with the intention of just staying for an hour or so to help her replacement do the Monday opening and send off all the reports they have to do. By 9:30, she was exhausted and home on the couch. I didn't say anything, but I was concerned. Of course I can't tie her hospitalizations to that but.... My guess is Barb is just trying to hold on to something that's still real.

For both PJ Hagler and her husband, Mike, the thought of her leaving work permanently represented a disturbing new phase in her illness.

I'm so tired by about noon that I just know I will probably not get back to work. I can't even imagine going back for a few hours. I have so little energy and so much pain—only helped by morphine—that work seems impossible to even consider.... I'm trying to face the reality that my life is changing.

After she agreed to long-term disability, PJ described her sense of finality on the day Mike picked up her things at work.

The hardest part was for Mike. Yesterday things were kind of quiet at work with Veterans Day and a lot of people off, so he went to my office during lunch and boxed it up. He was doing pretty good until Kathy, a lady I was secretary for, came in to see what was going on. She talked to Mike and then she ran out of the office, crying. Well, Mike finished boxing up my office and after he got everything in the car, he called me and we both started crying. He said he thought he was going to be all right with this and so did I but it just seemed so final. Then today I went through the boxes and I just fell apart. I know I won't get back to work and I feel so sad about it.

Joleene Kolenburg commiserated with PJ.

I have been retired for some time, since 1989, but I worked part-time as a bookkeeper for a travel agency for a year and a half. I quit just before I started chemo in January. I was at an anniversary party for the grandparents of my boss at the travel agency, and Barb, my boss, came running up to me and said, "Are you ready to come back?" And that was sad for me, because I knew I could never go back. I laughed and said, "My brain is dead, you wouldn't want me." She said, "We'll work around that." I know how hard it is to give up something that you enjoyed so much.

Not every employer is this understanding. In the down-sized corporate world, action taken against disabled or chronically ill workers can be devastating. For Lisann Charland, the break from work came abruptly, and from an unanticipated source that left her bitter and disillusioned at her former employer.

I had been doing very well physically and emotionally after eight months of chemo and was looking at returning to work. However, my whole world turned upside down after I received a phone call from the

Corporate Office the day before I was scheduled to start on a part-time basis. I could not return to work because the sale of my company had been officially finalized, and the new company's rules do not permit part-time status for people on sick leave. All the hard work I had put in to physically and mentally help me get well just went out the window. I was devastated. I had to re-evaluate my life and make new changes. My fifteen-year career had ended abruptly. Not only did I have to learn to be a non-working girl, but I had to accept that I had to live on disability insurance for the rest of my life. I had to do a lot of soul-searching and talking to myself and crying to get through this. I felt I was penalized by both the old and the new company. I could not believe how much this metastasis had cost me, physically and emotionally. I had to forfeit my raise and promotion effective two weeks after I went on medical leave by my old company, and unbeknownst to me at that time, I had been labeled a "liability" by the new company.

While Pam Hiebert's employer was generally supportive, there were moments when her changed status was difficult to bear.

I had to tell my boss last week that I needed to go in for testing. He quickly blurted out, "You get someone trained right away on your copier system," and I replied, "Even if the tests turned out to be bad, I would never leave without making sure someone could take over for me." This is the worst kind of dependency! I hate it that I am no longer seen as a dependable worker. I am marginalized, even as I live. I struggle not to let myself be victimized, but there's always this silent, subdued energy of dark clouds rising....

I know initially my actual job performance during treatment was grim and it has left deep scars. I felt like I was doing 125 percent of pure grit. But, then again, if grit has a value of .01 cent—125 percent isn't much. I always try to keep myself in a position of having to prove that I am well, rather than being caught in a situation of having to prove that I am sick.

I remember how I would struggle to my job where I would sit like a zombie, unable to process, unable to learn, unable to function. Yet I was there. Just getting there became my major focus. I joked and said, "Heck, I

*can be sick at work, or be sick at home." But secretly, I was terrified of
lying in bed and never getting up. I needed people around me. I needed to
have a schedule.*

Her partner, Sylvan, also remembers how the time during chemotherapy
treatment affected Pam's performance at work.

*Pam would go in some days and just put her head down on her desk,
finding that the effort to get to work exhausted her, but feeling that staying home and feeling miserable would have been even worse. People were
supportive at work, but she clearly wasn't able to contribute much.*

In treatment again after many years of remission, Barb Ragland wondered
how long she'd be able to continue to work.

*I had hoped to tough it out until retirement in December, but I'm so
weary now, I wonder if I can make it. With the stress from these things,
along with the effects of the drugs, radiation, etc., I crawl out of bed at
5:30 or 6:00 in the morning and don't get home until 5:30 p.m. when I
collapse and am in bed usually by 7:30.*

Barb found that her employer, a state university, worked with her in planning what was best, as she weighed the available options:

*I have discussed disability with my employer—the Dean—who says
I need to think of my health first although he sure hates the thought of me
leaving.*

*The university benefits counselor suggested I start right now, either
working just four days a week to use up my vacation time and sick leave,
or start disability right away. By the time I use up all my sick leave and
vacation time, the benefits counselor said that for the last seven weeks
that I won't have income, I could draw Catastrophic Leave.*

Long accustomed to self-reliance, Barb had some difficulty accepting this
kind of help.

*However, since I am a state employee, this plan looks good to me.
The benefits counselor kept stressing that it was a state benefit that I had
earned and I shouldn't hesitate taking it. I guess in the back of my mind I
envision welfare. My comforting thoughts now are that since I've just*

started my second week on medical disability retirement, I will have time to do things that I want to do when I want to do them. I don't like the reason that I've had to retire early, but I plan to enjoy it while I can.

Finding other interests

If you choose to, or are forced to retire from your work, on disability or otherwise, it makes good sense to strive to develop other meaningful activities, or to follow already existing interests, now that you have more time to do so.

The crucial thing to avoid is isolation and inactivity. Often, if you stay in contact with people, new possibilities will come about through opportunities and connections you hadn't anticipated. But you must be open to them. In exploring the Internet and participating in the Breast Cancer Discussion Group, Bob Stafford found a way in which he could make a real contribution, and eventually developed a website and discussion list for men with breast cancer. Other discussion lists for kids who were ill and who were dealing with a family member's illness derived from his concern as a father for his son and daughter.

> *I "retired" in January of 1993. And was almost immediately lost because I didn't have a whole lot to do. Bought a new computer system and started learning new things that I could do. Also played with the many radios I've acquired. And now I have a new "job".... So even if you don't go back to work you still need to find some activity to become involved in.*

Barb Pender describes herself as a "late bloomer," returning to college following her divorce and enjoying her work coordinating math and science camps for middle and high school students. This past year, she's had to let all that go, because of her health, but she hasn't let this slow her down.

> *My interests are many! I keep in touch with my "students" and we try to meet once a month for pizza and chit-chat. My 15-year-old son is involved in rodeo—he is a bull and bareback bronc rider. So I am busy traveling to his various rodeos around the western states, cheering him on and taking great pictures of him! I also spend the better part of my week caring for my grandchildren while their mother, also divorced, works to support them. I wouldn't change that for anything—they're wonderful!! I also make time for various crafts and projects—I make angels, do*

needlework, collect dolls, tea sets, Hard Rock Cafe pins, McDonald's and Burger King toys and anything else I can get my hands on. I have a terrific life!!

Barb's capacity to find the positive aspects in the adversity of her experience has also led to her being asked to speak on several occasions before audiences of breast cancer survivors. Barb, and others who have become involved with groups dealing with breast cancer advocacy and support, have transformed the experience of having cancer into a focal point and source of meaning in their lives.

Speaking out, in itself, can become meaningful work. The people who agreed to be interviewed for this book have inherited a legacy of activism, briefly evoked here by poet and feminist Audre Lorde, who lived with metastatic breast cancer for many years, and died in 1992. Two months after her diagnosis, in 1977, Lorde entitled her speech to the Modern Language Association, "The Transformation of Silence into Language and Action." Her words speak to those who find the courage to tell of their experiences, whether or not they call themselves activists.

> *I have come to believe over and over again that what is most important to me must be spoken, made verbal and shared, even at the risk of having it bruised or misunderstood. That the speaking profits me, beyond any other effect...In becoming forcibly and essentially aware of my mortality, and of what I wished and wanted for my life, however short it might be, priorities and omissions become strongly etched in a merciless light, and what I most regretted were my silences.10*

Of course, there are many avenues to be pursued. Many people will find the most meaning in continuing the work that was already theirs, before their illness. Some are able to stay at work until the final months or weeks of their illness. Caren Buffum, who taught until two months before her death, described her own relationship to her work at different times during her illness:

> *The year I was participating in a Taxol study at the NIH, I was also teaching full-time. I would fly down to Washington every three weeks for three days. To do this, I had to write out extensive lesson plans for a substitute, do some very tiring traveling, spend two nights at the NIH, travel back feeling rather sick (often with my flight delayed for bad weather), return to school and try to catch up on the loose ends from my absence,*

*visit the doctor three times a week for blood work (usually during my free/
preparation periods at school), and then start the cycle all over again.
Needless to say, I was completely frazzled by the end of that year.*

*I took the next year off from teaching, working instead at a friend's
law firm. It was work I had done for several summers, good pay, comfortable environment, somewhat flexible hours and semi-interesting work. It
was also extremely depressing—I realized then that I couldn't possibly
spend the rest of my life going to a job that wasn't meaningful to me. I felt
like if I had limited time left, this was definitely not the way I wanted to
spend it. Of course, financial issues meant I had to work, but at the end of
that year, I knew I had to return to teaching.*

*Thankfully, my husband got a new job along the way that allowed me
to return to teaching on a part-time (mornings) basis, which is what I am
doing now. But once again, as I look at my situation and that of others, I
realize that there are many women with breast cancer who must continue
to work long hours in jobs that are just jobs, and I thank God I go to work
each morning with eager anticipation*

Jenilu Schoolman worked as a psychotherapist until the end of her life,
going so far as to meet with her clients so that she and they could reach a
sense of closure during the final weeks of her illness. Some months prior,
she placed her choices in a larger context, using her experience to highlight
a need she believed that many women with metastatic disease deeply feel.

*I am thinking about the fact that we clearly understand that women
are most deeply moved by their affiliative needs (as opposed to achieve-
ment or competition). That fact must lay at the core of a new way of
thinking about how to mobilize women to deal more constructively with
their disease. I think that we look at the information on support groups
and think we have found it. But I think that is the tip of the iceberg. I
think we haven't begun to understand what happens to women when they
are diagnosed with a disease that potentially and actually isolates them.*

*For example, many people are impressed with the fact that I go to
work every day. They think somehow that is "brave" or I don't know
what. I go to work to be with people. I have spent my entire adult life
dealing with others and I need to be in a kind of emotional contact with
other people. Staying home and being sick is just plain isolating. Those*

times when I have had to stay home have been agony, partly because I am stuck in my home alone. Which is not to say that I can't enjoy my own company, etc., but that a fundamental need for affiliation is being ignored.

Now if you magnify this process because of increasing illness and people's reaction to cancer, you can get a woman who is really cut off emotionally from others and who then gets very depressed; not from the cancer or from the prospect of dying, but from the isolation.

Six weeks before her death, Jenilu spoke of the difficulty she had communicating her continuing sense of aliveness in relation to her life's work to those who should have been most able to understand.

Over the years, I consulted with three different hospices. When I got sick again last year, I resigned from all but one of them. I continued with the one in Troy because I particularly enjoyed them and they were doing some interesting things. Well, the last time I was there, one of the nurses, clearly having consulted with the rest of the nurses, decided to confront me. "Aren't you building sand castles? Shouldn't you be staying home, waiting to die?"

My response was first of all to feel very odd. I agreed that perhaps I am building sand castles, and I may be a lot closer to death than I think I am but...so what? As I explained, I really don't think I can handle daytime TV and quiz shows. Though I love spinning, weaving and reading, there is only so much of that I can do. And, since my entire life has been about being of service to others, it only makes sense to continue to do that as long as I can. Fortunately, my work is so physically non-demanding I can do it when I really feel pretty sick. And if I'm too sick to drive, Pauli gladly drives me to work. But, honestly, who I am is about being there for others, listening and caring. Why should that change now? How could I suddenly become this narcissistic person who says, "Everyone come pay attention to me?"

Is this courage? For me, this is simply living your life in a singular fashion. It also does say something about our institutions; one might think that hospice might be somewhat more sensitive to the issues of living as well as dying. But maybe they are so focused on the process of death (and that everyone must have a "hospice perfect death") that they miss that people live till they die.

CHAPTER 11

Final Gifts

Disease Progression, Hard Choices, Last Days

THIS CHAPTER WAS HARD TO WRITE. It will probably be hard for you to read, too, since it discusses what happens during the final stages of metastatic breast cancer, when the available treatments are no longer effective, and the disease, beyond controlling, overtakes the body and causes death.

Like most women who have had breast cancer, when someone I know and care about dies from the disease, I can't help feeling a cold shiver of dread along with the sense of grief. Losing someone I am close to brings my own death closer, making me wonder when and how it will come. Yet, facing death and dying head on can have its benefits, too, as I hope to show in this chapter.

The early sections of the chapter deal with the confusing and difficult end-of-life decisions patients and physicians must often make, and with the problems most of us have in confronting the dying process, making treatment choices, and allowing ourselves to talk openly about our own fears and wishes.

Gerry Wirth, whose wife, Cindy, died in February 1996, evoked the process as he experienced it: "This disease started like a mist, deepened into fog and ended like a tornado." At the end of this chapter, Gerry and five other husbands recount the final stages of their wives' illness and describe their deaths.

No one is talking about what everyone knows

Drawing up a will is hard enough, not to mention drafting an advance directive and health care proxy, where you have to make your wishes about life-sustaining interventions clear and appoint someone you trust to make medical decisions for you when you are no longer able to. Why, you may well ask, should this book even include a chapter on dying? Isn't the real point to focus on *living* with metastatic breast cancer as long and as well as you can? An open discussion about dying only seems to bring the reality of death that much closer, and to undermine the positive attitude and fighting spirit so many feel is important. Often, dying cancer patients and their families feel that by avoiding this topic, they will somehow avoid burdening one another further, and causing even more pain. And so they never talk directly about death and dying.

Yet the process of talking about dying, and planning for these contingencies, can also bring a sense of relief and connection, whether it is many months or even years beforehand, or when the person is in the final stages of illness. It's not as if these thoughts can be entirely banished from your mind, even if you would wish it. An awareness of mortality is a fundamental part of the human condition, and never more so than when you face death imminently. Avoiding these thoughts and discussions often drains away necessary energies, limits intimacy and increases feelings of isolation and depression.

Psychologist Froma Walsh, President of the American Family Therapy Association, is concerned about the impact on families when these feelings aren't communicated:

> We have social expectations that inhibit us from saying the "D" word, and we keep thinking, "I shouldn't say, 'are you dying' or 'you may die soon.'" Perhaps it's partly the fear that if I say it out loud he may think I want it to happen, or if I say it out loud maybe it'll happen sooner. It's kind of a superstitious belief.
>
> To say to someone, "You're dying, aren't you? or "Are you dying?" or "Do you think you're dying?" may help that person feel more comfortable. Often there's tremendous relief when the person who's dying can now say it out loud. What he may say is, "Yes, but I didn't know if you realized it," or "I didn't want you to feel worse by talking about it." Everybody avoids talking about it because they're afraid they're all going to break down in tremendous grief or it will be too painful for others. If there were a single message, it's for people to take that risk to talk about the unspeakable together.[1]

Dr. Fred Schwartz, Medical Director of the Visiting Nurse Service of New York Hospice Care, reports that his hospice team is sometimes asked by family members to withhold the severity of the prognosis from a patient, which they will agree to do, unless the patient asks directly. There's a price to be paid, however.

> When we go into the situation, there's often a sort of heaviness, because no one is talking about what everyone knows. Patients almost always know that they are dying. They may not want to talk about it, or they may not want to talk about it with family. But they almost always know, because they can feel the energy slipping from their bodies. They know they're not getting better. And they are protecting the family, often, by not talking about it. And the family, likewise, seeing the patient deteriorating, will not talk about it. So there's a sort of conspiracy that goes on. It really blocks the most heartfelt communication between people. Very often, I will come and during the visit with the patient, when the family's gathered around, the patient will say, "I know I'm dying. How much time do you think I have?" Or "Will it be painful?" And this is the first time this will have come up. It's often a real revelation to them, and breaks through a lot of barriers.

Another isolating factor often enters into the final weeks and months of a person's life. Very ill people often withdraw into their "inner circles," as sociologist Kathy Charmaz says.

> Immersion in illness shrinks social worlds. It forces people to pull into their inner circle while pulling away from others. They must try to protect themselves and to keep some control over their lives. They have little strength for anything beyond illness.... Pulling in permits ill people and their caregivers to tighten the boundaries of their lives, to reorder their priorities, and to struggle with the exigencies of illness.[2]

Necessary though this may be, Charmaz points out, pulling in "sets an empty stage for future social isolation."

As her illness visibly progressed, PJ Hagler felt the withdrawal of friends and members of her church keenly and wondered what to do about it.

> I have tried to let people know that should the time come, I'm okay with it. I still want to be part of life though. I wonder why the need to pull away is there other than maybe no one feels comfortable discussing this

topic. We are all given a death sentence when we are told we have cancer unless we are blessed with remission. So many of us with mets have to live with this idea of dying, yet we find it difficult to bring it up, even with each other. Do we try to avoid reality?

Bob Stafford agreed with PJ:

I know the fear people go through and the hope they so desire to have. And sometimes we have lied to them through silence. One of the freeing aspects, though, is the acknowledgment of our mortality. Then we really can begin to enjoy life.

Nancy Gilpatrick also sensed the need for openness in discussing this difficult topic. "Let us please talk about dying," she wrote back. "It will help us to live."

People throughout history have seen for themselves the seeming paradox Nancy alludes to: that confronting death leads to increased aliveness, and that avoidance only begets a diminished sense of self. The psychologist Carl Gustav Jung believed that "We do not become enlightened by imagining figures of light, but by making the darkness conscious."

Dr. Irvin Yalom, an existential psychiatrist who has worked for many years with terminally ill cancer patients at Stanford University, wrote:

*...death is the condition that makes it possible for us to live life in an authentic fashion.... A denial of death at any level is a denial of one's basic nature and begets an increasingly pervasive restriction of awareness and experience. The integration of the **idea** of death saves us; rather than sentence us to existences of terror or bleak pessimism, it acts as a catalyst to plunge us into more authentic life modes, and it enhances our pleasure in the living of life.[3]*

It is all very well to speak in vague terms about confronting mortality, but for the metastatic cancer patient whose illness is far advanced, these lofty issues take on real and immediate proportions, when patients have to confront decisions about ending active treatment and entering palliative care.

Isn't there something else we can try?

"When I think about this time, I have conflicting feelings," Gerry Wirth said, recalling the period between Cindy's high-dose chemotherapy treatment and the discovery of further metastases. "I remember it as a time of great hope, great anxiety, great joy and great disappointment. I also remember it as when I began to feel it wasn't a question of whether, only a question of when."

As we have seen, living with metastatic breast cancer frequently involves trying one treatment after another over an extended period of time, often a number of years. Each time a hormonal treatment or chemotherapy drug or combination of drugs is used, the cells of the cancer work hard to survive by mutating to become resistant to that and related treatments. In the later stages of the disease, metastatic sites also tend to become larger, and more widely spread, invading other organs, causing pain and interfering with normal functioning more and more.

At the same time as treatments are becoming less effective, their toxicity is likely to be greater as the patient becomes sicker. Since it's impossible to know for certain if a treatment will work until it is tried, many oncologists and patients are inclined to try one drug after another, until it is obvious that no other treatments make sense, the person is too debilitated to withstand further treatment and the disease is finally beyond controlling. This agonizing process often takes everyone involved through fluctuating cycles of hope and despair.

On Thanksgiving of 1996, after six years with metastatic disease, PJ Hagler was in despair, as one treatment after another had failed to reduce the size of the metastases in her liver:

> Last week we were told I don't have much longer to live and that this will most likely be my last Christmas. I'm still on 5-FU by pump, but the oncologist said I will probably only tolerate it for about one more week. We are asking him to try compassionate treatment with Her2-Neu or anything else he can think of. I'm still well enough to fight this thing. I'm not ready to die.
>
> Mike and I talked about it this weekend and I still have fight left in me if they would just let me try.... I know there is something out there that would help me live longer.... I'm so depressed right now because it feels like I should be able to do something to live if I'm willing to go through the pain of the treatments.

> *I'm only 46 and I want to live. Is there something so wrong with that? My friends were talking about retirement and I want to go to the place we always dreamed about in the mountains to retire.*

By New Year's day, after a hospital stay and an adjustment of medications, PJ was more philosophical as she examined the preceding year:

> *I have been on one type of chemo or another since last February. Not much has helped this year but I'm still here. So while I say the chemo hasn't worked, it has bought me time. My oncologist and I will use whatever we can find. I have a great deal of faith in him and also in God. I know I will die when I'm supposed to, and not a day early. So much has changed since 1983 when I first discovered my breast lump. The meds I've taken just this year didn't even exist then. God has given me almost fourteen years that I didn't expect.*

But later that month, PJ was in the hospital again with pleurisy, pain and difficulty breathing caused by the pressure of her swollen liver.

> *I'm in rotten shape right now, but I have been in rotten shape before. I don't know how to quit. I have heard all this praise and positive thoughts about how I am handling the latest bad reports. I don't know any other way to handle them.*

One month later, PJ finally had good news:

> *Dr. Nick was so excited today that he called me at home. Last Thursday I saw him and he took the tumor marker blood test. I had the last one in December and it was in the 80's, which is the lowest I've had in six years. Well, he called today to say he wanted to give me the first real good news he has been able to give me in forever. My markers are 10!!*
>
> *I have to give God the credit for how much better I am feeling. My oncologist even said, "I am good, but I'm not **that** good." But God is good enough to make you well. He does good work. He answers prayers.*

A few days after that, still filled with gratitude for this latest reprieve, PJ reflected in a letter to another woman who had been feeling desperate:

> *I would love to be whole and well again for one day in my life. But this is not going to happen. We all know that up front. But we can live each day to the fullest and if it's a bad day we just get through it until the*

next good day. We all have ups and downs, believe me. People tell me how courageous and strong I am. Well, I love my life and I love Mike so much I can't even think about our life together ending. And I have faith that God is using me and my breast cancer to help others realize it doesn't have to be a death sentence.... But the bottom line is I don't know how else to live. I can't imagine giving up and not doing treatments or whatever it takes to keep living. I don't want you to think I'm saying don't get discouraged or down or sad. That's impossible. It happens. But please keep fighting. Life is so worth living.

After a summer of nausea, pain and lowering blood counts, Kathy Stone wrote on Thanksgiving 1996 that she had been feeling somewhat better.

*Seems my red count along with platelets and other "things" that are looked at in blood tests have been steadily declining for the past five weeks now (I get a blood test every week, a fasting panel every three weeks). My white count on my last test dropped in half. I haven't been on chemo since the beginning of July/end of June...can't quite remember, I was so sick when we decided that chemo was no longer the route to go. Since I've had all the "big guns," as they say, and the mets are continuing to steadily grow, the doctors and myself felt that we would save whatever there is **left** to save in the way of chemo for when we need to really slow this sucker down again. Anyway, the doctor feels that the continuing dropping of the red counts is due to the cancer now being in the bone marrow. The drop in the white count is still unexplained unless they just caught me on a curve. I did have a sinus infection that day.*

As for how I feel, I haven't felt so good in a long, long time. This past spring and summer were pure hell with all the nausea and unknown illness I went through.... The bones are degenerating and I had lots of pain ...but now it seems that the pain medication is working. I have a good combo going of Dilaudid and MS Contin and Toradol, along with the steroids that help with pain also. Talk about appetite.... Two months ago I didn't want to hear the word food...today, I can't get enough of it!

Well, that's where I'm at...feeling good but knowing that this crazy, awful stuff is continuing to grow in me. I have several soft-tissue tumors in and around my clavicle, neck and left shoulder area, with some cutting blood supply and giving pain.

Three months later, Kathy's disease had progressed still further:

> I just got home from the oncologist's office. CT scan of chest wasn't
> too bad, but wasn't good either...showed up new mets and more mets in
> old areas. Still can't find the reason for so much crippling pain in left
> shoulder, chest area, rib area. Doctors think it is referred pain from my
> sternum and spine because they are so badly full of tumors. It feels like
> someone broke my ribs and then sat down on them. I was upset and mad
> that nothing concrete was said in the report of that specific area. Any-
> way...due to all the new mets in the bone scan and CT scan they are going
> to put me back on chemo...trying to help pain and maybe slow mets down
> some, but I think it is mostly for the pain so I keep doubting if I should be
> doing it.... The pain is bad, so maybe this chemo will help. Who knows?

> I am so confused this afternoon and all I want to do is cry, but am too
> tired to even do that for too long at a time.... I'm so sick and tired of it
> all.... When does it stop, or does it? I guess we just keep on fighting until
> there is no more fight left in us.

The next day, Kathy was reconciled to the thought of more treatments,
relieved that her husband, Chuck, would go with her to the doctor's office.
Through the support of family and friends, she had recaptured some of her
usual resilience:

> I do dread the new chemo, I'm tired of being tired, but ya gotta do
> what ya gotta do...right? And I never want to give in or up as long as they
> think there is a bit of hope to slow this sucker down. Life is too precious.

> If we can just stay sick long enough, a cure will be found and we will
> be able to get completely well and whole again with it. I'm going try to
> stay sick for as long as it takes...and in the meantime, no telling where
> you will find me because I don't plan on staying put in the house or in the
> bed when not absolutely necessary. I plan on living and enjoying every-
> thing I can.... My motto is you can hurt and be sick outside your home as
> well as inside, so why not go out and have fun if it's manageable at all.
> Anyway, as I've said before...it makes it that much harder on "ole man
> death"...he just might get tired of looking for me and give up!

When asked how they might come to a decision about when it wouldn't
make sense to continue treatment, most of the people I interviewed chose
not to respond, saying that they felt they were far away from that decision

point and found it too depressing to think about. Those who did talked about how difficult this decision would be for them. How would they know when to stop? they wondered. If there was any chance at all a treatment will work, how could they say no to it?

End-of-life dilemmas

However personal they may be, these decisions also touch on issues of medical history and ethics, as well as public health policy. Just as it helps to grapple with your feelings if you know they are shared by others, it may also help to frame individual experience in the larger medical and social context. Understanding the forces at work in our society against confronting the reality of death explains much of the withdrawal and avoidance many metastatic breast cancer patients feel coming from their health care providers. Daniel Callahan, medical ethicist and president of the Hastings Institute, focuses the question:

> Is death to be accepted as a part of life, or fought to the end? Most doctors, and most Americans, are just not certain what the answer to that question is—and it shows in the way patients are treated at the end of their lives, and sometimes in the way they (or their families) are treated.[4]

Part of the problem is that death, far from being understood by the medical establishment as a final outcome of many diseases, is usually defined as outside the proper scientific scope of medicine. *Cecil Textbook of Medicine*, the recently revised and classic primary guide for physicians, devotes only 25 of its 2,300 pages to death, and only five pages to pain.

> For a book filled with accounts of lethal disease and ways to treat them, there is a strikingly scant discussion—three pages only of treatment for those in the terminal phase of disease. It tells what to do to hold off death, but not what is to be done when that is not possible. That omission is a stark example of the way death is kept beyond the borders of medicine, an unwelcome, unwanted, unexpected, and ultimately accidental intruder.[5]

Ellen Scheiner has the uncommon perspective of being both a high-risk breast cancer patient and a doctor with a lifelong interest and experience in medical ethics. Ellen gave the first "death and dying" lecture to the experimental chemotherapy unit at Memorial Sloan-Kettering Cancer Center in 1968. "No one died there," she says wryly.

As a physician who always prided herself on her compassion, Ellen thought she'd understood before her own intensive chemotherapy what patients with advanced cancer felt. But her own experience with the "dissolution of self" that came with her chemotherapy was a revelation, and has caused her to reflect on her own wishes, should she have a recurrence.

> I'm a living example of a doctor who didn't want to keep patients alive beyond their time, who **still** didn't understand what it was like. At this time, at age 63, if I got a recurrence, I would take simple treatment. That's all that I would do. When I was first diagnosed I wanted a real crack at living, I wanted to give myself the best possible chance. I think I've been given this life and I am responsible for maintaining it. But I need not abuse it by overtreating myself.

> The simple statement, "You know you have a choice of doing absolutely nothing, and there's nothing wrong with that. You can live in a comfortable way, or there might be lesser treatment, and pain medication." I think these simple sentences are not said, often. If they were, people might say, "Oh, I don't want any more treatment, then. I'd rather have my grandchildren in my lap."

> I've already told Vicky [her oncologist] that if I get a recurrence, I don't want Taxol. It made me too sick. I told her at the beginning: "I don't want to be kept alive heroically. I'm going to take this, and I'm going to fight like hell to get through this treatment." I've told the people who have my health care proxy what I want. I know, because I am a doctor, that people don't need to have treatment. They need to hear it from somebody who will say, "You don't have to do this."

Ellen has thought further about the dying process she might seek for herself.

> I know that I might have painful metastatic cancer, for which I can foresee palliative treatment, and that I might need to enter a hospice for pain management until my death. Although sedated, I could be still surrounded by loved ones and enjoy a touch, a strand of Bach, the way light streams through a window. I would not seek death.

A "good death" is not always possible, as Ellen knows. There are some circumstances under which life would no longer be desirable for her.

> *The worst scenario for me is that I could no longer think clearly or enjoy anything much because my thinking apparatus itself was affected. Possible reasons include dementia or an encephalopathy, which is difficulty in perception because of a chemical derangement or brain metastases. In this context I would prefer not to live. As a physician I know well how to commit suicide.*

> *However, I might not have the mental capacity to act. I would not presume to ask a friend or colleague to assist me (assisted suicide), if indeed I could recognize my altered mental state, because that person would be guilty of murder under our present laws. I am familiar with cases in which assisted suicide has been attempted and the person has not died. My wishes are known in advance, and someone might seek help for me if I lost awareness. This, for me, makes a strong case for euthanasia, or a legally approved way of having competent people confirm the patient's mind state, and of carrying out the patient's wish to die. Laws would need to be amplified and, in all probability, physicians would need to administer the lethal agents. I hope that these laws are enacted before I need them.*

As a physician willing and able to discuss death and dying openly, even when it comes to her own predicament, Ellen represents a minority in her profession. Nowhere is the avoidance of end-of-life discussions on the part of doctors and patients more evident and more tragic than in the hospital care of the dying. The findings of a broad study of the care of critically ill patients, entitled SUPPORT, involving nearly 10,000 hospitalized patients in the advanced stages of cancer and other terminal conditions, in five leading medical centers, were published in the *Journal of the American Medical Association* in November 1995.[6]

"Many Americans today fear they will lose control over their lives if they become critically ill, and their dying will be prolonged and impersonal," the study authors state in the introduction, echoing the fears most metastatic breast cancer patients express. These concerns have given rise, the study authors go on to say, to a visible right-to-die movement and widespread concern about the "economic and human cost" of end-of-life treatment. They have also led to efforts by consumer and professional organizations to promote health proxies and advance directives, and to search for ways to facilitate better doctor-patient communication about end-of-life decision making.

Prior studies had indicated that "communication is often absent or occurs only during a crisis. Physicians today perceive death as a failure...and they provide more extensive treatment to seriously ill patients than they would choose for themselves." Consequently, this study was designed to look at communications between medical professionals and patients near the end of life, a time when doctors don't clearly convey patients' chances for survival, and patients and families don't discuss their wishes soon, or often, enough.

In fact, the outcomes of the first phase of the SUPPORT study, which involved 4,301 patients, led to some shocking findings:

- The SUPPORT patients were all seriously ill, and their dying proved to be predictable, yet discussions and decisions substantially in advance of death were uncommon.

- Communication between physicians and patients was poor: only 41% of patients in the study reported talking to their physicians about prognosis or about cardiopulmonary resuscitation (CPR).

- Physicians misunderstood patients' preferences regarding CPR in 80% of cases.

- Furthermore, physicians did not implement patients refusals of interventions. When patients wanted CPR withheld, a do-not-resuscitate (DNR) order was never written in about 50% of cases. Nearly half of the DNR orders were written in the last 2 days of life.

- The final hospitalization for half of patients included more than 8 days in generally undesirable states: in an ICU, receiving mechanical ventilation, or comatose.

- Families reported that half of the patients who were able to communicate in their last few days spent most of the time in moderate to severe pain.

To rectify these conditions, over the two years of the intervention phase of the SUPPORT study, specially trained nurses facilitated communication about risks, outcomes and choices with 4,800 patients, their physicians and families, in an effort to ensure that patients' wishes were followed and decision-making was informed and collaborative. But this intervention didn't make any difference: "Improved information, enhanced conversation, and an explicit effort to encourage use of outcomes and preferences in decision-making were completely ineffectual."

Dr. Joanne Lynn, director of the Center to Improve Care of the Dying at George Washington University, and one of the project coordinators, interpreted the disappointing results:

> The reasons for this are ingrained in our society. Physicians are taught to save lives, that death is a failure. Patients and families have come to expect miracles in every case. It's easier for everyone—professionals and patients alike—to follow the usual path of aggressive treatment, even when it's clear that it is leading nowhere. No one wants to give up too soon. That's one reason why everyone is so reluctant to discuss dying.
>
> Suffering while dying must become a bad outcome in the health care system. Everyone has a vision for living. Our society also needs to create a vision for living well while dying.[7]

Daniel Callahan, commenting on the failures of the SUPPORT study interventions, takes this back to a personal level:

> It has too often been presumed that people know what they really want, that they can know in advance what they want, and that clear choices—yes/no, on/off—will present themselves. Those seem to be wrong, excessively rationalistic presumptions. The only real surprise is that those who should be more perceptive about human nature have believed that what patients say they want is exactly what they do want. I wish I knew myself that well—and especially knew how I will react to the (by definition) once-in-a-lifetime circumstance of my dying. Where am I supposed to get that kind of knowledge about myself, much less certainty about what I think I know? Where is anyone to get it? [8]

When they are still healthy, people may be quick to say they would discontinue treatment as soon as recovery seems unlikely and significant loss of quality of life appears imminent. But in the moment of crisis, many—perhaps most of us—will accept treatment as long as it is offered. Panic and the physiological instinct to survive are strong influences, especially when these choices haven't been thought through in advance. These scenarios are all too familiar. An elderly friend of mine, dying of lung cancer, was taken to the hospital in respiratory crisis. Panic-stricken, she agreed to a ventilator, something she'd expressly rejected in her advance directive. "Terrible mistake," she was able to scrawl in a note to her husband after she was stabilized, and asked that he arrange for her to be sedated and withdrawn from the ventilator, so that she could die in peace.

In February of 1996, eleven years after her liver metastases had first been diagnosed, Jenilu Schoolman wrote her friends that her oncologist had told her "it is all over but the shouting."

> My liver is pretty well shot with tumors that are out of control. My back is filled with metastases to the point of bones being about to shatter from the weight of my own body. In short, things look very grim. I will spare you all the gory details of the past week because they haven't been pretty and I don't want to hurt you with my pain. Suffice it to say, I began chemotherapy on Tuesday with three drugs that are new to me. My oncologist said plainly he doesn't hold out much hope that they will do any good and he wouldn't blame me if I decided not to go on with treatment. But on the other hand he knows me, and he knows I'll try anything.

> The radiation oncologist feels she can do a good deal for my pain, but she is very worried that so much of the bony part of my lower back is involved that, as the radiation wipes out the affected tissue, there won't be enough bone to support my body and whatever is left will simply shatter. So I am wearing one of those belts that carpenters and men who work lifting wear, hoping that will provide enough support to get me through the time when I have little bone. We have also added more morphine to my regime, which seems like an excellent idea.

> Other than that, I am still working. The schedule for radiation is stable. It's the same time every day so I can actually plan! I am also holding an open house for all my patients, past and present, so I can say good-bye to them and let them say good-bye to me. This is not fun....

> However, I must admit that in spite of all the Cassandras in my life, I am still optimistic. Or crazy! I told my oncologist that if I could find a window in this nasty space, I'd climb out and run away. He looked at me quizzically. I explained that since childhood I have had a problem climbing out windows and running away; playing hooky. When I worked at Ellis Hospital this reached monumental proportions because I had a base-

ment office. Especially in spring, I'd lock my door, climb out the window and I was gone! Unfortunately I never told the secretary I was leaving and I know I caused havoc a number of times but...that's the wild woman in me that just can't be tamed. Well, I'm about to use that same wild strength to find another window and climb out of this mess. My doctor laughed and said he was sure that if it were possible, I'd do it. Remember I did it eleven years ago, so why not now?

Like many others, Jenilu coped by entertaining a dual possibility: making realistic preparations for her death, while at the same time still hoping that further treatment might give her more time. When Jenilu died two weeks later, at home under hospice care, my first thought was that she had been right about climbing out that window.

Hope and treatment choices

But what about hope? Doesn't giving up treatment mean giving up hope? Yale surgeon and professor Sherwin Nuland writes cogently about how hope can become transformed during the course of terminal illness.

> Hope lies not only in an expectation of cure or even of the remission of present distress. For dying patients, the hope of cure will always be shown to be ultimately false, and even the hope of relief too often turns to ashes. When my time comes, I will seek hope in the knowledge that insofar as possible I will not be allowed to suffer or be subjected to needless attempts to maintain life; I will seek it in the certainty that I will not be abandoned to die alone; I am seeking it now, in the way I try to live my life, so that those who value what I am will have profited by my time on earth and be left with comforting recollections of what we have meant to one another.
>
> There are those who will find hope in faith and their belief in an afterlife; some will look forward to the moment a milestone is reached or a deed is accomplished; there are even some whose hope is centered on maintaining the kind of control that will permit them the means to decide the moment of their death... Whatever form it may take, each of us must find hope in his or her own way.[9]

Most of the people I interviewed expressed a need to preserve hope through continuing treatment. But often, as time went on, and the disease progressed, their hope found other measures, more modest perhaps, but no less meaningful: for more time with family, to accomplish life ambitions, or to be present at crucial events. "I would argue that of the many kinds of hope a doctor can help his patient find at the very end of life," Nuland writes, "the one that encompasses all the rest is the belief that one final success may yet be achieved whose promise vanquishes the immediacy of suffering and sorrow."[10]

As the SUPPORT study suggests, many, if not most, people are willing to gamble against heavy odds and debilitating side effects for a slight chance at more of this precious commodity called time. This disturbs Nuland, who writes of the seductive lure of high-tech medicine for his late-stage cancer patients, few of whom, he reveals, were willing to say "no more" to treatment.

> *Almost everyone seems to want to take a chance with the slim statistics that oncologists give to patients with advanced disease. Usually, they suffer for it, they lay waste their last months for it, and they die anyway, having magnified the burdens they and those who love them must carry in the final moments. Though everyone may yearn for a tranquil death, the basic instinct to stay alive is a far more powerful force.[11]*

A further reason for this may lie in our capacity to accept death in the abstract, that it must come to each of us, but not in the particular, that our dying or that of someone we love may be *here* and *now*...and that it may be time to change one's focus from fighting the cancer to thinking about letting go. Easy to say, but much more difficult to do. The power of hindsight being what it is, Callahan believes that the way in which these decisions are often made is a complex process:

> *The answer often comes down to a series of subtle, small, incremental steps, none of which actually thwarted patient or family wishes in any obvious fashion, and each of which was based on some hopeful medical possibility, with both the hope and the possibility stimulating each other to the point of folly.*

> *More generally, we fail to realize how profoundly ambivalent most of us are about accepting death, not just because of the threat of death itself, but because we are heirs of the same tradition of technological optimism that has dominated modern medicine. Even if we say we can accept death, we believe in our hearts that the sting of death can be medically delayed, that fatalism is itself a source of fatality, that death is a kind of*

human artifact. No less than physicians have we laypeople come to believe that part of the success of modern medicine stems from a commitment to a zealous use of technology, a zeal no place better expressed than at the margins and against the odds.

We believe as a general value that one ought, with spirit, to fight death. We may with all sincerity mean it when we say we do not want clearly useless or futile treatment. But that is not of much help when clinical uncertainty or psychological ambivalence are present; then we may waver, unsure of ourselves.[12]

Though far from this stage in her own illness, Sharon Multhauf has stood by as many friends have faced these choices:

It would be awfully hard for me to say "no more treatment" as long as there was reason to hope that treatment could buy me more time with my family and friends. But my hope is that such time would have some measure of quality to it. In other words, I am willing to be in a wheelchair, I am willing to be bedridden, as long as I am not experiencing constant pain and nausea, which would make it hard to enjoy being with my loved ones. And if I'm so spaced out from narcotics that I can't communicate, what good is the time I have? I know that there is a lot that can be done to control pain and nausea, especially when addiction and long-term effects are not constraints. Therefore, I expect that I would want to try one more therapy, and one more, and one more, to squeeze some more time out of this life of mine, even if I was fully aware that none of these would cure me. The time when I would say "enough is enough" would probably be when the treatment's side effects could not be controlled enough to let me enjoy my loved ones.

I will rely on my doctors to tell me what they know, and on Lloyd to offer his support, wisdom and love, but ultimately, the decision is going to be mine. I'm the one living in this body, and if anyone on this earth is going to decide it's time to leave, I think it should be me.

For Nancy Gilpatrick, it is the sickening memory of how she had felt after her high-dose chemotherapy that leads her to feel she might stop treatment at a certain point.

I won't do chemotherapy until the end of my life. I want to enjoy my life until there isn't any life left in me. Those two sentences convey a lot of information in few words. Behind those words are lots of sleepless nights, conversations with Terry, and reading the words of women on the breast cancer list. It's also a promise I made myself after the high-dose chemo: no more chemo. I was so sick and weakened I didn't want to do it again. I may do more chemo; it's just that there will be an end.

Since I've been told I will in all likelihood die from the breast cancer or mets, as a relatively young woman I want to have a good quality of life, while trying to find a balance in quantity. I don't want to be bedridden any more than is absolutely necessary. My cancer has not responded well to chemo and so I'm not interested in running through the different meds to find the **one** *drug that will work. I'd be despairing and disappointed while having to recover from the side effects of chemo.*

Since facing death is painful for all of us, it's probably human nature that we instinctively turn away and try to ignore its reality when we can. A large part of the courage metastatic breast cancer patients ultimately find in themselves relates to this confrontation. Dr. Irvin Yalom quotes psychologist Otto Rank describing a neurotic as one "who refuses the loan (life) in order to avoid the payment of the debt (death)."

Contemplating one's own death and dying creates anxiety, which Yalom calls "the price you pay for being fully human."[13] Caren Buffum, like the others interviewed for this book, struggled with paying that price.

What is probably most prevalent on people's minds, the question they would really like to ask but rarely do so, is how do I deal with the idea of dying from this disease. How am I so calmly "facing death"?

I first dealt with this issue in a clear and conscious way when I thought about doing a "living will." I was asked over and over again at each admission at the NIH for my treatment back in 1992–93 if I had prepared a living will or advance directive. Each time, I told myself I probably should make one out, but each time I felt like that would be admitting that I was going to die soon and, in some weird way, I might even hasten the event's arrival. But I thought about all the people who have died totally unexpectedly. Of course the Karen Ann Quinlan case immediately came to mind because of all the media coverage. But hers was a classic case of the confusion caused by an untimely situation that no one was prepared for. It occurred to me that **everyone** *had to deal with the issue of dying, if for no other reason than to realize that it was a* *reality of life and there were things we each need to do that we may not have advance notice on.*

So I finally sat down and put my living will together, almost with a smug satisfaction that I had done a responsible thing that most other people simply put off until it's too late. I could deal with the reality of death as not so much the result of my having cancer but, rather, the result of my having life. It gave me a new way to look at dying—not as an imminent event but, rather, as an unavoidable one.

The problem with doctors

Doctors are no more immune to a fear of death than the rest of us, it seems—especially when they see death not as a natural and inevitable outcome of disease, but as a personal defeat or failure. Research suggests that some doctors may even be drawn to medicine by unusually strong fears of death, even a need to conquer it. "It's frightening for a lot of physicians to deal with dying patients," writes Yalom. "Physicians find lots of ways to get away from these patients quickly."[14] Because this abandonment can be devastating, and a close and trusting relationship with an oncologist is so crucial throughout the course of the disease, many of the people in this book have made a point of discussing these issues freely with their doctors far in advance, making sure that their wishes were explicit and would be honored, and trying to gauge their doctors' commitment to them.

Anyone facing end-of-life decisions concerning medical treatment would do well to heed Sherwin Nuland's cautions about medical arrogance and abandonment:

In an attempt to maintain control, a doctor, usually without being aware of it, convinces himself that he knows better than the patient what course is proper. He dispenses only as much information as he deems fit, thereby influencing a patient's decision-making in ways he does not recognize as self-serving.... The inability to face the consequences presented by loss of control often leads a physician to walk away from situations in which his power no longer exists, and this must certainly be an ingredient in the abrogation of responsibility that so often takes place at the end of a patient's life.[15]

The source is more than a matter of individual ego, Nuland believes. These attitudes are the spoils of a century that has indulged in the "conceit" of the mastery of science and medicine over the inevitability of nature.

> *Every time a patient dies, his doctor is reminded that his own and mankind's control over natural forces is limited and will always remain so....The greater humility that should have come with greater knowledge is instead replaced by medical hubris: since we can do so much, there is no limit to what should be attempted*—today, and for this **patient!**

No more poignant or instructive example of a doctor's vulnerability exists than Nuland's recounting of his brother's death, in which he admits how and why he withheld the truth that his brother was dying from him, regressing, as he acknowledges, to "the misconceived paternalistic dictum of the professors who taught me a generation ago: 'Share your optimisms and keep your pessimisms to yourself.'"

> *No one who has treated cancer patients will ever discount the power of the subconscious mechanism we call denial, which is both friend and enemy of a person seriously ill. Denial protects while it hinders, and softens for a moment what it eventually makes more difficult.*[16]

In his essay "Intoxicated by My Illness," the critic Anatole Broyard, dying of prostate cancer, issued this challenge to physicians:

> *Not every patient can be saved, but his illness may be eased by the way the doctor responds to him—and in responding to him, the doctor may save himself. But first he must become a student again; he has to dissect the cadaver of his professional persona; he must see that his silence and neutrality are unnatural. It may be necessary to give up some of his authority in exchange for his humanity, but as the old family doctors knew, this is not a bad bargain. In learning to talk to his patients, the doctor may talk himself back into loving his work. He has little to lose and everything to gain by letting the sick man enter his heart. If he does, they can share, as few others can, the wonder, terror, and exaltation of being on the edge of being, between the natural and the supernatural.*[17]

Bob Stafford relies on his doctors to be candid with him about the time when treatment will no longer make sense:

> I want my doctors to be deadly honest with me. I'll find the hope, I already have the hope that I'll need. But I want them to tell it like it is, even if they are wrong. I had a doc tell me in June of '95 that I had a good six months, probably a year left (and the guy was trying to encourage me). He was honest but he was wrong. I can handle the truth. And I know how important hope is. But sometimes we grasp for straws because the hope we have is based on false information. I'd rather have hope based on truth.
>
> I think there will come a time when more treatment doesn't make sense. I'll know when and it will probably be intuitive. I know I don't want to be bed-ridden for very long. Being comatose is not being "alive." And I don't want that either. When I see that coming then I will forego treatment and let God/nature take its course. I have a good doctor who respects my wishes and will tell me if he has anything more in his bag that will offer me what I want. I want to be active as long as possible. The best illustration you can give is Cardinal Bernadin of Chicago. He was active in his ministry until the last three weeks of his life. That's what I want. It will be my decision alone because my family and medical help are all hurting because of me. They want the same thing that I want. They are hurting watching me get worse and worse.
>
> Some will say we're not fighters, but you and I know that's not true. There comes a time when we recognize reality. When we know we've given it everything we had.

This chapter's emphasis on the failure of hospital medicine to deal with dying in a humane way is intended as cautionary, but there are still excellent resources out there. Many physicians are extremely sensitive to these issues, and are able to help their patients make wise choices, and come to terms with what is happening. And they understand the crucial importance of expert palliative care. As Dr. Kathleen Foley of Memorial Sloan-Kettering Cancer Center writes:

> In the real world in which physicians care for dying patients, withdrawing treatment and aggressively treating pain are acts that respect patients' autonomous decisions not to be battered by medical technology and to be relieved of their suffering.[18]

Caren Buffum wrote of the moment when her doctor gently raised the issue of stopping treatments with her for a second time:

> I sit in the doctor's office, perched on the examining table—my feet dangling like those of a child.
>
> "New tumors in the liver."
>
> Three times is not a charm—it's scary. Three scary reports. For the second one, I was in a hospital bed and Stephen [her oncologist] said that sometimes it's okay to let go. I know he wasn't telling me that I should, but he wanted me to know that I had permission.
>
> "I know," I said. We hadn't talked about this before. It had never been the right time. Was it the right time now?
>
> I then saw two clear paths ahead of me, cutting through the rest of my life. One was very short: the treatment didn't work. The other disappeared over a hill.
>
> The short one had a name: "Going home to die." But when I left the hospital, I didn't know which path I was on.
>
> Now comes the third report. Stephen once told me there would always be something else to try. But I guess he meant if I really wanted to … if it was worth it … if all things weighed in that way. Now I understood. It wouldn't always be worth it.
>
> Stephen asks me what I want to do next. He understands my need to make choices. He knows what I will say. But does he know why?
>
> He worries that when the time comes to let go, I won't. I will suffer because my fists are clenched too tightly on a life that isn't mine anymore.
>
> I worry that Stephen thinks this. I want him to know something—I want to see peace in his eyes.
>
> I am not desperate, I tell him. I am not afraid to die. I do not cling to life out of fear. But I have too many reasons for sticking around. I need at least two years to get my musical produced.
>
> Two years! I can see the horror on his face. Does she even know? he is thinking.

I want to laugh. Of course I know. So what? I want two years. I demand two years. So there!

At home, I realize what I have done. I have taken my life back in my hands again. In the hospital I had raised it to my feeble lips, like a dandelion puff, and blew it down the road to let the wind carry it along whichever path it drifted over. Then I had given the short road a name and dared to peer down it, thinking that if I saw its end, I could rest.

There is a peace in having looked, but I am not ready to gaze down that road. I have chosen the other path.

I'm glad Stephen and I talked about "things." Hopefully it has set his mind at rest.

From holding tight to letting go

In her next message, again philosophical, Caren updated her friends:

Four weeks ago, I was letting life slip out of my hands—God, I was so tired of hanging on so tight. Two weeks ago, I grabbed life back again. Yesterday I got some so-so blood tests. Slip—And scans next week—I haven't a clue what that will do. Even with symptoms, I find it hard to believe there really is in my liver a "thing" as big as the space between my doctor's hands when they are spread six inches apart. So the battle feels like it is really between my will to live and my willingness to die.

But a month following that, in late May of 1996, Caren felt sure that she was indeed entering a new stage in the process.

Last night I took another hard look down that other path. I have been having persistent pain in my right side, about where I believe my enlarged liver sits. My appetite has been seriously depressed, and with all the other symptoms, I have been wondering if I need to get serious about doing the things I know must be done in my lifetime.

I was feeling very discouraged and shared my fears with Dave. He agreed that the symptoms do seem to point in one direction (first time I wished he hadn't been so agreeable). And he found it scary too.

I was up very late—the pain made it hard to sleep. But also, I didn't want to let go of Dave. I do not feel ready to let go.

I understand more and more why Stephen keeps reminding me that non-treatment is an option. How many cases like mine has he seen? People who are undeniably on that path, and it is just a matter of time? He knows that in each case, the length of their lives was not seriously altered by the choices of treatment and that the main difference is quality of life. So he is wondering, I'm sure, if I will understand this enough to preserve my quality of life in the end and not sacrifice it for the dream of a miracle cure.

But still, he and I are investigating options. Doesn't every cancer patient hope there is that as-of-yet undiscovered cure just around the corner? And as I have told him, I enjoy so much in life—as long as I can continue to enjoy my life, I want to stick around.

Two months following that, in early July, Caren wrote that she and her family were beginning to prepare themselves:

I saw my doctor yesterday and he said all the signs point to liver failure, and there is nothing we can do. There will always be other treatments available, but either they are pretty wimpy at this stage or will make me very sick and impact seriously on the quality of whatever life I have left. I guess the bottom line is that he is talking in possibly weeks ... but sometimes docs get it wrong. And I do believe in miracles.

But Dave and I have talked openly and honestly with our sons and other family members and friends, that I probably don't have a whole lot longer. It feels weird to finally talk about it in practical ways. There are things we have to take care of. And then there are those things we want to do as a family and as a couple that we will aggressively try to accomplish. A dear friend in Seattle is trying to arrange a trip for me to visit them out there. My heart's desire is to go overseas one last time, primarily to Israel, but that certainly seems out of reach. So we are trying to come up with family things that are doable—a few days at the shore, a visit to old stomping grounds in New England, camping, a concert or show, special meals, etc. We've asked the boys for ideas for things they want to do with us all together. I have been very tired, a symptom from the liver problem. Typing this is very difficult—my fingers won't cooperate, and I keep falling asleep mid-sentence.

As the reality is setting in, Dave has become more initiating, more comforting. He's moved from being helpful to being heartful. If nothing else, this stage of the disease seems to be bringing us closer together. I am doing "okay." Surprisingly calm, and I think that is a supernatural gift from God. I have my "good" cries and then next minute laugh at my own morbid jokes. My faith is continually being strengthened, and while I don't know how I will handle tomorrow, I am thus far able to handle today.

Caren handled her remaining days with grace and courage. A month later, surrounded by her family and a couple of close friends, she died peacefully at home. At her memorial service, her husband, Dave, spoke about her last day, how members of their congregation and friends had come to say their good-byes, how the music Caren had composed was played and people came to sing her the songs she had written, and how their youngest son, Levi, pointed out to them all how his mother had died with a smile on her face.

It would be cruel to suggest that everyone can or should face the prospect of dying with such equanimity and acceptance. To believe this is only to perpetuate the "nobility" myth that pervades much of the literature on terminal cancer, the prettied up image of the brave, uncomplaining cancer patient who slips away quietly, determined to inconvenience no one. We all hope that when it is our turn, we'll be able to face death bravely and calmly—but in the interim there are many deep feelings of fear, anger and regret to be confronted.

Some of the anguish and bitterness felt by metastatic breast cancer patients as treatment fails and pain and disability increases is eloquently expressed below by Sandra Yandell. Now 33, and first diagnosed when she was only 27 years old, Sandra had just celebrated the first anniversary of a grueling fifteen-hour surgery to rebuild a spine shattered by metastases.

I went shopping a few days ago, and in the main aisle the store had a wonderful display of potted flowers. They were all so lovely, but I settled on a miniature red rose and a fluffy purple hydrangea. I thought it would be so nice to have some life around me, something bright and colorful and cheerful. They were looking a little sad late yesterday, so I watered them and hoped for the best.

Last night I had a terrible time sleeping. Everything just hurt—back, shoulders, pelvis. I woke up crying about 4:00 a.m. and took another MS Contin (I usually take one before bed). I was still pretty groggy when I got up this morning, and it made me a little late to chemo. The office was incredibly busy today, but I talked to my doc briefly after I finished my chemo (Navelbine since August). I took a bus home in the rain, and I was okay until I got home.

I took a look at my flowers and burst into tears. I can't keep a plant alive, how can I keep myself alive? My tumor markers have shot back up, doubling since my last test. My doc is additionally worried about the bone pain, which she says would be consistent with a failure of the chemo. I don't want to do this anymore. I'm so tired. A year ago I was still in the hospital, and back problems started almost a year before that. I can't remember what it's like not to hurt, not to be sick, not to be pale and tired and empty. The really sad part is that I was feeling so optimistic, hopeful that maybe it would stop for a while and let me go on with things. I even had the audacity to start growing my hair out again. I don't want to make any more treatment decisions, I don't think I can face nausea and neuropathy and hair loss and on and on. It's a horrible nightmare that I've been stuck in for almost six years, a nightmare that continues to cheat me and rob me of health and life and time. How much do they have to cut out of me, how many poisons do they have to pump into my body? How many pain pills will make the hurt go away?

But even anguish as wrenching as this, having found its expression, tends to be short-lived, especially when the loving support of friends and family is there. A few days later, Sandra wrote:

Just in case you're wondering, my hydrangea is hanging in there, and I'm going to put it in a bigger pot tomorrow. Sometimes a change of location and scenery can do wonders. The miniature rose, however, looks totally dead, but a gardener friend said that he can put it into dormancy and in three months or so I can have it back and blooming. Pretty amazing, if you ask me. I guess it helps to listen to an expert sometimes, because other people can see things in ways that I can't. A different perspective, a sunny window, a little care…it's incredible how things look when you change them around a bit.

Hospice and palliative care

In 1995, the National Cancer Institute spent only $26 million dollars, or slightly over *one percent* of its budget, on research into pain control, quality of life issues, palliative care and hospice. Although they are supposed to represent the highest standard of care, only half of the nation's fifty NCI-designated cancer centers even offer hospice programs. Only one third of the half million cancer patients who die each year receive hospice care, 90 percent of them at home.[19]

Hospice physician Fred Schwartz believes that attitudes are changing around such issues as:

> ...the rules and regulations governing insurance, health care in the last six months of life, who is appropriate to be aggressively treated versus not appropriate. These are money issues that will be looked at as money becomes the driving force in health care, because hospice is less expensive, as well as more humane.

> The comment that all of the health professionals on our team get constantly—nurses, social workers, doctors, home health aides—is "Why wasn't I told about your services six months ago, three months ago?" And it's the last day, or week of their husband's life or father's life. "Why wasn't I ever told that this existed?" they say, or "Why did the neighbor next door have to say, 'Gee, why don't you contact a hospice?'"

New York oncologist Dr. Samuel Waxman presents a physician's perspective on hospice, which reflects the inconsistencies of a medical system that doesn't handle these issues well.

> Most hospitals are not equipped for dying. You have to go through the legalities of signing a DNR, and other procedures. All of that gets in the way. There's just no simple answer. The best places to die are terminal care facilities. With home hospice, I am often dealing with an agency and nurses I don't know. It's a voice on the other end of the phone. Sometimes it's amazingly good; sometimes it's not. The family is the best source of knowing what's going on. When hospice works, it's fabulous, and I am quite relieved to have a patient being handled at home. I think it's better. But it's individual. With an older person with very little family support, it's too much to ask. With little children involved, it's very hard.

It's very easy for a physician to just turn things over and get out of your sight. You don't have to sit and explain things, and hold hands. It takes a lot of time, a lot of time, and I believe physicians are getting very disgusted with the system out there, by how they're being treated by the business community, being shown a lack of respect, a lack of loyalty. People whom you've taken care of for years are suddenly on a different plan and you can't even see them.

Hospice physicians are not generally that accessible to me. I tend to work with the nurses. I want to have the continuity with my patients, and handle their needs. I'm just saying that I don't like turning over my patients to terminal care facilities unless I know them. If they're in home hospice, I don't want to say good-bye until I have to. And it bothers my patients, too. Sometimes it gets a little complicated, because they are seeing other doctors, and they don't know the patient, they're just treating the pain. So it can be a problem, but it tends to be the best way.

Fred Schwartz explains his perspective as a hospice physician on the issue of which doctor is primary in this situation:

My role is basically symptom control. If somebody is well tied into their own doctor, either at the office, or if their doctor makes home visits, then we really don't directly interact, unless the physician asks us for some advice or to act as a consultant. This happens a great deal. Many times the doctor will say, "I don't know how to handle the pain, but I want to maintain a relationship with this patient. Can your doctor order the pain medication?" And usually I will do a home visit and just be a consultant on that patient. Other patients are just not tied into their doctors, or the doctors don't do home visits. Maybe some of their recent care was in a tertiary hospital like Sloan-Kettering and they live out in Eastern Queens and the trip is overwhelming. At that point, they will ask me to become involved. I get involved with about 50 to 60 percent of our patients. I become primary physician for them.

"Doctors keep doing things the same old way," says Dr. Joanne Lynn, director of the Center to Improve Care of the Dying at George Washington University, and one of the authors of the SUPPORT study, mentioned earlier in this chapter. We are only beginning, Lynn says, to deal "with the fact that no matter how long you save a life, there's still a death in store, and that that part of life should be good, too."

What services does hospice offer? Schwartz describes what his team does:

> *Once a family makes the decision to stay at home, they need that support, that physical support and emotional support—for patient and for caregivers and the larger family unit. For the patient, the first priority is symptom control. Get the pain, the nausea, the agitation, the anxiety, the constipation or whatever the symptoms are—get that under control. Nobody in agonizing, writhing pain wants to talk about God or what's going to happen to their spouse. From the patient's perspective, symptom control is the cornerstone that allows you to go into those other, deeper areas. We usually say that our hospice team can provide emotional, psychosocial and spiritual support. So what does that mean? It means that we try to see people holistically. It's not only that they have a pain where their liver is pressing on something, but also, what's going to happen to their retarded daughter when they die, or how is their wife of fifty-five years going to adjust to the new situation, or who's going to take care of their dogs when they die? Or whatever their issues are.*

Breast cancer patient Barbara Quirarte, a hospice volunteer in Bandon, Oregon, describes what hospice does, as she sees it:

> *The aim of hospice is to provide comfort to a dying patient and the family. This includes the physical, emotional, mental and spiritual aspects. There are so many areas: getting mental comfort for a patient by a volunteer attorney for legal matters, taking the patient's children to the newest movie, arranging for hospital bed and other items to ease the patient's home comfort, picking up prescriptions, taking the patient for a ride to the beach, and talking and talking and talking about whatever the patient needs to talk about, as well as the patient's family and friends.*
>
> *The most important job is pain management. If this isn't accomplished, hospice has failed. Intractable pain is often what traps a patient in a hospital. When a hospice nurse visits, one of the things she evaluates is the pain level and arranges for whatever is needed with the doctor. As a volunteer, it is my job to report pain immediately to the nurse. Not just the pain the patient tells me about, but the **unspoken** pain too. Often the patient doesn't want to "complain," or doesn't realize that there are other drugs to help, or can't take what she has because it upsets her stomach but doesn't want to say anything for fear of being a bother. Also, the body language of a patient gives one a clear indication of unspoken pain. We*

look for that, talk to the patient, call the nurse, the nurse contacts the doctor, the doctor prescribes, the nurse or volunteer gets the medication and delivers it to the pharmacy or patient. If it doesn't help in 12 to 24 hours, further steps are taken. Very often it is the hospice nurse who first realizes a morphine pump is in order, since he/she sees the patient much more often than the doctor.

Our hospice coordinator once told us that 90 percent of the patients that say that they "just want it all to end" are the ones in extreme physical pain. Once that pain is diminished, the quality of life immediately picks up, and the patient no longer wants it all to end.

Quirarte does express some cautions, however:

Unfortunately, not all hospice workers, doctors, nurses are good pain managers. Everyone in hospice gets to know who really cares about the patient's quality of life, and who doesn't. If the time comes that I am terminal, I know which medical personnel I want on my team. Unfortunately, a patient and family usually don't know, and go into this situation blind and pretty much at the mercy of everyone else for their quality of life—unless the patient has an advocate. We have the knowledge to advocate for ourselves, but there comes a time that we need someone else to step in for us.

Dr. Ira Byock, President of the Academy of Hospice Physicians, believes that dying can be a relatively gentle process, but only when there is sufficient support. For home hospice, this may mean that there needs to be a committed family member or friends who are willing to be full-time caregivers. The hospice team—nurses, physicians, social workers and pastoral counselors—are expert in the control not only of pain and other distressing physical symptoms, but also in relieving the emotional suffering that goes along with all the impending losses. There are five simple but powerful statements that every dying person can say to, and hear from, their loved ones, Byock believes. They are:

Forgive me, because in any relationship there are mistakes that need to be forgiven.
I forgive you, for the same reason.
Thank you.
I love you.
Goodbye.[20]

Final gifts: Six stories of dying

Death is the great mystery. We regard it with fear and fascination, as well as overwhelming grief. We deny its inevitability and avoid its approach. Despite the growing hospice movement, the dying are still largely hidden away in hospitals. Many of us have never seen a person die, nor do we allow ourselves to think about what our own deaths might be like. We are inclined to agree with Woody Allen, who once quipped: "I'm not afraid of death. I just don't want to be there when it happens."

Yet for our own peace of mind, it's important to demystify the dying process, to understand how ordinary families get through it. Six husbands of women who died of breast cancer have agreed to share their stories, reproduced here at some length.

Bob Crisp, talking about Ginger's death

Ginger had been failing rapidly when Bob wrote how she and he were facing the prospect of additional treatments:

> I'm not ready for this in several respects. My approach to problems is persistence and it's paid off for me in the past. I've never been close to a decision like this, so everything is new. I'm not ready to accept the "no hope" aspect of the decision. I know that many people in the past have tried to hang on for the possibility of a magic bullet cure. And, however remote, the possibility hangs heavy.
>
> Ginger is closer to the "no more treatment" decision. She has kind of worked up to this. It started with statements like "At some point there may be a time when the treatment problems and the chances of success are so low, that I will not want to continue." This statement has moved to ever stronger stages where now it's "no treatment unless someone can show me that it won't degrade the time I have left and it has a reasonable chance of success."
>
> I have to let Ginger get there in her own way. For my part, I can't go to her and say something similar to "Face reality, no treatment's going to work, the cancer is spreading, it's only a matter of time ...days, weeks, months..." Sometimes a person wants the response: "Don't give up, there's

always hope...." I would rather go down in flames trying something than to play it out for a few extra months. However (big however), I could never be sure until I face the situation and have gone through as many ordeals as she has.

As he had throughout Ginger's illness, Bob allayed his own anxiety by trying to research what they might face next. There wasn't much available that was specific enough for him.

The possible paths that may be taken, what they may look like, how long, how painful ... I could not find. Kind of funny that you can't find something on how a person dies from breast cancer. It would sure be helpful for me. I may go talk to her oncologist as he told our daughter (my step-daughter) that it might "get ugly." She did not ask and he did not give any more detail.

More and more, Bob was aware of feeling a certain sense of distance from Ginger.

I also see an emotional separation that angers me at myself. Yet I know it's my own defense system working to protect me. I have been grieving since April of last year.

I still see the future and she does not. This seems inescapable under these conditions. I can talk and dream of a trip, say to Russia, and know it's something I might do. She can't talk or dream of something like this, as she knows it's not likely. It's a weird place to be. Sitting around with friends, it's easy for me to say something about something I would like to do... but it's different for her. However, I do notice that she will talk about something on or for the house that may be in the future and it will hit me that I hope she is here to see it. When the reality is most likely: I live, she dies, then it's weird. Probably because you have always talked about the future from the same position. Now it's different. Just weird, can't give you a better description.

A month later, Bob reported their meeting with the oncologist.

She asked him about what was ahead and he talked about some physical problems she would encounter. He did not offer and she did not ask about time. If she had wanted to know, she only needed to ask. This is as much as she wants to know as of now. Or that is my reading of it. I think she wants to know what to expect physically in the next few weeks and nothing more. This was the product of months of working our way through this and sensing what Ginger wants and seems not to want. Ginger is not shy. Recall she can be a hard-ass lawyer: one of my friends described her (in legal work) as meaner than a one-eyed water moccasin (old Arkansas expression). So if she wants to know something or talk about something, then she can be quite forceful. We've had many discussions with doctors along the way. She has been detailed in asking about what/how long, etc., on treatments. Her mortality has been brought up on several occasions. Here, she does not ask for detail or more specifics. In the fifteen months of fighting this thing, she has been consistent in not asking about "how long do I have."

Ginger has not "stopped treatment." She is open to anything that might help and not have serious side effects. Not many options, but I think she prefers this to the "official stop procedures." I think that takes away the last glimmer of hope and she is not ready for this step. I think she will get there, but in her time, which is what I want.

She has withdrawn somewhat. She's afraid of losing it emotionally. She does not want to be alone. She wants to do this in the way she thinks it should be done: with dignity, with faith, courage, respect.... In doing so, she hides (suppresses) some emotions.

Two months later, Bob wrote that he was now ready to describe Ginger's death:

The days before Ginger died were very difficult. A week before she died, she started to lose contact with us. We only had a couple of short conversations after that. The last five days were essentially no contact. There were a couple of times where she seemed to indicate an affirmative to wanting some water or similar items. But she was still there internally. She would get very agitated at times and try to move and get out of the bed. At first, it was hard to restrain her. I know that she was in a panic state—not knowing what was happening. We would talk to her to try and calm her. This might go on for fifteen minutes or longer, even an hour at times. The frequency, duration and intensity of these episodes diminished with time. I'm sure the reason for the diminution was that she was too tired to exert herself for any extended period of time. Her pulse rate stayed in the 130+ range and sometimes went up to as high as 180.

We had someone with her around the clock and worked in shifts. I tried at first to stay up as I was afraid of being asleep when she died. After two nights, I realized I could not take this pace and started to sleep some, about four hours a night. The others promised me they would wake me if it looked like she was near death. The morphine pump was a problem in that we had to keep giving extras. It was the only way to keep her calm. They would increase it after we told them of what happened. But it always seemed to be too low to avoid agitation until about the last twenty-four hours.

She took nothing for about five days: no liquids, other than a few drops of water from a straw that we offered as much as she wanted. She had problems with congestion in her throat and lungs that caused difficult coughing. It was very difficult to watch her try to cough and not have the energy to clear the congestion. We had a suction pump to clear the congestion from her throat, but she resisted it and it was hard to get her to accept it. It helped a little.

Her two daughters, Kathy and Ann, and I took on the primary responsibility of any decisions regarding morphine, etc. They wanted her more sedated than I did. These circumstances are difficult as each person has an opinion of what should be done. I'm trying to forget the interpersonal aspects of this as they were done in difficult circumstances. It was a difficult time.

Bob was somewhat reluctant to describe what happened on the day Ginger died.

I don't know if this is something you will want to read. It's not pretty. The death process is ugly, but mixed with some items of beauty and love. I won't be offended if you choose not to read or stop along the way.

It was my first time to see someone die—never happened to me before. We had just a little warning as the person sitting with her noticed that her breathing was slowing. The rest of the family asked me if I wanted some time alone with her and I said yes. I thought the time was close but thought it might go on for awhile, and I told them that I would sit with her and then let them have a few moments alone. Her breaths were spaced apart by several seconds—long enough that after each one you wondered if she would have another. And then she didn't have another breath. I checked my watch and waited a minute and knew she had died. I checked for a pulse and nothing. She just stopped breathing— nothing else. I waited a few minutes alone with her and then went and told the others.

The hospice nurse came first. She is also a deputy coroner and can sign a death certificate. She was very good—knew exactly what to do and things went smoothly. It took about two hours for the funeral home to come and get the body. By that time, several friends had come whom we called. Before the funeral people came in, we sang and danced to the song "Lord of the Dance." It was spontaneous and seemed right. Then the funeral home people came and I asked to help load her body. We put a plastic type board under her body, wrapped the sheets around her and they covered her with a blanket. Then, again I asked to load her into the van, so I pushed her out and loaded the dolly into the van. I watched it drive away. Immediate cremation was her wish so I knew that was the last time I would ever see her remains.

My emotion was primarily one of relief—that her pain and suffering was over. That nobody would ever stick another needle in her arm, or cut on her, or do radiation, or chemo. This emotion of relief stayed with me for several days through the funeral.

Now, I've moved into the sad phase. The reality that she is gone is setting in. That all the dreams will never be. That she is gone from this life and I must go on.

When asked how he might advise others who are forced to face the death of the one they love best in the world, Bob reflected,

I think you show up and do what is needed. Be present in a loving and caring way. It will be emotionally and physically exhausting. Try to pace yourself, as it is a marathon and not a sprint. You can't stay at someone's side for that many straight days. Get some time alone, take long showers, sit outside alone, be close but get some relief. And, listen to your soul and do what you need to do, not just for her but also for yourself. You have to go on and it's important to follow the path where there will be less regrets. I have very few regrets, but I did a lot of things my way, which is not necessarily the right way.

Gerry Wirth, talking about Cindy's death

In September and early October, Cindy was getting severe head-aches. Somehow everyone thought that it was due to rotting teeth, and she even had two removed. But the pain persisted. It was discovered she had three large tumors in her brain. The whole illusion of normalcy started to crash down.

What happened during the following months was very perplexing and painful at the time. Cindy was preparing to die. She became very withdrawn from us. Her life consisted of doctors, hospitals, watching TV at home, and that was it. She was extremely hard on the kids, it was as if she was trying to raise them in the short time she had left. But the worst thing was that I did not see it for what it was. I just reacted to the actions, not the process. My love for her and compassion were at an all time low because I did not understand what was going on. I now believe that she was withdrawing from us so the process of dying and meeting God would not be as painful for her.

I still took the kids to Cub Scouts and gymnastics. I had to spend a lot of time outside of the house because Cindy's tolerance for the normal noise children make was very low. Cindy did not seem to mind being alone, and the kids loved being able to be children. Somewhere during this time the cancer killed my wife even though she still could breathe.

Cindy's parents had to come back. They felt extremely guilty about leaving. About as guilty as I felt for hiring such a lousy sitter. They were wonderful. They relieved my worry about child care and allowed me some peace of mind when I was at work. They also helped me to buffer Cindy better from the children. I am so disappointed in myself about not having the strength, wisdom and insight to allow me to demonstrate my love for Cindy to the end. I got tired.

I did not have much emotional support. I have been contemplating that for the last several weeks. I did not have support, not because people did not care, but because I did not know how to ask for or accept it. During the bulk of Cindy's illness, we relied on each other for support. It seemed like the rest of the world was much too pessimistic for our tastes. In retrospect, they were probably more realistic. Because of this perceived pessimism we only accepted "physical support." Help with the kids, house, cooking, etc. Emotional support was not allowed. When the time came when I could use it, no one was used to giving it.

It is a mistake I hope I never make again.

A few weeks later, Gerry was more philosophical about what had happened, although his regret about not saying good-bye is a litany that runs throughout his narrative.

I lost Cindy sometime in January. She knew the end was near and started withdrawing from the living and preparing to die. Many people I have talked to say that this is normal. What would have been tragic is if I would have lost her in October of 1991 when she was diagnosed. We both know many people who die on the day they are diagnosed with cancer and the rest of their lives are spent waiting to stop breathing.

Cindy, and I guess myself, did everything we could to live and enjoy the four years that followed. She raised her newborn daughter into a confident, caring four year old. She gave my son a love of nature and books. Most importantly, she taught me how to be a good, patient and loving father. We went camping, to Disney World, to museums, zoos, parks and theater. We enjoyed our friends and everything about life.

During the final weeks of Cindy's life, Gerry recalls not being able to comprehend what was really happening.

Cindy was becoming less able to walk or function. She would get from her bed to a chair in the living room and back to bed. Sometimes she was even too weak for that and stayed in bed. She had no patience for the normal noise and bickering that children do and she was very hard on both of them. Cindy's folks were staying with us, helping with her and the kids and letting me go to work enough so I would not get fired. I tried to have things as normal as possible for the kids while making things comfortable for Cindy.

I found out later that she said good-bye to some of the office staff who had been a special part of her treatment over the four years. They were not willing to accept it and admit the fight was over. I wish I would have been there so I could have picked up on this. It might have prompted me to start my good-byes.

Clearly, though, Cindy had prepared her family for her death in other ways. Gerry recalls Cindy's careful instruction about caring for their children and the house. In the last months of her life, she was teaching him how to cook.

*Cindy was extremely patient. She would tell me over and over how to do things. She would even write down checklists. Most importantly, she would never criticize in a negative way. It was always, "this is okay, but if you try **this** it might work out even better." I did not always do these chores cheerfully, I was trying to build a new career in the company, but Cindy rarely let my sullenness affect her gentle guidance.*

The last thing that she taught me was how to make pizza. Both our children loved her homemade pizza. She taught it to me in December. I had to carry her from the chair in the living room to the kitchen so she could keep an eye on me! I will never be one quarter the homemaker she was. But whatever I am I owe to her.

Gerry described Cindy's last week day by day.

Tuesday, February 6. I came home from work and visited Cindy. She was okay, lucid and had been given several neurological tests. I went home for supper and brought the kids back to visit in the evening. She was not all that interested in seeing them. Another sign I should have caught. We did not stay long, as she was tired.

Wednesday, February 7. I went home to eat, and returned with the kids. She did not even want them near her, as she hurt so badly and they were wanting to hug and hold her. We did not stay very long and I told the kids to say good-bye. I knew I would not bring them back as long as their mother was like this. I did not want them to have that memory of her.

Thursday, February 8. Again the same pattern, except at 9:00 p.m. the nurses called and said I should come to the hospital as her vital signs were weak. Cindy's mom and I rushed over. Her mom stayed until 11:00 p.m. She then went home so she could get the kids ready for school in the morning. We felt as much normalcy as possible was best. I stayed the entire night, just holding her hand and napping in a chair. I was not smart enough to talk to her.

Friday, February 9. On Friday morning her oncologist came in. He said there was nothing else that could be done. She should be sent home to wait. And he was going on vacation. I knew there was no hope left, but I did not want her to die at home in front of the kids. I convinced the doctor to check her into inpatient hospice. There is never a good time for an oncologist to take vacation. It just was so devastating as Cindy and I had so much faith in his compassion.

I went home and slept two hours and then tried to find an inpatient hospice. It was a nightmare. My insurance required hospice care to save money. Inpatient hospice is hard to find and thus limited to one week. Everyone thought Cindy would linger. Additionally, all the hospice "counselors" tried to make me feel guilty for not taking her home. Finally, one of the nurses in the oncologist's office used her connections to allow her to stay where she was at hospice rates. Cindy's father went home on the pretense of signing up for his Social Security retirement benefits. I believe he did not want to be here for the end.

Saturday, February 10. Saturday was my day to be with, and try to support the kids. I took Courtney to her gymnastic lessons. Matt had earned free pizza at Pizza Hut for reading thirty books, so I took them to lunch there. It seems ludicrous I did these things on the day Cindy died. I visited her in the afternoon and evening. She was drifting in and out of consciousness but never really lucid. I just held her hand and wept. I got home at 7:30 p.m., exhausted. I only had had four or five hours of sleep in two days. I was about to go to bed at 8:30 p.m. when the hospital called again. Cindy's breathing was labored, I should come.

I did not believe she would die that night. I was upset because I was so tired but went anyway. When I got there she was breathing very hard. I sat with her and held her hand. I whispered my "good-byes" and "I love you's" in her ear. I sat in the chair and dozed off until 11:00 p.m. When I awoke, I decided to get some coffee so I could stay awake with her. I was gone for ten minutes. When I returned, the room was very quiet. I thought her breathing had gotten better. Only slowly did I realize that she had died. I waited thirty minutes to ensure she was gone before I called the nurse. We had the proper DNR papers, but I wanted no arguments.

I was furious with myself. For four years I was with her through as much as I could, but I was not there at the end! Others have told me that *sometimes they wait until you are gone to die, especially if you have not let go of them. I do not know if this is true. But I wish I would have been there.*

I made the appropriate calls, her mom, my folks, and went home. As I left the hospital, a selfish sense of joy and relief came over me, as I knew it was over and I would not have to come back! But it was also a lonely walk to the car.

Looking back, six months later, Gerry's regrets were transformed into advice he hoped to pass on to others in the same situation.

Cindy took her last two chemo treatments to please me. She had given up. Those treatments were very painful and I do not blame her for not wanting them. The ironic part about it is that I encouraged her to take them because I thought that she was still fighting and just needed encouragement.

It is hard to know when to acknowledge the fight is over. I wish I would have so we could have said good-byes before she lost lucidity. Not knowing if she heard my final "good-bye" and "I love you" is one of the two things I regret still and probably will until I die. If you can somehow communicate this so others will not make the same error, it would be very helpful to those left behind. We focused so hard on fighting cancer that I waited too long to say good-bye.

Fight as hard and as long as you can, but know when to say good-bye.

The rituals Gerry observed on important dates, however painful, helped him to work through his grief.

I decided to go to mass in the morning and then stop at the cemetery to place a bouquet on her grave. I thought that marking the day in that way would help. It didn't. My pain and grief was as strong as it has ever been. I wept over her grave for an hour. It is a good thing it was 7:00 a.m. and the cemetery was really closed. I wept for all the times I did not understand her enough. I wept for all the times her children will not have a Mom at a special day. I wept for myself, and the loneliness that is always with me. And I wept because I cannot even order a grave marker that I feel is special enough to mark her final resting place! I am not used to indulging my pain in this way, but on that day I did.

Others have told me that there will be another in my life some day. I do not believe it will ever happen. How can I ever find someone with whom I have shared so much?

We celebrated her birthday, too. Because our anniversary and her birthday are so close, we always postponed the big celebration until the anniversary. But we always did something special on her birthday as well. Usually we went out for ice cream at a special store in town. Matthew really enjoyed telling the waitress it was his Mom's birthday. We went out for ice cream in the evening. Matt asked if we could. For some reason he wanted to celebrate. When he asked I did not think I would enjoy it. But I did.

Our anniversary, June 23, was much better. This year I took the kids to a water amusement park. I went with another couple, the Jacobs, from school. They knew it was our anniversary and would not take no for an answer. It was a day of total distraction. But seeing all the kids have a great time gave me a warm feeling. I am not sure I am doing a good job as a parent. I try the best I can, but there are always doubts. Seeing them have a good time, like before Cindy died, helps to give me confidence.

For me life goes on. There is a huge hole in my life, but the pain is subsiding. What I miss most is someone to share things with. Triumphs, decisions, work, quiet times. Many people who lose a spouse say they are not really gone, just there in a different way. I envy those, for Cindy is very far from me. But yet she is all around. The needlepoint pictures on the wall, the dinner recipes I cook. Her gifts live on, her companionship is missed.

Chris Tribur, talking about Candace's death

My wife had two recurrences, one shortly after HDC. Up until the last, I refused to acknowledge the inevitable. We never discussed it and, in fact, my wife quickly became incapable of discussing options and so I made all the decisions, including a final one to cease treatment that will haunt me the rest of my life. To the best of my knowledge my wife did not wish to cease treatment, and I certainly did not want to let her go. I think when the time comes, the choices narrow themselves and we do the best we can. These are extraordinarily difficult circumstances to find oneself in, but we do what we do and there is no value in second-guessing or beating oneself up after the fact.

I took her to the Cancer Treatment Center in Tulsa, where they ran a battery of tests. She deteriorated steadily. One night she had an episode where she flung herself out of her wheelchair and started shrieking at me incoherently. I took her to the inpatient floor of the tower comprising the CTC and they admitted her. She became incontinent, developed labored breathing and was in a near comatose state. The docs took me downstairs to x-ray and displayed the hundreds of CT scans we had brought from Denver with us. They showed me that one of her lungs was completely filled with fluid and the other was spider-webbed with tumor. She was admitted to intensive care.

Late the night of the 3rd of July 1995, they called in a pulmonary doc. He told me they could drain the filled lung, but her blood count was so low, that she could bleed to death. He recommended doing nothing. They put her on a morphine pump. I sat and stood by her bed frantically pressing the infusion button every time she stirred in discomfort.

On the 4th, I called my sister-in-law Helen, who was staying with the girls in Denver, and suggested they fly down. Helen stayed, and the girls came. Candace's oldest sister and her husband had already driven up from Georgetown, Texas. Zoe visited her mother one time in ICU and wouldn't return. Miri stayed with me up to near the end. When Candace started to go, Miri reacted rather violently and I grabbed her and left the room. My brother-in-law called us in our room to tell us Candace was gone. The girls and I departed the next morning for Denver.

When Chris read a message from another husband about the importance of discussing end-of-life decisions and saying good-bye, he expressed both skepticism and regret.

My wife and I never really dealt with this and she was the one who did the pulling away. I fault her for nothing, I only regret that we didn't really come together to face the inevitable. I think we could have emotionally held onto each other lovingly, instead of existing in "bubbles" of denial. Second-guessing in my situation is futile and destructive. I just wanted to say I admire you for your clarity and wisdom.

Every circumstance is different. I don't know what her choice was. She made no overt indications of her wishes. I speculated that she may have subconsciously or unconsciously thrown in the towel as early as April. Maybe earlier, I don't know. Without spoken direction from her, I was dragged reluctantly to the final stage. I didn't want to give up.

I had no help from anyone. I had a feeling that people (family, doctors) were stepping back from us. I felt kind of abandoned. I agreed to no more treatment a couple of days before she died only when it was spelled out in black and white for me. I suppose everyone should have a "living will" or something comparable. But I saw no clear-cut place prior to the time of my decision where one could, in good conscience, "pull the plug." If she had looked into my eyes and said, "No more, Chris," it would have been different, maybe. I don't know. Calculating intellect has very little place in this scenario, in my opinion.

She had the services of a pain specialist while in ICU. At one point after the morphine pump was hooked up, a nurse said they wanted to make sure she didn't get "too much." I snapped back, "You've got to be kidding!" I had already agreed to no further treatment, and the attending physician said several times to me "I have a bad feeling."

I don't think you will find two circumstances or two individuals who will react the same in such circumstances. I regret I didn't do more at an earlier time. I go back over the whole chronology and second-guess everything! Her favorite oncology nurse reacted to the news of her death, "but her prognosis was excellent!" My wife's older and favorite sister holds her oncologist responsible for letting her cancer get out of control. I don't know what to think. The only comfort I have is that my wife was tired of fighting and seemed to let go on her own. She slipped slowly into a childlike state of mind, where she looked forward to almost fantastic, dreamlike plans for the future and stopped looking back at the harsh road she had traveled.

All in all it was not a neat and tidy affair by any stretch of the imagination. I felt out of control most of the way.

Scott Kitterman, talking about Mary's death

As Mary's cancer worsened, Scott, who had researched exhaustively and played a major role in treatment decisions, was finding it hard to let go. Describing his state of mind, he wrote that he was coping with "plenty of denial."

> *I'm still subconsciously convinced that there's a way out of this. When my mother died of breast cancer in '83 we had a good six months warning that the end was coming. I was convinced that I had prepared myself emotionally for her death. I was really wrong. Hit me like a ton of bricks anyway. So, each time a brick lands on my head I just do my best to shrug it off and move on to the next one. It's not easy, but once again what other choice do I have? You can't really cushion yourself from the blows.*

Although he'd encouraged Mary throughout to continue in treatment, and fight the cancer aggressively, Scott was also aware that there would come a time when further treatment would be futile.

> *We knew a month or two ago that the chemotherapy regimen she was starting then was the last one it made any sense to do. We had looked through things then—there were some things in Phase I trials, but nothing that was even in an NCI sponsored trial. Mary wasn't interested in an option that bought her a few days or weeks. If it wasn't measured in months, she wasn't that interested in it. She would have liked something measured in years, but it didn't work out that way. That's the first thing, in terms of how her wishes went. She was very aware of how this was likely to turn out, and had thoughts in her mind about what was reasonable to do and what was not.*

> *We didn't always agree 100 percent on that, and there were several times during the last seven months since she was diagnosed with recurrence that she'd say, "Well, it's time to give up." I'd say, "No, not yet—these things it makes sense to do." And she'd say she'd go on.*

> *The problem is that when you are undergoing some form of chemotherapy, and it looks to be effective, you just don't know how long it's going to be effective.*

What finally happened was that about three weeks before she died, she got what turned out to be her last chemotherapy treatment, and that night started having some unusual pain.

The doctors discussed with us going back to methotrexate, which was the first intrathecal (in the membrane surrounding the spinal cord) chemo which she'd had back in March. She'd been on that until the disease had gotten resistant. So they said, "We can go back to that, and give it three days in a row, rather than just one, and see what that does." Based on her feeling, she didn't want to suffer if it was going to just give her a few more days.

It was the news of this latest recurrence that caused both Scott and Mary to make their decision.

When they gave her the news that the cancer had come back, she looked at me and said, "I'm ready." And I said to her, "It's time." One of the things that amazes me in my own reaction to all of this is how quickly I flip-flopped. I was always the one banging my fist on the table, saying, "We need to go on, we need to do the next thing and keep going." But based on what we'd agreed on, about how you made these decisions, it was obvious that we were at the point where we were done. There was no doubt in my mind that that was the point where we were at. There wasn't any in hers either. We'd always been researching and looking for options, and we knew that the chemo she'd been on was the last one that made any sense. We hoped we were going to get more time out of that, but we didn't.

Mary said she wanted to die at home. I didn't know how I felt about that. My only prior experience with a close family member was when my mother died of breast cancer in 1983, and she had died in the hospital, so I had never dealt with that.

I was a little worried about having Mary here. She wanted to come home so that's what we did. End of discussion. Once she got home, it turned out to be just fine. I really felt quite comfortable with it. We both slept in our bed. It seemed almost normal a few moments at a time. It was certainly physically and emotionally easier not to be divided between taking care of Mary at the hospital and taking care of Sylvia (our daughter) at home. One of the things I'd been going through was that when I was at the hospital, I wanted to be home with Sylvia—she stayed in day care during the day, and I saw her in the evenings. When I was here, I wanted to be with Mary. Bringing Mary home ended that feeling of being divided. That was an important thing for me. It gave Sylvia a chance to see her mother again.

The one difficult problem we had in getting Mary out of the hospital was in the area of pain control. She was on the morphine pump with the button you push to get more, but the thing that kept happening because most of her pain was spasmodic, she was on a very low basal rate, and then most of the morphine that she got was in bolus form. Because her disease was progressing fast it was very easy to get behind the power curve on that. They had ordered additional morphine for IV push. When you needed that, it told you it was time to raise the amount of morphine in the box, but then you had to get orders written for that, and that takes time. On top of that, she'd have really bad ones, where no amount of morphine was going to make any difference. So in those cases, they had Ativan, which is similar to Valium, and that just put her out, to sleep. Sometimes that was the only way to get her out of that pain. That was fairly successful. There was kind of a step hierarchy that you walked through to try to manage it, and you always knew if you gave her the Ativan, that within thirty seconds she'd be asleep, out, and at least not feeling the pain. But that's the problem. Morphine and Ativan are closely controlled substances, and they don't like to give out morphine, except in the PCA pump, and they certainly don't like to give out Ativan either. That was the one area where we had trouble with the going-home part of it. In the end, we worked it out okay.

Hospice was very helpful. As it happened, we didn't need a huge amount of help. Mary's mother came and stayed with us, and I was here, and my father came and stayed as well. There were plenty of people in the house to help out and do things. I am very comfortable, more than most people would be, in doing a lot of the medical things that needed to be done.

Before we brought Mary home, I had a little talk with Sylvia. She's not even three yet, so she has a limited understanding. She really doesn't talk much yet—she's got a little speech delay. Something to do with stress in the family, I think.

She'd been to see Mary in the hospital. Whenever Mary would feel like giving up, I'd always take Sylvia to see her and she'd change her mind. Not particularly fighting fair, but it worked. She understood, and had been sick herself in the hospital, so she thought, well you go to the hospital and you get better.

I said, "Sylvia, this time Mommy's just not going to get better." She got very sad, but then, like any two year old, five minutes later, her mind was on something else. So when we brought Mary home, Sylvia was a dear. She went up to her Mommy and hugged her, and lay down with her and wanted to be with her. Sylvia was scared by her, and she couldn't stay there for a long time, but she spent as much time as she could deal with.

She wanted to know what she could do to help. It really impresses me how well she has dealt with all of this. I felt it was important to keep her as informed and involved as could be, given her age.

By the time we got home on Friday, Mary really couldn't talk anymore. She was awake and aware, and obviously knew where she was. She could occasionally get a word out. There was some confusion. She was on a fair amount of morphine by then and the cancer was progressing. She was Catholic, so we had the priest come in and give her last rites, while she was still aware of what was going on. We made sure that the spiritual aspect of it was taken care of.

People called and said, "Well, maybe I'll come by next week." I said, "Look, this disease has always been very aggressive. It's moving fast. I don't know how long it's going to be. So if it's important to you to see her before she's gone, I wouldn't wait. Come now." It got progressively worse over the next several days, with less time when she was conscious and more time when she was basically asleep, although even when she was not obviously conscious, you'd see evidence that she was aware of what was going on around her. Until the point she died, I think she was aware.

By Monday, she had fluid in her lungs. First it sounded as if she was snoring, then it got heavier from there. We sat her up and that seemed to help. She had IV fluids, to keep her hydrated. Her kidneys were starting to shut down as the disease progressed. Tuesday she was worse, and we put her on oxygen that morning, and just about 1:30 she stopped breathing, and her heart stopped beating and she died.

At the end, it was very quiet and peaceful. One of the things she had told us was that she wanted her mother and me with her. Just a couple of minutes before she died, she opened her eyes just a slit, for the first time in about 12 to 18 hours. It was almost as if she was checking to see who was there. I'd been downstairs because her mother was saying a rosary with her, and I left them their privacy for that. Something just told me it was time to go upstairs. I'm not sure why. But she opened her eyes a little bit, and her breathing just gradually got a little more ragged, a little more ragged, and just stopped. Then a couple minutes later, the color went out of her face and her heart stopped.

I called the hospice people and the funeral home and they pretty much took care of everything from there. I'm sure that some of how I feel right now is masked by shock, because it's only been just over a week. But I do feel surprisingly at peace with the whole thing. I miss the hell out of her, and I cry sometimes.

The key thing is that now, looking back, I don't have any feeling of regret: damn, if only we had done this. We did the things that there were to do. We researched the hell out of it, to make sure we had explored our options and knew what all of them were. It tears me apart, what happened, but it was going to happen. There was nothing else that could have been done about it. That's another thing that makes this different than my mother's death. There are some things that should have been done differently in her case. So much has changed in pain control. Then it was, "You can't have your shot. It hasn't been four hours yet." Morphine's been around for a hundred years.

The person going through this has a lot of ups and downs. It's very easy for them to get despondent and depressed and give up. One of the things that's important is, even if you know how things are probably going to turn out, to keep some hope alive that maybe, that's not going to happen. What Mary had was rare and there wasn't a lot of current research about it. We had to do research by analogy. We always had a hope that if we could just get this thing beaten down pretty thoroughly, there was something that might produce some kind of durable remission. Hope was present with every kind of chemotherapy we tried. It was only the week before her death when we realized that the last chemotherapy had failed, that we realized that that wasn't going to happen. And so throughout the whole seven months, we knew what was probably going to happen and what we hoped was going to happen. Keeping that hope alive is critical.

I'd always heard people say about dying, "Oh, it was nice and peaceful and she was surrounded by her friends," and so forth. I never believed that was possible. But that is basically what happened. It was surprisingly calm and peaceful.

Somebody asked me, "How are you going to feel if she dies in your bed?" I thought, well, I'll just buy another bed—Mary wants to come home. I haven't felt the need to do that yet. I may change my mind over time, but I slept in the bed that night after she died.

Chris Leach, talking about Pat's death

Pat was anything but a stoic cancer "patient." Her medical knowledge (she was a psychiatric nurse) of course was a mixed blessing. It kept her busy and gave her a certain degree of satisfaction to be informed on the different options that were available and under research. But that same knowledge also reinforces some aspects of the disease that might better be pushed back into the recesses of the mind somewhere.

Regarding her "calm" reaction on hearing the news of her brain mets, I don't think she changed in any significant way during the last months. Although now that I am reflecting on that thought, I think it is safe to say that she did seem to change somewhat as far as her acceptance that she (we) were running out of options. But once again, she did not change at anytime to the extent that she became someone else. Her reality in all its splendor was with her and us right up to the second she died.

Pat and Chris, who loved to travel together, had decided to take a final trip up the California coast, visiting friends and family, and stopping along the way for the constant transfusions Pat now needed as the cancer spread through her bone marrow.

That would have kept me from going on any trips. But with Pat it was different. Since we knew pretty much where we were going, I and she made phone calls with her oncologist's help, and set up appointments for blood transfusions in San Diego, San Francisco and Eureka, California.

As we traveled up the coast of California, I would stop to tank up the rental car and drop Pat off at a hospital to have her blood tanked up.

We left San Diego and flew up to Marin County. Pat received a couple of units of blood at Marin General Hospital. We visited relatives, and visited a woman that Pat had met on the Internet. Again, I noticed that Pat seemed to be moving a little slower, getting tired more frequently, but still getting the most out of each day. She even seemed to be enjoying dining out but not with the same gusto as in the past. By the time we got up to where our son lives in Arcata, her blood counts were dropping to the point that it looked like it was dangerous to go more than three days or so without a transfusion.

On or about August 13, she called Dr. Susan Rabinowe, her oncologist in Hartford, Connecticut. Based on that call her doctor said we better get home as soon as possible. Susan tried to keep a positive spin on it by suggesting that we were already gone for three weeks and had seen everyone so that should lessen the disappointment. Actually I was glad we were going home, I was nervous to say the least. We drove the 280 miles from Arcata to San Francisco, caught a red-eye to Hartford arriving at about 12 noon the next day, Thursday, August 15. We went directly from the airport to St. Francis and Dr. Rabinowe. I thought at the time that she would examine Pat, give her a couple of units of blood and send us home with the expectation that we would come back in a few days or so. That was not to be. Pat was admitted to St. Francis that day and there she stayed until I brought her home on September 5. That first night was the only time she was alone up to the day she died on September 11.

The next day I went back to St. Francis, and with the exception of two nights when one of the children relieved me, I camped out in the hospital room with Pat. As I said earlier, she was never alone. She had a steady stream of visitors. It was actually peaceful at night when just she and I were alone. The nurses and nurses aides loved her. I learned some nursing skills myself. Pat was pretty much incontinent, I took care of everything 90 percent of the time before the nurses ever responded to the bell. We actually had some tender moments, if you can imagine that.

A critical event, by the way, is the issue of pain. Pat, understandably, had said on several occasions that her biggest fear was pain and suffering. Mercifully, she never experienced significant pain. Shortly before we left for California she had been having some fairly annoying pain in her neck, shoulder and hip areas. Even that disappeared. Her demeanor became relaxed, even when she wasn't on Ativan or other medication. In fact she did not take much in the way of medication the last couple of weeks at all. The memorable thing is and was her sweet smile. One of the reasons they all loved her in the hospital was that she was incredibly solicitous of others, especially with that sweet smile that was her lifelong trademark.

The attending physicians were very helpful. It became pretty obvious that Pat probably was not going to get better. I knew it, they knew it, but it didn't matter in the end, we simply loved her, stayed with her and waited. It was, I think, a case of mutual understanding that we were on the homestretch. We never really said, "Well, I guess this is it, honey." We just knew, and simply stayed close together the whole time.

I had, by this time, talked with several of the doctors, given them Pat's living will. It was her and my intention that extraordinary intervention not be used just to keep tissue alive. She, myself and the children agreed that we did not want Pat to wind up being a medical experiment. A CT scan of Pat's head was called for to see if her mental fogginess was caused by the low blood counts or possibly cancer impinging on her brain. Pat and I were alone in her room when the doctor announced that the CT scan confirmed that the cancer was, in fact, now pressing into the brain. Pretty heavy news, I'm sure you will agree. In the past Pat had reacted, again understandably, pretty strongly to far less devastating news. This time she looked at me very calmly and simply said, "Well, that's not what I had hoped for." And that was the extent of that.

The kids were driving up to Hartford every day. Not surprising, they and, needless to say, I loved her to an unimaginable degree. Stephen flew home just a few days after we did, by the way. He canceled the whole semester at Humboldt State so that he could be with his mother. We were happy about that, not that it would have been any other way.

Back to the results of the CT scan. It was at this point that we made the collective decision that no further treatment, other than palliative medication for pain if necessary, would be given. Pat wanted to be at home, so on September 5 I took her home. We got home early afternoon, it was a beautiful day. She sat outside in her wheelchair with the sun, kids and dog for a couple of hours. We set up the hospital bed in the living room, facing the picture window, trees and birds. The next day, Friday, we were able to get her outside again when the hospice nurse came by to do her interview. She almost completed it when we had to bring her in because she was getting tired. In the meantime, friends, neighbors, relatives were streaming in and out all of the time. More food than we could eat. We allowed anyone that wanted to be with her to do so. By the time Monday rolled around, Pat was pretty much sleeping all the time. It was getting harder to get her to take any liquids. But again, thankfully, there was no sign of suffering. We kept her comfortable. But still it was the worst time of my life. The feeling of helplessness was overwhelming.

We kept trudging along, waiting. We had reached a point where we were whispering in Pat's ear to let it go, that it was okay, let it go. On September 11, Wednesday morning, my oldest daughter was alone at Pat's bedside when she called to me that Mom was breathing strangely. I listened to her chest with my stethoscope, checked her pulse and told Kathleen that I think this is it. In a matter of minutes after saying that, Pat simply stopped breathing. I held her hand, caressed her head in my arms and cried my eyes out.

Pat died at 11:20 a.m. I called hospice, and they came over in a short while. In the meantime all of the children, Pat's mother, the hospice nurse gathered around, and an hour or so later I escorted Pat to the van, and from there she was taken to the crematory.

Hospice was wonderful. By their own admission they did not have to do very much because the kids and neighbors had things so attentively under control. They told me they had never seen such love and family support. If they weren't just trying to be nice I guess that is a very nice compliment. But they sure were there if we needed them. They have been following up to see if I need any support as well.

Pat's physicians were honest and straightforward. Other than that I did not feel they had any real involvement, certainly emotionally anyway, other than assuring me that they would be sure they did all they could to keep Pat from suffering.

What was helpful was the care, concern and relationship we had with the hospital staff, and, of course, the love and support—ongoing, I might *add—of family and friends. I honestly cannot think of any significant things I would do differently. We are just very lucky that we have the kids and friends that we have.*

The advice I have for others is just that: invest your love now and you will not have any regrets later.

We bought a little plot at the local cemetery. I brought a small tarp. They let you dig your own hole for ashes. I took an antique family silver teaspoon, gave each of the kids a clear plastic 35mm film container and half filled them, using the spoon, with Pat's ashes. That way they could each take a small portion of their mothers remains and do what they liked. I then put the remaining ashes in the hole, put the silver spoon, Pat's wedding band, and, removing my wedding band, placed that in the hole also. Then each of us sprinkled soil over the ashes and objects, Father Kevin said the burial prayers, and we all went to breakfast.

Seven months after Pat's death, Chris sent this update on their family.

Our daughter Maura had a beautiful baby boy on December 19. He is now almost four months old and the cutest, most lovable little creature that God ever created, or however those things happen. So I am now a grandfather, consequently my accolades for my grandson may be some-what biased. My oldest daughter, Kathleen, is due to deliver her first baby this July 12.

The only really sad part about the new baby is, of course, Pat's mem-ory. It was the one major "milestone" she did not make. I have to admit, I am starting a few tears writing this part. When Ryan was born, we all had the same thoughts, namely, "If Pat could only have been here for this." Knowing how she felt about her own kids, we knew all too well how she would have reveled in joy over the grandson she never got to see or hold.

But life, as they say, goes on, and you can be sure that any grandchil-dren we have will hear much about the wonderful grandmother they never got to see....

Glenn Clabo, talking about Barb's death

As I was finishing the final editing on the manuscript of this book, Glenn Clabo wrote that his wife, Barb, had fallen ill with very rapidly progressing multiple tumors in her liver, that had recurred after some months of remission following her high-dose chemotherapy. After consultation with her oncologist, Barb decided to seek no further treatment and to die at home. Within a few weeks, she was gone. When I went to pay my respects at the funeral home five days after her death, Glenn and their close friend Phyllis Dalby, a nurse who had been with the family throughout, sat down with me and recounted what had occurred. Although Glenn and Barb's children, Jamie, 20, and Chad, 18, didn't take part in the interview, their role in her last days was central.

Glenn spoke first of what led up to the last day of Barb's life.

> In my eyes, how we got to the day was basically our life. It wasn't just a moment of discussing our feelings with each other. We were spontaneous most of our life in our relationship. What really got me to that day, and how it all evolved, was this: When Barb got diagnosed, when we found out the cancer was in her liver, we were talking about treatment and how far she really wanted to go. One of the things that really got me upset was that she was concerned she wouldn't do enough, or that I wouldn't think she did enough. That really made me mad. We talked about it, and never really resolved it.

> Three or four months later, after the bone marrow transplant, when she was pretty much well, we sat around for a day or two and forced ourselves to talk about a lot of things. One of the things I told her was that I was really mad about that. I told her it was okay with me when she wanted to die. It was like this huge thing came off of us, and she said, "I promise you, when it's time, I'm going to go. But when it's time, it's my time." I said, "Fine, I want you to understand...don't stick around just for me...don't fight on for me."

> How the day evolved will help you to understand a little better. I basically knew what was going on. I had done a lot of research, finding out how this process happened. We talked with the doctor that Monday, and he told us, step by step, what was going to happen.

The night before, I stayed up, just talking to Barb. She was in and out. She would stay awake for a few minutes and then just fade off for a half an hour, or an hour. It was hard to wake her up, and at about 4 o'clock, I couldn't feel a pulse. She wouldn't respond to me. I got up, went out and got a drink of water, and came back. I kept talking to her. Her pulse would go real low, and then she'd just come back. Then about 6 o'clock, she woke up and started cracking jokes. That's when I realized she was fighting it, that she just didn't want to let go. We needed to do something to make her comfortable, to make it okay.

She was in our bed, and she just didn't want to be there. She wanted to be out in the living room, on the couch, in her favorite place. The sequence was: we went from the bed, then we took her and put her in a chair and sat her in the middle of the room, in a chair with wheels, because we never got the wheelchair, then we moved her to my chair, the Lazy-Boy. We basically had to carry her. We put her in that chair and she didn't like it. So finally, I just picked her up and put her on the couch. She wouldn't lay down. She was still in and out, and when you moved her, it really brought her down. Her pulse just basically went to nothing. She just sat in her spot on the couch, sitting up, for five hours, semi-comatose.

Phyllis came in when I was in the computer room, taking a break. She told me Barb's medical status, and said, "Glenn, maybe you need to talk to her." So I went out into the room, and talked to Barb, but I never really had the feeling that she wanted me to talk to her. She really didn't want to hear what I was saying, that it was okay, that she could let herself go. I never really felt comfortable with it. There was something wrong. And this is where it starts getting really weird. I still haven't figured it out.

One thing that was bothering me was that everyone sat in the living room, just crying, moping, touching. It seemed like they were even embarrassed to laugh. Jamie came up one time and said, "This is not what Mom wants. We've got to lighten this up."

I sat on the couch for a long time, got very tired, and finally got up and said, "It just isn't time." I went off with Phyllis and another friend out on the deck and we talked for maybe half an hour. During that time, Barb was comatose, I would say. She was moaning, a continuous moan, which was probably her voice box relaxing. Then Jamie came out of the house and said, "Dad, she's calling you." Maybe she was...I don't know if she was, but she looked like she was just saying "Glenn" very rapidly.

So I sat in front of her and hugged her. Chad was on one side, and Jamie was on the other side. And I very slowly said a bunch of things. It wasn't planned. It wasn't a thought. It just came out. It was how I felt. I think the real key to the whole thing was that I kept saying everything was okay, "I'm okay, Jamie's okay." But what really was the key, what changed things and let her relax, was when Chad said to her, "I'm okay, Mom. I promise I will be okay."

I say it was cosmic, and it really felt beyond human...because she very slowly just stopped moaning, as I kept talking to her. I told her, "Barb, everyone's going to cry. We're not going to cry for very long, and we're all going to be happy again. I promise you that." And she stopped breathing, and some of the people in the room began sobbing and screaming. And I just sat there—and she started breathing again. It was almost like they scared her awake. I kept on saying, "Please, I told you...please...everything is okay. I told you they were going to cry. Don't let them scare you. Everything is okay. They're going to cry, but they're going to laugh again." And she basically calmed back down, and she stopping breathing. She just died, sitting up.

I got up, and to be honest with you, I didn't know where the hell I was. I still don't know what I was feeling. Probably I felt every emotion in the whole world. I didn't even feel like a human being. I went in the bathroom and I was just sitting there. When I came back out, the kids were on the deck and everyone was saying good-bye. I went up to my kids, and I said, "Let's not treat it like it's the end. Let's treat it like it's the beginning. Just carry on with what she wanted us to do." And we are. I see a huge difference in my kids. This whole thing has changed us altogether, especially my son.

It was perfect. I almost feel it was out of some kind of romance novel...

At this point, Phyllis offered some of her impressions:

Glenn asked me if he was romanticizing what happened. And I said, "No, not in my opinion." I have never seen anything like this. I feel privileged to have been a part of it, really. The amount of love and trust between Glenn and Barbie was something so rare in life, to see that between people. Glenn loved her enough to be able to let her go, to do what he had to do. And that Barbie trusted him enough to listen to him, and to believe him, and let go. That was so obvious.

The first time Glenn talked to Barbie, they weren't ready. Maybe he wasn't ready, and she could sense that. But then, as things got worse, to me she seemed very torn. She wanted to go, but she couldn't. She was hanging on. There were no vital signs at this point. She was moaning...and the people with her, the family, were getting very upset. People kept asking me, "Is she in pain?" I said, "I don't think so. I just don't think she wants to let go."

Glenn just kind of walked over to her. I had the feeling that he was a man with a mission. He knew what he had to do. He knelt down between her legs and put his arms around her. He said everything right. I don't know where the words were coming from. Even when he was talking to her at the end, it was not morbid at all. He even made a few jokes. As he talked to her, you could see her visibly relax. That sense of torment that she seemed to have just went away. He said to her, "Relax, take it easy, go with it, it's okay. We love you."

I just feel so blessed to have been able to see something like that. I don't think I will ever see something like that again—that kind of love and trust between people. Glenn was so open and welcoming all the time. That's not always true with families. Any friend who wanted to come by and see her and spend time with her, the door was open. She did have good friends come by and hold her hand. She was surrounded by love.

They say that the hearing is the last sense to go, and that it's very intense when someone is dying. In the three days I was there, we joked and called her "satellite ears" because she'd be in the bedroom, and people would be talking quietly in other parts of the house, and she'd hear them. Friends would be visiting, and she seemed so out of it that they started talking a little bit louder, and she'd say, "Oh, stop talking so loud." I've seen that with other patients, that their hearing became much keener.

One of my fondest memories was the night I got there, she was lying in their bed, and I lay down beside her. She kept going in and out, falling asleep. But she said to me, "This is the end, isn't it?" I said to her, "Barbie,

*you have a little bit of time, but not too much. I guess you know that."
"How much time do you think?" she asked. I said, "I really don't know, but
if there's anything you want to tell me...." She started talking to me about
Glenn. She said, "I know nobody will ever take my place with Glenn.
We've been together for so long." (He was 13 and she was 15). She said,
"I want you to make sure he gets some companionship. He'll need a
woman. And I want you to talk to Jamie. Don't let Jamie scare her away."
I said, "Have you already talked to her about that?" She said, "Yes, I
have. But you might have to talk with her, too." I said, okay, and I will
encourage Glenn when he's ready.*

*Such incredible love. That night, she was in the bathroom, having a
hard time. She was very yellow, and her stomach was swollen with ascites
at that time. She could hardly walk, and she couldn't toilet herself. She
was crying and saying, "I'm sorry" and "I look so terrible." It was what
any woman would feel with her husband. He put his head in her neck,
and nuzzled her, and said, "How beautiful you are to me. I love you." And
he meant it. And she settled down and let us help her. In his eyes, she was
still beautiful.*

As the interview ended, Glenn reflected:

*I am sitting here and amazing myself. I'm doing okay. Twenty
months ago, I thought I was going to go nuts. I've been preparing for this,
I think, for a long time. But it's weird. Everyone's telling me what a beautiful thing it was. But I just talked my wife into dying. It's a strange feeling. I just talked my wife into dying, and everyone is telling me that's
beautiful. If you had told me that two years ago, I would have called you
absolutely crazy. But I'm not the man I was then. It's amazing how my
whole mindset is different.*

*I prepared myself for her death, but I didn't prepare myself to be
doing that. I've been trying to figure it out. I know what I said. It wasn't
planned. It just came out. Phyllis had mentioned earlier: "You know, you
may want to talk to her." But I don't know how it all came about—it just
happened.*

*But I'm also torn, sitting here saying my wife is dead. For thirty-four
years we were together. And I am feeling relief—well, it's not relief, but
kind of like I'm at peace. To me, that has to be what people work for. It's*

something that they have to work for before it all happens. Don't wait until the last second and try to cram it all in. That's really what happens. It's never a good time to talk about death, no matter when it is. When you're first diagnosed, you don't want to talk about death. When you're feeling well, you don't want to talk about death. When you're not feeling well, you don't want to talk about death. We forced ourselves to do it.

People look at me a little funny when I say, "Everything went perfectly." But if I am going to die, that's the way I want it. We were there. Her best friend was here. Her father and brother were here. And there she was, sitting in her place.

I realize that I've been very busy for the last week. I was alone in the house one day...and, well, Jamie's going to leave eventually, and Chad doesn't live there anymore. I know it's going to be hard. I haven't prepared myself for that as much as I tried to prepare myself to make sure that everything was resolved. All the little things we needed to say, were said. Her last words were, "I love you." I will never forget that, and neither will the kids.

CHAPTER 12

Still Here

The Anatomy of Courage

I have woven a parachute
out of everything broken.

—William Stafford
 "Any Time" from *Allegiances*

PEOPLE DEALING WITH METASTATIC BREAST CANCER and those closest to them become true experts on how to cope with the disease. In this chapter, they will share what they have learned, and some of the advice they have offered to others.

Here are some of the common pathways these people have walked. Walking with them, you will see how they have learned to accept their feelings, allowing the contradictions and complexities of being human. Seeking control where it is possible and finding acceptance where control cannot be found has been crucial to each of them. So has living in the moment, taking risks and pursuing their dreams. Reaching out to others, both giving and receiving, has lent them strength and a sense of community. They have allowed themselves to laugh at their affliction and all that it entails. They've kept hope alive through fierce determination and a reframing of the illness experience. Although each person's spiritual beliefs are unique, these women and men are united by the common bond of having sought some deeper meaning in their lives and in the illness that brings them together. In all these ways and more the anatomy of courage is revealed.

Illness and the human condition

Of course, illness and death have posed life's fundamental predicament since human history began. A vast body of literature and art exists that examines the basic questions of the human condition. But for now, perhaps one example from Existential psychology will suffice.

Interred at Auschwitz for three years at the hands of the Nazis, Viennese psychiatrist Viktor Frankl observed that the concentration camp inmates who survived this unthinkable ordeal psychologically seemed to be those who were able to find some meaning, or transcendence, despite the horror around them. In his best-known work, *Man's Search for Meaning,* Frankl stated his belief that meaning is essential for life, and that the struggle to achieve meaning was, in fact, the most basic motivational force in human beings. In contrast to the Freudian "pleasure principle" in current favor at the time, advancing the pursuit of pleasure as the dominant motivator in human behavior, Frankl spoke instead of a "will to meaning" present in all people. As he put it, "Happiness *ensues;* it cannot be pursued."

There are three potential sources of meaning in life, Frankl believed. First, what a person offers to the world, through his or her creativity; second, a person's experiences in living and encounters with others; and third, a person's relationship to suffering and with that which cannot be changed. Survival in extreme circumstances means being able to locate some meaning in suffering, Frankl wrote, and went on to state that the most important human freedom, "to choose one's attitude in any given set of circumstances, to choose one's own way," could never be taken away.

In the little "space" that remains in the most wretched of circumstances, there is still some maneuvering room for connection, imagination, dignity and love. Frankl used the word "freedom" mindfully, and not with irony, because he knew that it was precisely the courage concentration camp survivors possessed that enabled them to find a certain psychological freedom, and to determine what was still under their control, despite their extreme circumstances.

Frankl felt that others in crisis could learn about the freedom of the human spirit from these examples. Though their circumstances may differ, people with life-threatening illness also face limitations, pain and the sense of being out of control. They face annihilation and uncertainty. They, too, must struggle with despair and demoralization and loneliness.

Dr. Rachel Naomi Remen, Medical Director of the Commonweal Cancer Help Program in Bolinas, California, told interviewer Bill Moyers:

There is nothing romantic about illness. Illness is brutal, cruel, lonely, terrifying. You have to understand that anything positive that emerges out of a real illness experience is not a function or characteristic of the nature of illness but of human nature. People have a natural capacity to affirm and embrace life in the most difficult of circumstances, and to help each other despite their circumstances.[1]

Common pathways

Since each person facing metastatic breast cancer brings to her experience memories, beliefs, strengths and strategies particular to her, and her alone, there can be no universal clearly marked road for her to walk, with acceptance and relief of suffering as its destination. There are common pathways, however, along which many have walked, presented here as a loose trail map to follow. If there is any lesson here, it is that these trails intertwine and co-mingle, that no clear route exists and that the forest, for all its beauty, is deep and full of thorns.

In the midst of that dark forest, sustaining private moments of light and warmth and deep faith come in spite of disease progression. As PJ Hagler wrote:

> *A quote I just love, that hangs in my office, shows a beautiful stream with rocks and trees. It says, "If it weren't for the rocks in its bed, the stream would have no song," by Carl Perkins. I love listening to the song of the stream of my life, rocks and all.*
>
> *I tell everyone that this is just my journey. I love that thought. I have taken this trip through the woods. There have been rocks, boulders, large logs and other obstacles along the way, but there has also been a beautiful stream with rocks that play a wonderful soothing song. There have been fields of wild flowers and when I'm still and just sitting alone the wild life comes all around me. I have been given an awesome sense of peace.*

Nancy Gilpatrick also found a way to integrate all that has happened to her into an unfolding sense of her life.

> *For me, the cancer is a journey. It's not one I chose to take. I don't believe in the "I caused it" stuff. I believe shit happens in this life. When it happens we make what we make of it. Each person finds the meaning in it their individual way. We encounter one another on the path, some going*

the same direction, some walking, some driving. We are all on the path called life and want to live. I'm clearer now than ever in my life. I love my life, even when it doesn't go well. When I have something come up with Terry, or my kids, I may rail against it at the time, but later I love having had the experience. This journey brings me so close to people and to my spirituality, I feel in awe sometimes.

Accepting emotions: Holding on for the ride of change

Most of the people I interviewed found it helpful to identify and express what they were feeling, whether this meant confiding in friends and family, to other breast cancer patients or to professional counselors, or simply writing in their own private journals. Psychiatrist Arthur Kleinman says that strong emotions flow easily from the deep losses of illness:

> The fidelity of our bodies is so basic that we never think of it. It is the certain grounds of our daily experience. Chronic illness is a betrayal of that fundamental trust. We feel under siege: untrusting, resentful of uncertainty, lost. Life becomes a working out of sentiments that follow closely from this corporeal betrayal: confusion, shock, anger, jealousy, despair.[2]

While striving to maintain a positive outlook, you can also learn to accept your periods of depression, fear, anger and even despair as normal under the circumstances, as Dr. Naomi Remen said in an interview with Bill Moyers.

> People talk about how love and cheerfulness and optimism are positive emotions, and sadness, fear, and anger are negative emotions, and negative emotions are dangerous. But my experience is that all emotions, to the extent that they engage you in life, are positive.[3]

Like the people interviewed for this book, you can learn to ride the emotional ups and downs, asking for the support you need and understanding the impermanence and natural changes of emotion. Witnessing what other people go through helps immeasurably with this. Every one of the people I interviewed for this book made contact with others in similar predicaments, both giving and receiving information and support. This has helped them to endure the darker moments and lent them hope and inspiration, providing a realistic context for the nature of their journey.

As a social worker, retired from her private practice as a therapist, Nancy Gilpatrick observed her own process.

I've let myself cry and have the down days that have come with all the unknowns and surprise information. I've grieved each step, each loss, or each piece of the cancer puzzle as it was revealed. I've practiced my Buddhism and mindfulness concepts... and practiced living in the moment...practiced letting go of expectations...and just letting go.

My spirituality has offered enormous comfort to me emotionally. It helped me manage my emotions in the sense that I knew from experience any feeling I had would pass with time. Whatever was happening with me would change. I simply needed to hold on for the ride of Change.

I'm a recovering alcoholic and drug addict with ten years of recovery behind me. Those years taught me from the ground up how to deal with my feelings, how to listen, keep what works for me when listening to others, and to let go of what doesn't work in my life. I've done that since diagnosis to the best of my ability. I put into action, once again, the tools of recovery that have taught me to live these past ten years.

Looking back at his wife's illness, Chris Tribur recalled the cyclical and sometimes chaotic nature of the emotional experience.

We grieved, we despaired, we hoped, we denied, we planned, we gave up, we hoped some more. We were caught in a maelstrom of emotional turbulence. I don't know what to advise others. My "rule of thumb" would be to fight to the end. That's an imperative of life, I think. You do what you "have" to do. You feel what you feel. Living is not subordinate to intellectual planning.

Allowing for contradiction, complexity and mystery

Maybe you're disappointed, having come to this final chapter, at not having read more in the way of direct advice, at not finding the kinds of lists, exercises and affirmations you might expect to discover in most self-help books. It's human nature to long for simple solutions and clear directions about how to proceed.

Yet, there aren't easy answers when it comes to facing a life-threatening illness. We've been discussing nothing less than one of the most problematic and fundamental of human dilemmas—how we as human beings can learn to contemplate and accept our own illness and death. Poets, theologians and philosophers have been ruminating about these issues for thousands of years. It would not do justice to the humanity of those I interviewed to simplify their process and experience. Like it or not, contradictions and ambiguity are as inherent in the course of disease as they are within our own psyches.

Throughout this book, you've seen that successful coping with disease has rarely followed a linear path, but instead has involved repeated struggles with accepting and adapting to a complex mix of emotions, choices, realities. If there is one "simple" message throughout, it has to do with preserving and supporting awareness, for as long as you're alive to feel and think and wonder. Be open to the paradoxical unfolding of your life.

At 33, Sandra Yandell has found it difficult to find any positive dimension to her illness. And yet, as she states, the complex bad and good of it coexist and are intertwined:

> Somewhere there is a balance. Yes, cancer is ugly and messy, a greedy demon bent on theft and destruction, sometimes insatiable. It takes me apart piece by piece, and eventually it will take the whole.
>
> But there is a nobility as well. Other people see me as strong, brave, "noble." They ask how I can do what I do, because they don't think they could. It's only because they've never had to. I don't feel particularly brave—I only do what's necessary. But I do have a strength I wasn't aware of before. If someone feels better by seeing me as an example, I'm not sure that that's so bad. It's funny in a way, because I used to be a "tough bitch," but now the same thing that made me "tough" has become "strong and stoic."
>
> Maybe I'm a **balance**. It's an ugly, messy, angry, tearful story tucked behind a pretty face and a strong spirit. I can't hide from the story anymore than I can stop worrying about keeping the pretty face.
>
> Now what did I do with that lipstick....

Letting yourself be open to *all* aspects of your experience can lead to a larger perspective. In *Remembrance of Things Past*, the French writer Marcel Proust, a lifelong asthmatic and shut-in who died tragically young of pneumonia, wrote: "We are healed of a suffering only by experiencing it in full."

Gaining control: Holding tight

The undercurrent of chronic illness is like the volcano: it does not go away. It menaces. It erupts. It is out of control. One damn thing follows another.

—Arthur Kleinman
The Illness Narratives

The struggle for control begins with differentiation. It is as simple—and as difficult—as Reinhold Neibuhr's oft quoted "Serenity Prayer," a centerpiece of the recovery movement.

> *God grant me the serenity to accept the things I cannot change,*
> *courage to change the things I can,*
> *and the wisdom to know the difference*

For someone with life-threatening illness, it becomes crucial to distinguish that which is within your control from that which is not. Sometimes, as with choosing late-term treatments, this is nearly impossible to do. In the can-do battleground of high-tech medicine, where a fighting attitude is admired and rewarded, it becomes important to keep in mind that acceptance does not equal passivity. Maintaining a sense of autonomy and control over the choices you do have, it is possible for you to learn, as a matter of course, to question your doctors, research your disease and treatments, make clear decisions about how you want to spend your time and resources. You can learn to contain the helplessness of uncertain treatment outcomes and disease progression by focusing on what can be accomplished and controlled. You can make plans and carry them out.

Pat Leach, insistent on following her travel plans until shortly before her death, advised a simple way to maintain hope:

> *Always have something planned that you can look forward to—this has been one of my basic philosophies since diagnosis. Planning a trip, short or lengthy, is great, but we can't always do that. So I've made sure there was always an event, in the future—a concert, a visit to an old*

friend, dinner out (even pizza or a lovely breakfast). My family caught on and now they plan things for me and make me get involved, even when my mood is lousy.

Kathy Stone had waited a long time to take a vacation to Reno, Nevada, and when she returned, she was elated, she wrote her friends on the Internet:

> I'm so proud of myself, I have to brag. When we went on our mini vacation this past week, I took an old wooden cane with me for an art project, to have something to do if I couldn't get out of the hotel room. I decapitate it with material that had all kinds of gambling motifs...dice, roulette wheels, cards, words, money, etc. It is fantastic and did I ever get a lot of compliments on it when I used it one day. I'm going to make it my **Reno** cane. Now I'm going to get me some more canes (about $15 each) and decoupage them to match different outfits. Who knows, maybe I'll go into the cane business.

> I had also bought myself a clear acrylic cane to use for dress up. We had a semi-formal dinner to go to last week and I took my cane, but then decided while I was out shopping to go by the craft store and pick up some "jewels" and sequins and some of that tacky stuff that you can use on appliqués to reuse them over and over again. Anyway, I put the tacky stuff on the back of the rhinestones and jewels and on the back of some pretty sequined trim and after it set, I placed the stones in some nice strategic spots and took the trim and covered the rubber tip of the cane. What an elegant, sparkly cane I had for the dinner. Not too garish, but not just a plain cane either. I felt like Cinderella at the Ball. I even used some of the leftover trim at the last minute to highlight my handbag to match. When the evening was over, it just all peeled off...the cane is back to being a plain clear acrylic (ready for a bow, a bell, a flower or whatever the occasion calls for) and the "sparkly goodies" are packed away and can be used again when I want.

> I've decided that if I have to use a cane, I might as well go in style...I'm too **big** to hide in a crowd anyway, so I might as well stand out loud and clear. The big, bald, one-breasted woman with the loud cane...but at least I'll be recognized!

Seeking surrender and acceptance: Letting go

Many of the people I interviewed sought peace of mind through surrender to a will greater than their own. They accepted that death and pain and loss were a part of living. They let go of illusions of immortality and entitlement and found comfort in the contemplation of natural cycles of living and dying.

At a meditation retreat nine months before her death, Mary D'Angelo reflected on her own struggle with acceptance and control:

> I've always felt that I was a self-made person, that I planned my life. Because I did things the way I did them, they turned out so well. So I used to congratulate myself and thought that I was a very strong person, that I could handle things. Cancer really taught me, or humbled me, that I couldn't, that I was vulnerable, that I couldn't "will" my life to be the way I wanted it to be. I think this control thing was probably a very good lesson for me to learn, but a hard one. I still want to be in control.
>
> But I also feel a sense of surrender. I'm not a religious person but I am, I think, spiritually connected. I feel that some spirit or something is directing my life and will take care of me. I think that gives me the confidence that I have about myself, and about living and dying. And that somehow everything will be all right. I think that's what makes me hopeful.

Nancy Gilpatrick wrote that it was often the natural world that brought her back to a sense of order and acceptance:

> Last week Terry and I drove to the desert outside Salt Lake City. We took a picnic and our binoculars and bird book. We saw some birds I'd not seen before. We saw a very large red-tailed hawk swooping down to catch a meal and then soar across the land. The wing span was at least four feet across. I got such a strong hit of how precious this life is. It is also a cycle: of Birth and Death. It's as normal to die as it is to be born. We do these things that keep us in touch with the land and with the timelessness of life and death.
>
> This is not to say I don't have incredible sadness about it all. I don't want to leave my children. I know it will affect them the rest of their lives

to have their mother die before they reach adulthood. I have come to love a wonderful man, I want to spend a very long time living and loving with him: I won't have that opportunity. We hold each other at night, look into each other's eyes and whisper our love to each other. I think of all the things I want to do still in my life and I won't be able to do them.

It doesn't make me angrier to want to "fight" this thing. I feel acceptance of it. I have breast cancer. I also have acceptance of wanting to do each and every treatment necessary to kill the cancer and give me time to live. Acceptance isn't giving up ....The Buddha said pain is part of life, that we all experience pain. It's a given. What we have a choice about is suffering.

Living in the moment: Paying attention

It is not hard to live through a day if you can live through a moment. What creates despair is the imagination, which pretends there is a future and insists on predicting millions of moments, thousands of days, and so drains you that you cannot live the moment at hand.

—André Dubus

The people I interviewed spoke often of the importance of living in the moment, of how they had learned to savor time with the people they loved and to seek out experiences that had meaning to them. Like them, you may have discovered that a focus on the present lends an intensity to life, permitting an appreciation and awareness of both inner and outer worlds. You may already be pursuing meditative and prayerful practices that help you to focus attention in the moment. You may also have begun to revise your goals to those which are short-term, and achievable, and to understand that worrying and regret represent unnecessary and painful trips to the future and past.

As medical sociologist Kathy Charmaz found in her study of people dealing with chronic illnesses, a moment-to-moment focus is related to the issue of control.

Living one day at a time is a strategy for managing chronic illness and structuring time. Moreover, it also provides a way of managing self while facing uncertainty. It gives a sense of control over one's actions and, by extension, a sense of control over self and situation.[4]

Existential psychiatrist Irvin Yalom found that his patients, too, had evolved this method of coping, which he encouraged.

> *Many patients with cancer...realize that one can really live only in the present; in fact, one cannot outlive the present—it always keeps up with you. Even in the moment of looking back over one's life—even in the last moment—one is still there, experiencing, living. The present, not the future, is the eternal tense.*[5]

In discussing her perceptions of how cancer patients, including herself, could best come to terms with what was happening to them, Dr. Rachel Naomi Remen told Bill Moyers:

> *My sense is that the worst thing that happens in life is not death. The worst thing would be to miss it. A friend of mine, Angeles Arien, says all spiritual paths have four steps: show up, pay attention, tell the truth, and don't be attached to the results. I think the great danger in life is not showing up.*[6]

Many of the people interviewed for this book have come to this understanding on their own. For some, like Ellen Scheiner, the capacity for focusing in the moment came from a conscious cultivation of the meditative state, which she analyzed for its elements.

> *If there is awareness and concentration, there's a suspension of expectation because you're not anywhere else: you're here. In that way, it has helped me profoundly. The combination of awareness and concentration are extraordinarily helpful with life-threatening illness.*

Others, like Barb Clabo, make this realization through the direct discovery that when they anchor their awareness in the present, their emotional distress becomes more manageable—at least as long as their "now" doesn't include a great deal of physical distress.

> *Staying in the moment is fairly easy for me to do. This is the only way I can survive. Thinking and dwelling on what the future might bring is too difficult and depressing, so I try not to let myself dwell on it. It helps when I am feeling well and working or doing things I enjoy. When I'm not feeling real well is when I tend to have bad days and think that I'll never feel good again.*

Nancy Gilpatrick tells a story about her diagnosis that illustrates how a shift of focus into the present, combined with the companionship of people she loved, offered her relief in the midst of crisis:

> As I drove home, I cried. Just let the tears flow. When I got home I didn't want to be alone, so I called my sister and told her. Even though I had prepared her by telling her of the appointment, she was stunned and cried. We cried together. I felt less alone talking to her. She immediately said she would be there for the surgery whenever I scheduled it. I was comforted knowing she would be with me.
>
> When Terry arrived we talked about this potential cancer diagnosis (I had some residual denial in place) and about our plans for the evening. He wasn't sure I would want to go out. We had plans for dinner with people we didn't know well. I decided that there wasn't anything we could do staying home, and meeting someone new might be a good distraction. We also decided not to tell them. There would be no talk of breast cancer. The evening was wonderful and stands out to me vividly as a true gift from the universe: we laughed and laughed, belly laughs, laughing in a way I hadn't done in a long time. We played cards and just had a great time. I learned from that first night to laugh when I could, when any opportunity for fun arose to participate, and second, I learned the value of being in the moment.

Determination and self-trust also played an important role for Mary D'Angelo, as she learned to combine the uncertainties in her prognosis with a newfound and poignant pleasure in daily life.

> I like to deal with one thing at a time, so I don't project into the future. I like the fact about my illness that even though there are statistics, my doctor doesn't really know what will happen with me. That makes me feel that I'm a partner with him in a way, that he helps me, but he doesn't have the answers. So why should I get worried, if there's no answer? If he were to say to me, "Well, you're going to die in three months," then I would get very worried—for a week, and then I would try to plan my death. So planning the death would be what would keep me from being overcome by sadness or anxiety. There's always something to do and to plan for.

*I think life is so rich and so full, you only really understand that
when it's threatened. It's a terrible thing to waste any time feeling
depressed or anxious or anticipating outcomes that may never happen.*

All people with metastatic breast cancer face a shortened life, and so time comes to seem precious to them. Many express concern about spending their remaining time engaged in meaningless activities or in states of fear and grief. Sue Tokuyama saw this as a preparation, whether or not her remission continued:

*Suddenly, the pace of my life must be accelerated. Saving for retire-
ment is an absurd idea. Waiting for anything important is a mistake. And
rarely a day goes by that I don't think to myself: What has my life meant
if I die today? I spend a good deal of what little alone time I have ponder-
ing what I want my life to mean. In the spirit of the idea that one is born
alone, and one dies alone, I am trying to create the expression of* me, *that
is not wife, mother, or friend. What am I in the universe? And I continue
to try to find that perfect expression with words, and in clay, and even in
the enthusiastic remodeling I am doing of our house. I am planting a garden. I am hungrily seeking wisdom, because I am not sure I have time to
wait for it to find me.*

*Breast cancer has made me roll up my sleeves, and get my hands
dirty in the business of living. If I live to be 90, I'll be richer for this experience. And if I die tomorrow, I hope I won't say that I'm unprepared.*

Cancer patients and their families often dread the future, fearing debilitating treatments, pain and the indignity of dying. But these are really only fear-laden fantasies and memories—the reality, when it comes, is bound to be something else, something that can be planned for in practical terms, and then met and managed, moment to moment. The British writer CS Lewis, who chronicled the death of his wife, the American poet Joy Adamson, in *A Grief Observed*, articulated this clearly:

*When the reality came, the name and the idea were in some degree
disarmed. One never meets just Cancer, or War or Unhappiness (or Happiness). One only meets each hour or moment that comes. All manner of
ups and downs. Many bad spots in our best times, many good ones in our
worst. One never gets the total impact of what we call "the thing itself."
But we call it wrongly. The thing itself is simply all these ups and downs:
the rest is a name or an idea.*[7]

Pam Hiebert recalled a similar realization:

> Last year I was having one of my long and valuable conversations with my father. I was going into much detail surrounding my thoughts and fears of death. At one point he interrupted me and said, "Pam! You are talking like this is a linear thing. You are talking like you see death as an end. Pam, don't you yet know—there is no death! There is no death, there is only life. Life is all there ever is!"
>
> At that moment I felt a burst of insight. He was right! My concepts of trying to draw boundaries with each event were only adding to the tension in my life. These linear lines of perception I'd developed for greater certainty, were in fact setting up potential battle lines. In reality there is no boundary as such. I was planning a war because it served to boost my feelings of security. His statement reminded me that the world is actually a seamless coat of no boundaries. I was confusing my map of boundaries—drawn lines set between sickness and health—as the territory. And what I actually desire is to find my certainty in the security of the territory and not the boundaries that I imagine.

Glenn Clabo, advising the husband of a cancer patient who felt he was caught up in a nightmare of treatment and uncertainty, put it concisely:

> Don't let the unsure future be the enemy of the now. We need only learn to enjoy now while it's here.

Risk taking: Dancing with uncertainty and challenge

A critical illness is like a great permission, an authorization or absolving. It's all right for a threatened man to be romantic, even crazy, if he feels like it. All your life you think you have to hold back your craziness, but when you're sick you can let it out in all its garish colors.

—Anatole Broyard[8]

You may already have had a glimpse or two of illness as an opportunity— perhaps as an imperative—for facing old fears and taking new risks. If so, you are in good company, for many of the people I interviewed felt this way. There may be a new sense of permission, as Broyard suggests, and less concern over what other people think and feel. It becomes easier to say "no" to obligations and conventions. Perhaps you feel freer to say what you believe and take new chances in letting yourself be known to others.

Despite her pain and disability from bone metastases, the medications and treatments and the morphine pump she was wearing, JB Boggs gave herself fully to a new beginning in her life, not knowing how much longer she would have to live.

> *Right now I am planning to be married in two weeks, on November 11. It is filling my whole world, almost, all these plans, and even displaces the thoughts of illness. Oh, but putting on that wedding gown was transformational. I am not sick at all. I am a fairy princess who has a lace gown and satin slippers and can only stand tall and proud as I float on this cloud of a dress and leave all awareness of having cancer behind me.*

> *How long will I live with this cancer? How long? I don't know but I am full of life and joy and hope.*

It is a risk to live fully in the face of death, when the impulse may be to withdraw from life. Sandra Yandell, wrestling with a marriage decision herself, felt tormented at the pain she knew would be coming for her husband to be:

> *I told Jim when he mentioned marriage that I was afraid that it would be too painful, because one day he is going to wake up and I won't be there anymore. He said, "Sometimes I already miss you and you're not even gone," which has to be one of the most heart-wrenching things I've ever heard. It tears me up to know how much this hurts those I love and there's not a damn thing I can do to make it stop.*

> *I'm not religious in the sense that I go to the building and do the rituals, but I do have faith in God. I will be in a place with no more pain, and there are dark moments when I wish I could just discard this brutalized body and go there, moments when I'm too tired to draw another painful breath. But there are still things to do before I leave.... Jim said that there will be a time to cry later, but for now we should live as much as we can. I'm trying, but I do wish that it all didn't hurt so much.*

At first, Sylvan Rainwater was frightened by her partner Pam's intensity, and the way she plunged into her cancer experience.

For my part, I knew that death and dying were things I knew little about, and needed to know about. On the other hand, Pam's way of embracing it, going to meet it head on, filled me with fear for awhile. I was afraid she was willing herself to die, believing what the doctors were telling her (and I myself was not convinced that they really knew what they were talking about). I was angry at her for being so willing to leave me. She tried to make plans, took out another life insurance policy, considered running up credit card bills. She talked as if she were certain to die in two years or less.

But as time went on and we began to realize that she wouldn't die immediately, that we would have warning and time to prepare, we both began to mellow out a little bit. We gradually learned that life is a gift, not a guarantee, and that though death comes to all of us, no one can really predict when. We learned to be grateful for the moment, to live life to the fullest right now, and that right now is all any of us really has. Wbegan to understand that the concept of the future is a construct, an illusion, not a solid reality that we can depend on.

For Lucie Bergmann-Shuster, risk-taking was a way of life long before her cancer.

I think some of us rather like living on the edge. It seems nutso and difficult for some folks to understand. My hubby and I like sail boat racing. It is not a pastime for those with impaired hearts or stress-related ulcers. Once a friend came with us, and we guaranteed that she would not have to do anything except be rail meat. It was a fierce race in the big boat series around Long Beach. Not only was my friend asked to lend a hand as we were trying to avoid a collision while keeping our competitive edge, but she got totally soaked in the process. There was a lot of yelling as we tried to unsnag fouled lines and twisted spinnakers. Afterwards, she said the folks on the other boat were doing just as much shouting during the hectic activity as we were. She just couldn't understand how anyone would pursue that kind of crazy sport and said that she'd just as soon defer her sailing experience to cruising.

What it comes down to is an insatiable curiosity to explore our limits in the world we live in. When we push ourselves to the edge, there is that fear and then, that amazing transformation to reach beyond the terror and survive by tapping into our inner resources and ingenuity. Such experiences make us stronger and more confident about who we are and how we function. Of course there are boulders and there are pebbles, and there are steep cliffs. Rising to the occasion does take a bit of prudence and prior experience.

Studying to be a physician in an era when her disability and sexual orientation were unacceptable, and there was a seven percent quota for women in medical school, Ellen Scheiner knew all about challenge and persistence.

> I did maintain control in the most dire of circumstances, but I've now learned that I don't have to, that the energy or force or spirit, if you will, is there. I don't have to create it consciously, because it is there. It's like when I went to medical school. I didn't think about it at all. It was simply so profoundly what I wanted to do, that I went ahead and did it. My notion is that if you really want with all of your being, then you do, and if not, you don't. Obstacles don't matter much. Sometimes the joy is simply in confronting it, in seeing it. That's why I say I've been staring into the abyss.

For Ellen, the real challenge of her cancer came from her willingness to entertain uncertainty and impermanence at the level of direct experience.

> I am different than I was a year ago. I've experienced the true knowledge that I am going to die, so I have no illusions about immortality—I can't project into the future, pretending I'll be alive, because I just don't know. I've developed my own little exercise, when I think that I'll have a recurrence or I'll not have a recurrence. I just bring my mind back to here, and I say, "I don't know." It's a meditative exercise. When I found out I really was going to die, in the visceral sense that you know that, it left me with nothing to stand on. I felt as if I were in free fall. Because, what was there to plan for? After awhile, it's extraordinary: I got used to standing on nothing. It's very freeing to stand on nothing. You don't have to have any illusions. I make my plans and I live the way I want. It's very different.

> I'm awed by how well I coped. I can't believe that this woman, who couldn't do one lap around her own living room, is running up and down Third Avenue. It's depressing and it's divine. There's something that's beyond us, as far as I'm concerned. I used to say: "I'm not doing this can-

cer treatment; it's doing me." I used to liken it to white-water rafting. *Sometimes your head's above water, sometimes under water. Sometimes you're in the boat, and you think you're steering but you're not really. That's the way I am beginning to feel about my life: that the force, the energy, the motivation was given to me. I don't sit there in the morning and say, "Well, today I'm going to do this." I don't do this. It does me.*

None of us knows what will happen in the next breath. We think we do, because that's how we live.

Living dreams deferred: Priorities and time

Something we were withholding made us weak
until we found it was ourselves.

—Robert Frost

Many people with metastatic breast cancer, rebounding from the identity losses of disability retirement, discover that they still have the time, and the need, to reinvent their daily lives, pursuing activities and relationships their careers had put in the background. The imperative of limited time gives them permission to put themselves first.

Lisann Charland, once a management analyst, describes her life now:

I live a plain and simple life, and keep no set schedule. I do what I want to do and when I want to do it. I continuously educate myself on getting well and living with metastatic breast cancer through books, support groups and various meditation/relaxation tapes. I have re-entered college, and become a full-time housewife. I have dedicated a lot of my time doing volunteer work as an auxiliary person at the hospital in the Cancer Unit and the Cardiac Unit. I spend time talking with patients about medication, side effects, questions to ask the doctor, and share what I learned from experiences and support groups. I take time for me.

My passion is gardening, and I spend countless hours weeding, planting, replanting, talking to my plants, etc. I find pleasure in the tiniest of things. I can be guaranteed total relaxation when I am in the garden. I talk and play with my animals and take walks with them. I also stay in close contact, and occasionally go out to lunch with my new friends from church, who include me in all their family gatherings.

Daily, I tell myself that "Lisann comes first." I am No. 1 in this life in each and every way. Living with metastatic breast cancer and all the problems I encountered has taught me to be good and kind to myself. I look for the good side of everything, throw pennies in water fountains and make wishes and pray for miracles.

For Barbara Ragland, her recurrence has spurred plans for travel and the pursuit of long-term interests.

I have always wanted to travel to various parts of the country where my ancestors once lived. Then I want to write accounts of the kinds of lives they lived and adventures they had, challenges they were able to overcome, etc. I have a good start on this already.

With my illness, I plan to do as much traveling as I can now. If my health doesn't permit much traveling later on, this will be the time I start using my notes and tapes to write about what I've found. I have done quite a bit of genealogy research, but have discovered that it's not the dates and names that are interesting, it's the intriguing lives these ancestors have led.

My illness has very much affected plans for the future and an attempt to live more in the present. I no longer say, "someday, I am going to—" I seem to be rushing ahead with household projects. I accept invitations to do things I've never done before. With home improvement projects, I no longer consider a twenty year guarantee. In my financial planning, I have decided to enjoy myself more now and save only the bare minimum for my old age.

I also have learned to enjoy the moment. I am learning not to defer my own wishes. I've started saying "no" when I'd rather not—(whatever). I'm practicing saying "why not?" instead of "why."

Bob Stafford wasn't ready to stop helping people when he retired on disability, so "Mr. Breast Cancer," as he likes to be called, set out on a campaign to educate the public that resulted in national network television coverage and an ongoing discussion group on the Internet for men with the disease.

The biggest thing is to inform people. It used to be absolutely nothing was said about male breast cancer and we were lucky to get a paragraph or even a sentence in breast cancer books. It's starting to change because there are some men willing to be identified with the disease and enough women have embarrassed themselves by saying we weren't survivors. We are though. I might have to wear a pink hat but if one guy catches his breast cancer early because of it, that's great.

From a shared concern about the well-being of their teenaged children, he and Caren Buffum started discussion groups for kids facing illness and death in themselves, a family member or a friend. Another discussion group he began focused on the needs of parents of critically ill children. Despite diminishing energy and increasing pain, Bob persists in his new interests, even though being in touch with many seriously ill people means constant reminders of mortality. When asked why, he says:

Being surrounded by so many hurting people really stresses our own resolve to continue on. But then we must go on so that others might know that there is hope and that it isn't always just death.

Reaching out: Connection and activism

The living of life, any life, involves great and private pain, much of which we share with no one.

—Barry Lopez

By virtue of their involvement with this book, and through the Breast Cancer List, support groups and personal contacts, all of the people I interviewed reached out to others, especially to those who were experiencing the same problems they were. They shared ideas, feelings, information, and helped one another solve the problems they encountered. They tried not to allow themselves to become isolated. While they felt disappointed and rejected when some friends and family withdrew from them, they came to understand that this was not their problem, and that there were people out there who were not afraid of intimacy with someone whose time might be limited. They asked for help when they needed it, allowing themselves to rely on others when necessary without feeling diminished by dependency. They made their needs clear, rather than expecting others to know.

For Bob Stafford, the sense of love and community he found after his cancer diagnosis was a revelation.

> *One of the great difficulties I've endured in the past as a child is never quite feeling loved. What I have found is another family. I've found people who genuinely love me. No strings attached. They love me. Now I have new men and women who are like parents. I have new brothers and sisters. And their love is overwhelming. That's why I'll put up the pictures and cards on the wall of my room. Reminders of all the love and warmth I've received over the years from people. For so very long I hated people and would strike out for no reason at all. But now, but now hate has been bound by love. You don't know the number of days I weep from the joy I feel because someone has shown me an act of love and kindness. That's why it is hard to let go.*

Barbara Ragland felt that her work to help others was crucial to maintaining her own equilibrium and perspective.

> *I was a Reach to Recovery volunteer for eleven years, and I'm sure one can't give encouragement to others for that long without having positive attitudes and philosophies rub off. They say that one of the best ways to get your mind off your own problems is to help someone else.*

> *My family always was important to me but now they are* **most** *important (my three children are all grown). I think most of us with mets have discovered a new joy in things like watching a beautiful sunset, sitting by a crackling fire while the snow drifts down, smelling the smoke of a campfire, etc. I guess one learns to appreciate the simple things.*

For some people dealing with metastatic breast cancer, the personal is inextricably linked to the political. Reaching out to others expands to social action. Breast cancer activism has flourished over the last decade as more and more women have found their voices. Impassioned and persistent efforts for increased research funding, as well as legislative and educational initiatives, have been fueled by the outrage and determination of breast cancer patients who are living with recurrence or with the fear of recurrence, and who have lost far too many friends to the disease. Their contribution is profound and powerful. For them, activism is a way of making a real difference, of transforming the lack of control and helplessness they may feel over a personal situation into social action that will benefit an entire society.

At the heart of activism is speaking the truth. Poet Audre Lorde, who died of breast cancer in 1992, spoke of silence and truth-telling twenty years ago, at the time of her diagnosis:

> Death...is the final silence. And that might be coming quickly, now, without regard for whether I had ever spoken what needed to be said, or had only betrayed myself into small silences, while I planned someday to speak, or waited for someone else's words....I was going to die, if not sooner then later, whether or not I had ever spoken myself. My silences had not protected me. Your silence will not protect you. But for every real word spoken, for every attempt I have ever made to speak those truths for which I am still seeking, I have made contact with other women ....And it was the concern and caring of all those women which gave me strength and enabled me to scrutinize the essentials of my living.
>
> ...And, of course, I am afraid—you can hear it in my voice—because the transformation of silence into language and action is an act of self-revelation and that always seems fraught with danger....In the cause of silence, each one of us draws the face of her own fear—fear of contempt, of censure, or some judgment, or recognition, of challenge, of annihilation. But most of all, I think, we fear the very visibility without which we also cannot truly live.[9]

Laughter in the dark

Few who spend any amount of time under medical care, particularly in a hospital setting, with its legendary foul-ups, delays, indignities and invasions of privacy can endure such an assault without a sense of humor. High-tech medicine, by its very nature, embodies both irony and a sense of the absurd, and, given a chance, patients are quick to pick this up, and exploit the dark humor that lies therein. The deteriorating physical self provides an irresistible, if somewhat bleak, source of amusement. People who are not themselves ill are often surprised—and perhaps even shocked—to find out about the amount of irreverent laughter cancer patients share with one another, and what delight they take in it, no matter how dark the content.

Poking fun at themselves, allowing themselves the freedom to laugh at the sometimes horrific disabilities and treatments illness has forced, is a hallmark of many cancer patients and an indicator of existential strength—diffusing awkwardness in those around them and indicating their own larger perspective.

Bob Stafford, who suffered castration as a treatment for his hormonally sensitive breast cancer, spoke freely of his "nutectomy" in a recent message, and signed himself, "Bob the eunuch 'Safe around any woman.'"

Sandra Yandell, forced to walk with a cane because of her bone mets, spoke of herself and a similarly disabled friend as the "gimp sisters" and signed a recent letter concerning new radiation treatments, "The Glow-In-The-Dark Princess." When a treatment was delayed because of low blood counts, she wrote philosophically: "The story of my life (heavy sigh)—slicin' & dicin', nukin' & pukin'."

Everyone who participates in face-to-face or online cancer support groups is familiar with the wildly funny "sick" and absurdist humor that accompanies discussions of the side effects of treatment, and the welcome relief it affords. Though such jokes often don't translate well out of context, here's a smattering from the Breast Cancer Discussion List on the Internet.

This was one response to a message discussing alternative treatments:

> I've heard about using a coffee enema for aggressive system detoxification, and I'm just wondering: I take mine black, two sugar—would it be okay to use a frosty Coke on a hot day for a change of pace?

A discussion concerning vaginal dryness, one of the menopausal effects of chemotherapy, led to a debate on the relative merits of certain products. "Just what is Astroglide, please?" a List member innocently asked, provoking the following responses:

> Astroglide is a KY jelly type lubricant one uses when having sex with aliens.

> You, too? I thought I was the only one having sex with aliens.

> Jeez, I thought it was a brand of reclining-chair! I guess I've been living too sheltered a life....

> I thought Astroglide was a ski exercise machine.

> So bummed to have missed the Astrogliders...did you say they were from Houston?

Another List member, Sue Hunter, marked holidays with satiric verse. Here is her "tasteful valentine for my chemotherapy friends:"

> *My head is bald,*
> *My face is green,*
> *My whatsy's dry*
> *(You know what I mean).*

> *My blood is thin,*
> *My veins are shot,*
> *But my chin is up,*
> *And I love you a lot!*

Although we intuitively sense its value, it's worth pointing out some reasons why laughter is such a great help and comfort. Psychiatrist Viktor Frankl points out that humor allows us to create perspective, to put a certain distance between ourselves and whatever it is that confronts us. "To detach oneself from even the worst conditions is a uniquely human capability," Frankl writes, adding that detachment is a hallmark not only of heroism, but also of humor. "Humor is said even to be a divine attribute. In three psalms God is referred to as a 'laughing' one." Tongue in cheek, Frankl agrees with theorist Konrad Lorenz, "that we do not as yet take humor seriously enough."[10]

Keeping hope alive: Grace and determination

"Hope" is the thing with feathers—
That perches in the soul—
And sings the tune without the words—
And never stops—at all—

> —Emily Dickinson

Keeping hope alive is both an active process of will and a matter of spirit. One way to keep hope alive is by redefining your goals and expectations to more closely match the realities of your illness. With mortality no longer in question—what *can* you hope for? Can you transform the uncertainties of your illness and treatment into open-ended possibilities? Is there an unfulfilled dream or a special event for which you can plan? Although often the unpredictable course of illness means living from day to day, especially during periods of crisis, it's still important to make room for special occasions.

Kathy Stone felt that remaining hopeful was an active choice that she made.

> *I have decided that whatever takes me and whenever it is will still be a mystery to me...the chances of it being breast cancer over something else are, of course, very, very high...but none of us is guaranteed the next moment. Therefore, I am trying my best to treat this beast as a chronic illness and live as full a life as I can while still trying to do my part to make this world a bit kinder place to live. In some ways it has given me a freedom I didn't have before...but it is hard to put into words. I intend to be making plans for a fun-filled life, enriched with many friends right up to the moment the bells start clanging for me. I hope I can pull it off. With all the love and support in my life, I know I can.*

JB Boggs displayed an equal determination to resist the domination of despair.

> *I just refuse to live in fear. I don't know what will happen, but I do know what will happen if I give over to the dark side. There's an expression I use, "Don't let the dark side pick you off." I think that there is a lot of choice. I think it's a matter of will. You can choose what you think and feel. You really can. Even when my thoughts are churning, going round and round, I can stop, I can look for some peace, some centered place to come from. I've learned that even when I am churning around, I can write. I am looking for peace. If I just keep writing, peace is going to come to me. Peace is right here, if I can just let myself go through it. I think it is a real choice. I think we can, just by force of will, get hold of our thoughts and not be so frightened. I think the way the brain works is that once you let yourself be frightened, it can just build and build and get bigger and bigger. And then you can't get out of it. You lose all hope and you lose the moment.*

Even when the hope for survival no longer seems tenable, the will to fully live for as long and as well as possible inspires patients and their families. Gerry Wirth recalls how he and Cindy kept their focus on life, even as death approached.

> *We held up by knowing time was precious. We could spend it living life or grieving. We chose to live it. Yes there was lots of pillow talk about the future and the uncertainty. There were many tears shed. But we knew to dwell in those tears was dying while we still could breathe. We just kept going and didn't give in.*

Transformation: Reframing a larger landscape

Nothing so concentrates experience and clarifies the central conditions of living as serious illness.

—Arthur Kleinman
The Illness Narratives

Many of the people I interviewed became expert in reframing their experiences with illness as challenges. Even in the most dire of circumstances, without denying or diminishing the pain and fear, they also sought out the benefits that were there to be found. They opened themselves up to new insights. They saw their lives with cancer as both a journey of discovery *and* a struggle to maintain themselves in difficult circumstances.

Psychiatrist Eric Cassell, a renowned expert on pain and suffering, spoke of the human capacity for transformation:

> *Persons are able to enlarge themselves in response to damage, so that rather than being reduced by injury, they may indeed grow. This response to suffering had led to the belief that suffering is good for people. To some degree, and in some individuals, this may be so. We would not have such a belief, however, were it not equally common knowledge that persons can also be destroyed by suffering.... The ability to recover from loss without succumbing to suffering is sometimes called resiliency, as though merely elastic rebound is involved. But it seems more as if an inner force is withdrawn from one manifestation of person and redirected at another.[11]*

The assignment of meaning, Cassell goes on to say, is one thing that permits people to cope well with destructive forces in their lives.

> *Meaning and transcendence offer two additional ways by which the destruction of a part of personhood or threat to its integrity are meliorated. The search for the meaning of human suffering has occupied humanity on an individual and cultural level throughout history. Assigning meaning to the injurious condition often reduces or even resolves the suffering associated with it.... Transcendence is probably the most powerful way in which one is restored to wholeness after an injury to personhood. When experienced, transcendence locates the person in a far larger landscape. The sufferer is not isolated by pain but is brought closer to a*

transpersonal source of meaning and to the human community that
shares that meaning. Such an experience need not involve religion in any
formal sense; however, in its transpersonal dimension it is deeply spiri-
tual.

Often, people will draw on their former life experiences for strength, and use what they have learned in another context to reframe their current experiences, as JB Boggs does here:

I was an avid sportswoman. I used to teach aerobics. I did a lot of
surfing and hiking, and I am used to being very, very physical. It was a
big loss. But I find that even now, when I get up to walk, when I take my
walker outside, and walk around the yard, I can feel the same physical
challenge. I can challenge myself. It's still a workout, and so if I look at it
the right way, I can still say I'm getting my workout. I'm going 20 feet fur-
ther today than I did yesterday. I'm less out of breath. I try to be happy
for the little gains. This year, I am a lot more well than I was the first
year. In these last two years, I've been in the hospital 15 different times,
averaging 15 to 20 days each time, by the time they get my ports in, get
my chemistry back in order. I know about hitting the wall, and I know
about pushing through it, and I know about training: it's frequency, inten-
sity and duration. I know those things in my own head, so that if I can't
do the intensity, I try to go for the frequency, or the duration. I try to use
my training and knowledge, and I cheer myself on. I do my exercises
every day with my bands. The doctor's really amazed that I am able to
keep up with my weight training and endurance and flexibility.

Lucie Bergmann-Shuster associated the extreme fatigue and sickness of intensive chemotherapy with the development of new powers of perception.

After being ever so close to death and so excruciatingly wiped out, we
begin to see life and its minutiae through a totally different perspective
and treasure it. We treasure the small gains, and the big gains or insights
as never before.

Among the people I interviewed, Barb Pender, laughingly referring to herself as "Pollyanna," was the most single-mindedly determined to find something positive in everything that happened to her throughout her illness.

I have been blessed with being able to find the good in every circum-
stance. And I believe that cancer (the original diagnosis and metastasis),

for me, is another test, adventure, experience. I am not angry. I am glad it was me and not my mother, sister, daughter, friend, neighbor because I **know** *I have the patience, perseverance and faith to get me through, because there is a greater plan for my life and I have the torch!*

The day that it was made clear to me that breast cancer was part of a greater plan for my life, I relaxed and knew that my experience was going to be "good for me."

I have never asked, "Why me?" I knew from the beginning that there was a reason—I have never felt randomly selected to get breast cancer but rather hand-picked. I believe we are selected for our strength of mind and character, for our courage and perseverance. Once the initial numbness wore off, these thoughts got me through with a smile.

I feel that getting cancer was one of the luckiest things that has happened to me. It taught me how to love myself for what is inside. It taught me to respect myself and others for who they are and not what they look like. Cancer has taught me to love life and to live and love each day to the fullest. It taught me to stop and smell the roses and to make sure my children and grandchildren know they are loved each and every day in words and deeds. And my cancer experience brought me back into the loving arms of my Savior—and that is **wonderful!!**

I do not think of my cancer as a "beast" that dwells within but rather as a gift, a learning experience, a part of a greater plan for my life. The cancer is a part of me—it is a part of who I am.

Caren Buffum, also seeking meaning and purpose in her illness, wrote:

I think some people are afraid that by allowing themselves to find anything good in the cancer, they are somehow surrendering to it and allowing it to have power in their lives. But the way I see it, cancer is destructive and dark, and when I draw something constructive and light from the experience, I am having power over **it.**

Bob Stafford reflected on the transformations in his life:

There have been a **lot** *of positive changes that have come about through cancer. My wife learned what intimacy is really about, that "things" aren't so important, and that having a spotless house isn't a necessity of life. I've seen her grow so much. My kids (whom I am* **very**

*proud of) know what the important things in life are and aren't. Did it
have to be cancer? No. But so many people are coasting along in life with
their hearts and minds in neutral that a crisis is necessary for them to
begin to value what life really is composed of. I think that is what was
happening here...we were coasting along and, quite frankly, I think had
we coasted along to this point, things would be much worse than they are
now. Is there heartache and pain? Yes, but then nobody promised me an
easy life.*

*This is not to say that if I look at this in a positive light then I haven't
felt anger or sorrow. That I haven't shed tears. That's not true. I'm trying
not to attribute any glory to it. I got cancer, I can't change that and neither can any of us. How we respond is another thing.*

Identity: You are not your illness

We sing inside our own little boat.
> —Kabir, translated by Robert Bly

The progression of their disease strips people with metastatic breast cancer
of many of the ways in which their identity had been formerly determined,
before they got sick. You may not be able to drive your children to school or
their ballet lessons, for example, or prepare meals for your family. You may
not be able to dance or to move without pain. With the hair loss of chemotherapy, and weight loss or gain, and surgical scars, your sense of yourself as
feminine and attractive to your partner may be compromised. Your stamina
may be so compromised that work, as you once knew it, becomes impossible. As these aspects of self slip away, the feelings of loss are inevitable. Yet
new self-definitions can come to replace these roles and activities, as you
struggle to identify your sense of self in terms that are larger than body and
illness.

Kathy Charmaz details the difficult process of coming to terms with immersion in illness:

*Transcendence of self means that the self is more than its body and
much more than an illness. Thus, illness does not fill or flood the self, even
though it may fill and flood experience. Transcendence implies self-accep-
tance, rather than any acceptance of illness cloaked in stigmatized images
and expectations of resignation. In addition, transcendence implies*

reevaluation and renewal. Achieving transcendence requires making choices and taking action.

Both loss and transcendence emerge from the experience of illness and the respective meanings that people confer upon it. Yet loss and transcendence are not static states of being, for one individual may experience both—sometimes dramatically, although at different points in his or her illness.... With each episode, another physical loss. With each event, another possibility for knowing self.

Certainly not everyone gains transcendence. Experiencing loss after loss can produce numbness and a shrinking of self. Transcendence is something of a fragile state, for affirming it may rely largely upon the person who experiences it. Further, ill people may feel that they have transcended their illnesses at certain points only to plummet into loss at other times.... Nevertheless, transcendence is possible if ill people have time for reflection, gain the tools to do it, and define essential qualities of self as distinct from their bodies. Encouragement from others to reflect and to define a valued self beyond a failing body supports transcendence. Moreover, others' acclaim of the ill person's perseverance, courage, or strength may prompt his or her definitions of transcendence. Suffering an onslaught of troubles without flinching often gives ill people a sense that they have faced the worst and have transcended it. Hence, transcendence may develop from suffering tremendous physical, psychological, and social losses.[12]

In the constancy of her sense of self, and her values, JB Boggs found ways to preserve her identity, despite the losses of illness:

I am still JB. I still recognize myself. I do not need to start from scratch to develop a support network or revamp my values. I cared for my humanity all along. I am not suddenly religious. My spirit has been with me all along.

My eyes are not now unexpectedly open to the meaning of things like Scrooge. No ghosts have come to visit to warn me, "Change before it's too late!" It is not suddenly Christmas to celebrate. I celebrate all along.

I do not feel I suddenly need to go climb Mount Everest. I do not suddenly feel the new urge to be human and real. I have been human and real all along.

I am still someone: What I want to do is continue to be at home and have my life. I am not crumbling into pieces. I am hurting, yes, but I still believe in myself as far as having skills and insights to help me. All the jobs and people and experiences and beliefs and values are intact and in place. I have tools to use.

JB used the memory of a movie seen in childhood to explain the changed world of serious illness.

In the "Incredible Shrinking Man," he ends up down in the basement, and goes out into the grass. The blades of grass are huge, towering over him, and the bugs are there. He cries, "But I'm still a man. I'm still myself. I still have all my feelings and I still exist. There's something to live for." It really affected me a lot. I must have been ten or eleven. I thought it was wonderful that he still had hold of himself, that though his world was chaotic, he still had a sense of himself. I think of that sometimes.

Faith, spirit and the search for meaning

When pain is to be borne, a little courage helps more than much knowledge, a little human sympathy more than much courage, and the least tincture of the love of God more than all.

—CS Lewis
The Problem of Pain

Clearly, the strong religious faith that many of the people I interviewed share affirms that spirituality plays a vital role in coping with metastatic breast cancer. In their view, there is a place for human suffering, dignity and transcendence in God's plan. There is order and purpose in the universe. This belief plays an important part in helping them to endure and transform their pain and loss into something deeply meaningful. A firm belief in the afterlife offers a further sense of hope and enlargement. For those who share beliefs with a spiritual community, a church or temple congregation, being cared for by this extended community supports the family and the patient at a time when isolation is more the rule than the exception.

Faith is not a given, however, and the struggle to achieve peace and acceptance is often hard-won, as Caren Buffum writes:

The most basic premise of my faith is that there is more to human life than a physical body—that we have a spirit that can and will exist apart from that which is now earthbound. Well, that sounds all well and good until one has to deal with the very real possibility that earth may not exist much longer for this one individual (or to put it the other way, the individual may not be long for this earth). So that has been the greatest challenge of all to my faith, and one that truly would not be able to be answered on an intellectual level. I don't know how it has happened, but somewhere along the way, my brain was able to let go of its need to understand eternal life and the spiritual side of existence. I firmly believe it has been an act of God's grace that I now experience a greater peace in my life than I had before I encountered cancer. I don't mean that life is easier—Lord knows it is not easier. But I live day to day without that underlying fear of what lies "beyond."

PJ reports how her faith has helped her to let go of her bitterness:

My spirituality has seen me through the pain and anger at breast cancer. I fight to keep my spirit up and my energy levels up and to not get too discouraged, which happens to all of us at times. My Michael has given me all that I need to wake up each day and pick up where I left off the day before. We have just celebrated our 27th anniversary last Friday, and for 13 years of that 27 we have lived with the fact that I have breast cancer. We changed our priorities and decided what was really important in life to us and then realized that this journey, while not what we planned, was a journey we could take together and still love every minute of every day. I have tried, and will continue to try everything that comes out there to continue to live. I try to keep the pain under control and my state of mind high among the stars and my spirit at peace. I have good days, super days and bad days, but I have been given another day and another part of the woods to explore with the one I love.

Some may think this is an unrealistic view but I have discovered to continue with the anger and the feeling of fighting against something brings me down. This is just the way I have found I can live with cancer and not rave about how much I have been cheated out of, or rant about what I might be missing. Things in life just happen and how we handle them is what can make or break our spirit. I'm honestly not always 100 percent positive but I do try to be and I feel better about everything if I turn it over to God when things get rough. God, Mike and a sense of humor are the three magic ingredients in my life that make it all worth living.

I have great faith, that is my first source of comfort. I believe I will only be given what I can handle. Sometimes I feel as if I'm at the limit of what I can handle. I get scared and I cry and pray for strength. If I need help at home, I have a wonderful church family that will provide meals, cook and clean or do just about whatever else I need.

Gerry Wirth reflected on the ways in which the faith he and Cindy shared sustained them during her illness, and after.

We believed that there is a God who is loving and good. We also believed that there is life with Him after death. With those two beliefs firmly rooted in our hearts, facing Cindy's illness and death was not over-powering. I know Cindy is with God right now. I know there is a reason that she was taken from us and some good shall come of it. Knowing these things has not made the experience painless. But it has allowed me to know all the suffering is not in vain. I do not understand the reason, but I know there is one. Our parish pastor said that Cindy was more well-pre-pared to meet death, one of the most prepared he had seen. Cindy also often told me not to let her sickness weaken my faith. It has not weak-ened it. It has tested it.

Pam Hiebert discovered a new sense of spirit through her illness.

Am I dying? Of course I am. And I have simply found a higher con-sciousness of this fact. Yet I also find, in this state of greater awareness, that for the first time in all of my life, I have such a keen appreciation for the small and endearing things about life. I wake with joy in my heart. I smile more deeply at the sight of a young baby. I am much more aware of the suffering of others and the frailty of existence in our world.

Somehow in this profound and devastating experience of the last three years, I have actually begun to identify myself as a person of faith. It is that faith that will continue to be an influencing factor in my cancer journey. It is this faith that will bring me home. I believe each one of us follows our own path to wholeness, yet the ability to pool our discoveries enriches the sacredness of our experience.

Certainly our resources and our connections with others provide the consciousness of living in community. Our friend Barbara wrote this: "A community is where a warrior returns to lay off her armor and let in the light and warmth of the sun. A place where wounds can heal and scars be displayed. A place that makes it all worth fighting for."

And Jenilu Schoolman wrote:

I have been asked how I could achieve such calm while facing death. What is the alternative? This is not a glib reply. The only other choice I can think of is to cry, to scream and yell, and just give up—but all that would be a waste of this precious gift of time. For me, the only way I can conceive of living is the way I am living.

Where does my strength comes from? Nature: trees and hills, snow and flowers, the little animals. All these have been a source of solace for as long as there has been a me. As a kid, I often found peace and comfort in the city park. Once I confided to my amused schoolmates that the trees and lake were my friends. And it is still true. Whenever I have turned to the natural world for guidance, I have not been disappointed.

In this crisis, I watch the cycle of the seasons. The trees do not mourn their autumn as the leaves fall at the appointed time. New ones are ready to replace them. Death and regeneration exist together everywhere I look in nature. Why should I be different?

The anatomy of courage

We would rather be ruined than changed;
We would rather die in our dread
Than climb the cross of the moment
And let our illusions die.

—W. H. Auden

Through their words and actions, the women and men who have animated these pages have laid bare the anatomy of courage. Courage implies, in Webster's definition, "The attitude of facing and dealing with anything recognized as dangerous, difficult or painful, instead of withdrawing from it."

These people have been able to summon the strength to turn *toward* what is most frightening, rather than to turn away, as our culture of denial encourages us to do. They have chosen to embrace the "full catastrophe," as Zorba the Greek termed it.

In doing so, they have sought out new sources of meaning and joy, as their lives unfolded moment by precious moment. They celebrated and they mourned. They let go of illusions and revised their expectations. They held tight to those they loved, forging real intimacy through honest expression, and they reached out to help others. They weathered the physical and emotional distress of treatments and disease progression with compassion for themselves, expressing emotion yet not drowning in suffering. They informed themselves and sought out the best of care, at times raging at the unfairness of the system and fighting for their right to treatment. They made conscious choices and plans. They sought transcendence and beauty in creativity—through poetry, music, art—and often through the writing they did for this book. They sought a communion with the natural world, sensing their own place in the flow of the seasons and in all of life. They passionately pursued a connection with God or whatever spiritual force they understood for themselves. From all these sources, and many more, they kept on keeping on—reinventing the strength day by day to live fully for the time that remains to them.

They are ordinary women and men just like yourself, possessed of no special heroic capacity before illness came into their lives. Put simply: they rose to the occasion. They did not accomplish this alone, without help. They learned, often from other patients, to assert and inform themselves. They depended upon the love and support of their families and friends. They relied on the skill and compassion of their doctors and other care providers. With the help of their spiritual communities, they sought comfort and meaning. By telling their stories, and sharing their insights, it is their hope and my own that your own journey will have been made less lonely and frightening.

It is they who should have the final words in this book. First, Caren Buffum, responding to a letter from a woman newly diagnosed with metastatic breast cancer, who questioned how she would ever be able to cope with this disease.

> I want to encourage you to focus on each day you live rather than trying to "know". I can't tell you how long it takes—I think it is more of a gradual process—each day gets a little easier. I guess you will have to

trust those of us who have come through it—that's what we're here for, to tell you we are on the same journey as you are and have just made it down the road a bit further. We are like scouts, trotting our horses back to tell you what's on the other side of the mountain. Of course, everyone's experience is different, but I do believe we share similar stages or cycles in our process.

If you can't rest in your own lack of knowledge, at least know that we know that it can happen, and no doubt will happen for you in time. Meanwhile, do your best to learn what is most important in life for you right now. How do you want to spend your time? What haven't you done yet that you have dreamed of doing? Whom do you want to get to know better but haven't taken the time? What places bring you the most peace? What time of day are you most relaxed? What memories do you enjoy recollecting? Since you can't know your future and a lot of other things about the disease, take the time to know yourself better and find what gives you greatest meaning and deepest joy. Then focus on those things. You might try keeping a journal of what you learn and feel, if you don't already. Don't try to do it all at once—a little every day.

At the closing of the year, Sandra Yandell offered these reflections:

This morning I was thinking about the Solstice—the shortest day and longest night—and I realized that's what my life feels like. Then I started thinking about my seventeenth winter, when temperatures at Christmas time were in the 50's and 60's, and I was in love with the younger version of the man I love now. And I can't stop crying, because I feel distilled into a moment in time—a bright, warm, too-short winter's day. I remember walking around the lake in the park with him, young love passionate and unsure of myself. One of those intense days that you don't want to end. That day went on into evening, but this "winter's day" ends with the light. Unseasonably warm and too brief, too few hours left of light. My first love becomes my last love in another winter.

There is another light waiting in that darkness, an unending season of joy. It would be so easy, sometimes, to slip away, to let go into that place where there will be no pain, and I will no longer need this body that has become my prison. I remember that seventeen-year-old body almost seventeen years ago, so self-consciously aware of myself in the presence of a *young man I adored. Some days I am again self-conscious, this time of the ravages of this disease on a once beautiful body.*

Today was a bright, warm December day. My love's kiss tastes the same as it did then, and though I live in my winter, it too is bright and warm. And I am not ready to watch the sun set on this winter's day.

One of the definitions of survival is "that which endures." I think I fit in this category. I've been battling this enemy for five years, through numerous surgeries, lots of radiation and now my second regimen of chemo. Sometimes I feel like a soldier who keeps getting shot, then patched up and sent back on the front lines. I know it's hard to hear stories like mine—it could have been, might have been, one day may be you. I pray that it will never be so, for anyone, but the fact remains that, although I am not disease-free, I am alive, and I will do whatever I can to keep going. In spite of the fact that I have serious bone mets, and my prognosis is not very pretty, still I can say I am a survivor, I have endured, I will continue as long as there is breath.

Profiles

EACH OF THE PEOPLE profiled below are quoted at some length in this book. They and the other metastatic breast cancer patients quoted more briefly in the text have consented to having their real names and identifying information used. Unfortunately, while their stories are accurate as of July 1997, it is in the nature of metastatic breast cancer that their disease may have progressed since these profiles were written.

Kim Banks

Kim, 36, a freelance magazine writer and would-be mystery novelist, lives with her husband, Richard, in a suburb of Denver. Lovers of the outdoors, they moved to Colorado to partake of the great skiing, hiking, camping and cycling here. Kim is rarely without a good mystery novel in her hands.

Diagnosed in 1992 with Stage IIB breast cancer, Kim underwent mastectomy with reconstruction, and CMF chemotherapy. Despite the fact that her tumor was hormone sensitive, she was unable to take tamoxifen because it made her migraine headaches much worse. Two years later, a new tumor was found between her pectoral muscles. While she was undergoing chemotherapy with CAF, new evidence of tumor was found in her lumbar spine. Radiation treatment and Taxol seemed to stabilize the growth of new tumors. Currently on Megace, Kim has had some difficulty controlling her pain, due to an allergic reaction to opiate pain medication.

> *I'm frustrated at the limitations my back pain puts on my travel, but am trying to enjoy each day to the fullest. The coming of spring has helped. I bought a new Winterking Hawthorn tree yesterday and the Newport Plum I planted two years ago is loaded with blooms. Planting*

the slow growing trees is reassuring. I feel like I'm sending myself a message that I'll be here to see them grow and mature. I hope to grow and blossom with them.

Lucie Bergmann-Shuster

Married with no children, Lucie, 52, lives with her husband, Cy, in Northern California. A former computer programmer and consultant, Lucie retired to work part-time as an acupressure massage therapist, and to pursue her interests in gardening, gourmet cooking, skiing and sailboat racing.

First diagnosed with breast cancer at age 38, Lucie experienced a recurrence to her ovary and surrounding tissue in 1995, more than twelve years later. Following abdominal surgery and chemotherapy, her disease appeared to be in partial remission for about a year, with possible spread to the bone. Now that the cancer has spread to her liver, Lucie is back in treatment with Navelbine, which has slowed but not stopped the progression of the disease.

I am facing death and have told my friends and family that I am dying, which in fact has been happening to my body since the beginning of this year. Granted, I am not yet in hospice but I have continued to steadily decline due to my liver mets. I have had quite some time to prepare for it. I knew I would be dealing with this dilemma once I was diagnosed with aggressive metastatic spread to my ovary a year ago. I asked questions then in terms of how long, and I was told anything from six months to five years. So I did a lot of planning then for what is going on now.

JB Boggs

JB Boggs, 47, a former receptionist, and her husband, Bob, a computer programmer, live in Southern California. Before her diagnosis, JB enjoyed athletics and was an avid sportswoman. She enjoys making crafts and taking them down to the children's wing and the cancer wing at the hospital. Married after her diagnosis, she took great joy in planning for the ceremony and making wreaths and other decorations.

In the process of x-raying and examining her back and ankle after a fall in August 1994, JB was diagnosed with a Stage IV breast cancer, which had already spread to her bones. Having been treated with several courses of chemotherapy, she is currently taking Arimidex. While she's been hospitalized repeatedly over the past two years, for pain management and other complications, and must wear a morphine pump for pain control, she remains hopeful that her disease is progressing slowly and feels her quality of life is still good.

> *I am still someone: What I want to do is continue to be at home and have my life. I am not crumbling into pieces. I am hurting, yes, but I still believe in myself as far as having skills and insights to help me. All the jobs and people and experiences and beliefs and values are intact and in place. I have tools to use. I can see others in the hospital and it gives me courage to see their courage. We help each other. Before I was sick, I was still basically the same person. I feel the movement to the future and I am a pilgrim on the path. I am okay. I am safe. I still have hope.*

Caren Buffum

A teacher in a private school, Caren lived with her husband, Dave, and two sons in Pennsylvania, where she also wrote songs, sang and played the piano and violin, and was active in her Temple congregation. At the time of her death, Caren was working on a musical version of Acts, adapted from the Bible.

Caren was diagnosed with Stage I breast cancer in 1985, and six years later, multiple tumors were found in her lungs and liver. After failing to respond sufficiently to an induction regimen to have high-dose chemotherapy, Caren took part in several clinical trials, of retinoids and monoclonal antibodies, and standard chemotherapy regimens, including 5-FU, Taxol, Adriamycin, Cytoxan and Navelbine. Eventually all treatment options were exhausted. She was able to teach until a couple of months before her death, in August 1996.

> *First, believe that there are good days and bad days. When you feel lousy, believe that it is not a permanent state of mind or necessarily going to persist every day. Believe that you may wake up one morning and feel better. And when you do have a good day, don't question it, like, "I shouldn't feel this way—I have breast cancer." Fact is, you probably also have a lot of other stuff—good stuff. The more you focus on the people you love, the things you like to do, etc., the more you will have to celebrate and feel good about. Try to plan events that you can look forward to.*

Lisann and Leo Charland

Married with no children, Lisann, 44, lives with her husband, Leo (Buddy), two dogs and a parrot in Northern California. Her parents still live in the Seychelles, where she was born, and she returns to visit whenever she can. A management analyst, now retired on disability, Lisann enjoys gardening, cooking and reading.

Lisann's breast cancer metastasized to her hip, sternum and chest wall in 1990, six years after her primary diagnosis at Stage IIB. She was treated with radiation and tamoxifen at this time. Four years later, a large tumor found in her liver was treated with intensive Taxol and Adriamycin, with 5-FU and leucovorin, followed by an innovative chemoembolization process, where the drugs were delivered directly to her liver. After a lengthy remission, she is currently being tested for disease progression.

> *Death and dying is all around us everyday. My very own mortality certainly crossed my mind as I felt so low this month. My worst fear is that I would become incapacitated and will not see my family. After I finished crying, and reasoning with myself, I did some gardening and cleaned up my fish pond. I felt much better after that. As the days progressed, I think I handled it pretty well—the best way I could. Things are getting better and I feel much better.*

Glenn and Barb Clabo

Glenn, 47, and Barb, 48, made their home in a Virginia suburb of Washington, DC. Barb worked as a computer operator for Home Depot and Glenn works as a business manager for the Department of the Navy. Their daughter is away at college, and their son has recently moved out on his own. After retirement from coaching baseball and softball for many years, they spent their spare time remodeling their house, working in the yard and taking long walks observing nature. In the past year, travel to meet new friends and renew old friendships became a priority.

Barb's primary diagnosis was Stage IV in October 1995, with all lymph nodes positive and metastases to the liver and spine. Following induction chemotherapy, Barb underwent high-dose chemotherapy with autologous bone marrow transplant. After some months of recovery, Barb was back at work full-time and apparently in remission when the tumor recurred in multiple fast-growing sites to her liver. Knowing that her tumor was likely to be chemo-resistant and that treatment options were few, Barb decided against further treatment. Barb died at home, peacefully, in June 1997, surrounded by her friends and family.

> Glenn: First...I wasn't prepared for the roller coaster ride. At times you'll feel like you're running at full speed with one shoe nailed to the floor. At times you'll find yourself saying and doing strange things. Wondering if anything makes sense. Completely confused by the amount of information....yet overwhelmed by the lack of clear/direct information. Nothing fits perfectly... yet what everyone does is right for them. You may have people tell you what's right for you and especially for your wife....soon you'll both understand that what she decides is right for her... and that's all that counts.

Bob Crisp (Ginger)

Bob, 56, a professor of computer systems engineering, lives in Arkansas, where he and his wife, Ginger, an Associate General Counsel for the state university, made their home. Together, they had five daughters by their previous marriages. They were both very active in church and civic affairs, and enjoyed traveling together.

Ginger was diagnosed in May of 1993, at age 51, with Stage IIB breast cancer that had spread to two lymph nodes. She was treated with a mastectomy with TRAM reconstruction and four cycles of CA chemotherapy. Eighteen months later, a tumor appeared in the armpit on the opposite side, and a skin rash turned out to be inflammatory cancer. In July 1995, HDC was performed, but Ginger relapsed with inflammatory disease within three months. This was followed by extensive radiation treatment that caused severe burns to her entire chest area, shoulders to waist. Further treatment was tried to forestall the spread of disease, but a pleural effusion left her short of breath, and the tumors and rash spread relentlessly. Ginger died in August 1996, with her husband and daughters beside her.

> This is an up/down process with some days (hours, minutes) better than others. And to learn that we will be sane again, but never the same again. The sanity must come from recognition, identification and acceptance of a new reality. A new reality where some things we took as certainty are no longer certain, that we are all terminal but some know more

about the time and possibilities than others, and that our dreams and visions of the past must be replaced with new dreams and visions. With this new reality and dreams and vision, some things emerge. That every day is a gift and to cherish the day. That every day I've had with Ginger is a wonderful treasure and to give thanks for what I've received and not obsess over what might not be.

Mary D'Angelo

Mary, a high school English teacher, lived with her husband, Charlie, in a suburb of New York City. A close-knit family, they spent much of their time with their three grown children who live and work in the New York metropolitan area. Mary and her husband enjoyed good food and fine wines, and loved traveling in Europe.

By the time Mary's breast cancer was diagnosed in 1988, it had spread to several lymph nodes. Her recurrence, some four years later, was in the liver. Strongly estrogen receptor positive, the tumor was successfully treated for over a year with tamoxifen, then with Megace. Since a course of Adriamycin failed to stop or even slow the tumor, Mary was concerned that she would not respond sufficiently with Taxol induction therapy to qualify for clinical trials in high-dose chemotherapy at the medical center where she was being treated. She decided on unusually aggressive high-dose chemotherapy at another hospital, administered outside of a clinical trial. Following six months of debilitating induction chemo with Taxol and cisplatin, and an ethanol infusion to shrink her liver tumors, she underwent high-dose chemotherapy with melphalan and thiotepa in April 1995. Despite multiple platelet transfusions, Mary died thirty days later from the effects of the treatment.

My philosophy is that there's always a way to make it right. No matter how horrible it is, or what you have to deal with, there is a path you can go down that enables you to be grateful in some way. That it can enrich you, instead of destroying you. You just have to keep seeking and finding the right door.

Bonnie Gelbwasser

At age 53, Bonnie works as assistant director of a news service at a small technological university, and lives with her husband, Herman, in Massachusetts. Their three children are now grown. Bonnie is an active member of the Cancer Center Advisory Council at the University of Massachusetts Medical Center, where she has been a patient. She is a member of a committee preparing the Breast Cancer Resource Guide for Massachusetts, a comprehensive, statewide guide expected to be published in the summer of 1997.

Bonnie was diagnosed with inflammatory breast cancer, Stage IIIB, in 1993. This form of breast cancer is rare and aggressive and historically has had a poor prognosis. After chemotherapy and a mastectomy, Bonnie's doctors recommended an autologous bone marrow transplant, which she underwent in 1994. Though she is closely followed, three and a half years later Bonnie is free of any detectable disease.

> *In May, I faced the possibility, for the third time since September 1995, that my cancer had metastasized.... I was told that I would live the rest of my life on a rickety bridge and that, essentially, I had been living an illusion because I expected that the ABMT would give me several more years, and here it wasn't even two years post-ABMT and my cancer had probably come back. And then the bone biopsy came back negative. And I thought about how my conversation with my doctor made it perfectly clear that I did not have the luxury of believing that I would live a long time—that, in fact, I could "light up the bone scan" in a couple of years and be on a track for death. So now I know (as if I didn't know before). And nothing has changed. I thought about this and went back to being my old, upbeat self.*

Nancy Gilpatrick and Terry Houlahan

A 43-year-old mother of twin teenage sons, Nancy lives with her recently-married husband, Terry, a postal worker and aspiring writer, and her sons in Utah. Before her diagnosis, Nancy was a social worker in private practice. She and Terry take long drives in the desert and enjoy bird-watching.

When Nancy was diagnosed with Stage IV breast cancer in November 1995, widespread metastases to her bones were found, and two breaks in her pelvis within a few months left her unable to walk. Recovering from recent high-dose chemotherapy with stem cell transplant in September 1996, Nancy was looking forward to being able to have surgery to repair her pelvis in 1997. A few months later, her disease recurred in the bones of her pelvis, and Nancy is back in treatment and experiencing further disease progression.

> I have a whole mixture of feelings about death. It kind of depends on what my brain is telling me about my death and that's a whole range of things. For instance, if it says "We all die. That is one of two certainties in life: birth and death," then I have serenity. It will happen to everyone and I don't feel chosen or picked on. If my brain is saying, "You are going to miss out on your kids' lives. Look, you just found the love of your life, Terry," whew, then I go through so many feelings. Mostly grief and a huge feeling of loss. I fear missing out on all these wonderful experiences that are possibly ahead of me. Then I cry and am sad. There's anger, too, when I feel picked on. Why me? Then my brain can say, "Why not you? You aren't special, less likely to die than anyone else." Then there is serenity again—the shorthand version of what takes hours and days to go through.

PJ Hagler

A 46-year-old mother of one grown son, PJ lives with her husband, Mike, in Maryland. Until she was forced to retire on disability, she worked as a secretary. PJ loves to read and travel, is involved with her church life and has been very active in counseling other cancer patients.

In 1991, PJ had a recurrence to her lung, with pleural effusion, seven years after being diagnosed with Stage II breast cancer in 1984, at age 34. In 1996, she was diagnosed with metastases to her liver. At the present time, her disease is progressing, and she has exhausted most available treatments.

> My oncologist told me when he signed my paper for a handicap sticker for my car that he never thought he would get to sign two of those in my case. The sticker is good for two years and he thought one would be my limit, when we started this adventure. I've told him I'm not afraid to die, I'm just not through living yet. I don't live with the idea that I might not be here tomorrow or next week or even next year. I still plan for the future. Mike and I talk about retirement days. But, realistically, I also talk about when or if I'm not here. And I'm okay with that.

Pam Hiebert and Sylvan Rainwater

A 49-year-old mother of an adult daughter, Pam lives with her life partner, Sylvan, in Oregon, and works as an electronic publishing technician for a community college. A self-described "spiritual growth seeker," she augments her medical care with naturopathic and Chinese medicine and visualization.

Pam was diagnosed with Stage IV breast cancer in 1993, with metastases to her left femur found at her initial diagnosis. Her disease was stable for over three years on tamoxifen. At the current time, she is again in remission on Arimidex, and delighted with the unexpected gift of more time.

I'm living in the here and now. I don't have a vision for the future. I deal with gathering information and continue to trust the natural process rather than demanding that I try to control these events.

Scott Kitterman (Mary)

Scott, 34, and Mary, 43, lived together in a Washington, DC suburb with their two-year-old daughter. Scott works as a systems analyst and Mary worked as an aerospace engineer. Scott enjoys traveling, reading history and science fiction and playing with his daughter.

Mary was diagnosed in the spring of 1995 with Stage IIIB breast cancer, and received an aggressive course of induction chemotherapy, high-dose chemotherapy with stem cell transplant and a course of radiation to control local spread. During the radiation, it was found that the cancer had spread to her cerebrospinal fluid and to her brain, indicating she had carcinomatous meningitis. Scott researched this rare fast-growing form of metastatic disease and all treatment options that made sense were tried. Despite chemotherapy administered intrathecally, and whole-head radiation, Mary died in the fall of 1996.

I don't pretend that patients can or need to know as much about medicine as their doctors. They had four years of medical school and years of follow-up training to learn what they know about a broad spectrum of medical topics. What you can do, and I believe must do, is learn a lot about the specifics of the case at hand so that you are in a position to make the decisions that need to be made. Doctors may have more information, but they don't necessarily make better decisions.

Joleene Kolenburg

A 66-year-old mother of two, and grandmother of three, Joleene lives with her husband, Jack, in Indiana. Retired from her administrative post at a nearby college, Joleene enjoys socializing and is active in her church.

Diagnosed in 1992 at Stage IIB, Joleene was treated with Cytoxan and Adriamycin, and took tamoxifen for three years, until a recurrence was found in her lungs. She enrolled in a trial protocol with Taxol combined with an experimental drug. After six months of treatment, she experienced a remission that lasted about ten months. Currently, Joleene is back in treatment with CMF, and is struggling to recover from pneumonia.

> *When I was first diagnosed with cancer, I really fussed and cried. I was 62, and I wanted to live until I was 72. I don't know why I picked that number. Now that I'm 66, I think maybe 72 is too soon. My youngest grandchild is 12 today and I'd like to see her graduated in six more years. I think if we love life, we can never really say when we will be ready to leave. I am not afraid of dying, and am ready to die, but as some have said, just not ready to leave yet.*

Pat and Chris Leach

Pat, 53, formerly a psychiatric nurse, lived with her husband, Chris, 59, in Connecticut, where he retired recently. Pat enjoyed running, completing two marathons, and liked doing volunteer work. The couple raised four grown children, and enjoyed traveling together.

Pat was diagnosed in 1984 with invasive Stage I lobular cancer. She was free of disease for five years, when she developed bone mets to her hip, treated with tamoxifen and radiation. Two years later, a liver tumor was found, and was treated for nearly two more years with Cytadren, another hormone. In 1995, with tumor in her bone marrow and several new bone metastases, Pat chose high-dose chemotherapy. Within a year, however, her red blood cell counts began to drop again, and the cancer returned. Although she needed frequent transfusions, Pat and Chris enjoyed a trip together to California only a few weeks before her death in the fall of 1996.

> **Pat:** *I just think that if I could deal with the fact of my dying and death, come to terms with it, so to speak, I'd be better able to face having this disease and just maybe wouldn't fall apart each time I get any bad*

news. It helps when the issue is being openly addressed. My family and friends are very uncomfortable whenever I raise the issue—they change the subject or say, "Don't talk like that/about that. You have years and years to live yet." So I push it to the back of my mind, but it is one subject that surfaces frequently.

Sharon and Lloyd Multhauf

A 54-year-old mother of a teenage son and daughter, Sharon lives with her husband, Lloyd, and her children in Northern California. She is a full-time mom and homemaker, active in her church and community, with particular interests in desk-top publishing and genealogy. Lloyd works as a nuclear physicist at a large laboratory. They enjoy sailing together on San Francisco Bay.

Sharon was disease-free for over seven years after her initial diagnosis in 1987 with Stage II breast cancer. In 1994, she experienced a local recurrence in her breast and concurrent metastases to her sacrum, pelvis and hip. Her disease had been stabilized on tamoxifen until this year, when the tumor in her sacrum began to press on her spinal cord. Sharon is currently undergoing a course of radiation treatments to stop this tumor from further growth, and relieve pain and numbness.

> **Sharon:** *I know that this "waiting for the other shoe to drop" anticipation can be horribly frightening for some people. The effect it has on a person's life depends on the way she/he handles stress, fear and worry in general. The real challenge is to do everything you can (within your own self-imposed limits) to work against a further recurrence, while at the same time living your life to the fullest without cowering in fear of the unknown.*

Barb Pender

A divorced mother of three, and grandmother of two, Barb, 46, lives with and cares for her elderly mother in California. Returning to college after her divorce, Barb coordinated a math and science camp for children, and still keeps in touch with her students, after retiring on medical disability. She loves doing various crafts. Recently, she has done some public speaking about her breast cancer experience. It is her face that graced the cover of the first edition of this book.

When Barb's breast cancer was first diagnosed in 1992, at Stage IIIA, she was treated with intensive Cytoxan and Adriamycin. When lung metastases were detected a year later, she entered a trial that involved induction chemotherapy with Taxol followed by two high-dose chemotherapy treatments with stem cell rescue/bone marrow transplants, a month apart, and a later course of radiation when the cancer metastasized to the skin. In the past year the tumors in her lungs, while still active, have been well controlled with Navelbine. Most recently, small tumors have been found in her eye and brain, which have been treated with radiation. It is too soon to know if the tumor progression has been halted for the moment.

> Almost four years later and still on chemo for metastases, I constantly update my definition of "who I am." Now I do let those that love me share in my joy and in my sorrow, but it has taken me awhile to do so. I know now that I am a beautiful woman. I try to be loving, caring, and kind. I also try to take every negative situation and find a positive somewhere—and I have been fortunate to find those positives.

Barb Ragland

Barb, 64, is divorced and has three grown children. Recently retired from her work as student coordinator at a university school of journalism, Barb lives in Nevada, and is currently pursuing her interests in genealogy, hoping to write a family history. She has always enjoyed working with young people, as the local director of a youth organization, teaching Sunday School and teaching in Alaska for a year. She was a Reach for Recovery volunteer for 11 years.

Barb was diagnosed in 1974 with Stage II breast cancer that had spread to 3 lymph nodes. A Halstead radical mastectomy and a course of cobalt radiation left her symptom-free until 1994, when she found two tumors in the mastectomy scar. Surgery, followed by a course of radiation and tamoxifen, appeared to put her into remission. In 1995, metastases were found in her sacrum. Since the tamoxifen had evidently stopped working, she was put on Megace. Another primary cancer was found in her remaining breast, for which she had a second mastectomy in 1996. While Barb is currently hopeful about achieving another extended remission, she is also at peace about whatever the future may hold.

> *I'm feeling good now and I think the mets may be stabilizing. It took almost twenty years before the recurrence came and then mets the year after. In the back of my mind I'm thinking that my cancer might be a slow-growing kind. I don't consider this denial—it's just the way I feel at the moment....I'm guessing I'll need some kind of treatment indefinitely. If it comes to pass that treatment causes severe side effects and risks, I may not choose to continue treatment. I'm a believer in the* **quality** *of life.*

Ellen Scheiner

Ellen, 65, recently retired from her private practice as a psychotherapist in New York City, which followed a thirty-year medical career as a nephrologist and specialist in internal medicine and medical ethics. She is a passionate music lover, student of meditation, poet and aspiring writer, currently working on a memoir about how illness has affected her life. Ellen's right arm was paralyzed due to a birth injury, and scoliosis ultimately forced her retirement from medicine.

In February 1994, a biopsy of a swollen lymph node revealed the spread of carcinoma, presumed to be from the spread of a breast cancer, though no lump was apparent and mammography was negative. Though gross pathology revealed nothing, microscopic examination showed multiple foci of in situ and invasive lobular carcinoma, which had spread to all fourteen lymph nodes. The odds of five-year survival with conventional chemotherapy were only 5 to 10 percent. Too old for high-dose chemotherapy, Ellen elected the intensive ATC protocol. The nine treatments given biweekly, involving as many hospitalizations, made it necessary for her to employ home health aides for over six months. Three years later, Ellen shows no evidence of recurrence, has regained most of her strength and is enjoying her retirement.

> *I did maintain control in the most dire of circumstances, but I've now learned that I don't have to, that the energy or force or spirit, if you will, is there. I don't have to create it consciously, because it is there. It's like when I went to medical school. I didn't think about it at all. It was simply so profoundly what I wanted to do, that I went ahead and did it. My notion is that if you really want with all of your being, then you do, and if*

not, you don't. Obstacles don't matter much. Sometimes the joy is simply in confronting it, in seeing it. That's why I say I've been staring into the abyss.

Jenilu Schoolman

A weaver and psychotherapist, Jenilu lived on a farming collective in upstate New York, where she enjoyed caring for her animals, from whom she procured natural fibers for her weaving. Her work as a therapist fulfilled her, and she took great satisfaction that her narrative of cancer recurrence, entitled "Within Measured Boundaries," which was published on the Internet, was meaningful to so many. Jenilu's story can be found at:

http://www-med.stanford.edu/CBHP/Personal_Stories/Jenilu.html

Diagnosed with breast cancer in 1982, Jenilu's cancer recurred to her liver three years later, in March of 1985. Told she had only a few months to live, she defied the odds by responding to chemotherapy and going into a remission that lasted until September of 1994. Adriamycin, Taxol and a pump that delivered the chemo directly to her liver gave her an additional year and a half. Jenilu died in February of 1996.

> *It is hard to say which changes in my own perspective come from living eight years longer, or which are a direct result of my close brush with death. I know I have become even more non-judgmental. I am also easier with the minutiae of life. Fewer little things really bother me. I find it relatively easy to keep a perspective on things. As the kids say, "If it ain't fatal, it's no big deal." That's not entirely true, but when you are able to look at life from the edge, it seems that only loving and honesty are really important.*

Bob Stafford

A retired pastor for a small rural congregation, who also worked in a psychiatric hospital on a pediatric unit, Bob, 46, lives with his wife, Sherry, and teenage daughter and son in rural Indiana. Since his diagnosis, he has worked hard to raise consciousness about male breast cancer on the Internet and on television.

Bob's cancer was diagnosed in 1988 at Stage I and was treated with mastectomy and CMF chemotherapy. Three years later, the cancer metastasized to his hips, ribs, spine and other bones. Orchiectomy (castration) was followed by hormonal treatments with tamoxifen, then Megace. CMF was discontinued when lung metastases were found two years later, and Adriamycin and Taxol have been tried. While his tumor markers have steadily risen, Bob is currently being helped by Navelbine.

> One thing I have thought about in the past is that there are no lessons on dying. For many death is not the problem, but rather the process of dying. No one can teach you that and it's an unknown territory. We hear stories of those who have supposedly died and returned. But nothing is said about the transition.... Those are the fears people face. How much pain will I suffer? Will I be able to let go? Will angels show up to carry me away, or will I have to walk?

Kathy Stone

Kathy, 54, and her husband, Chuck, live in Northern California and have four grown children, and four grandchildren. Retired on disability now from her job as a fiscal administrator, she considers her real accomplishments to have come from her efforts as a good mother, wife and friend. She enjoys camping and the outdoors, cooking and crafts projects.

Kathy's breast cancer had already spread to her supraclavicular lymph nodes at the time of first diagnosis in 1994. Aside from her mastectomy and radiation, she was treated with a course of Adriamycin, then CMF (Cytoxan, methotrexate and 5-FU). Multiple bone metastases were found upon completion of her CMF regimen, showing that the chemo treatments to date had not slowed the cancer down. The next year was spent trying three months of Taxotere, then ten weeks of continuous 5-FU and more radiation, with very little results. Starting into the third year of the disease growing, Kathy is on a regime called TEMP that employs (t)amoxifen (although she is ER/PR negative), (e)toposide, also called VP-16, (m)itoxantrone, also known as Novantrone and (p)latinol, also called Cisplatin. Kathy is also taking Aredia every month to help strengthen her bones.

> I think those of us with mets probably all feel the same...we are confused...we want it to be understood that we can have strong thoughts, questions and feelings about dying, but that it doesn't mean we have given up...and what is giving up anyway? I don't think anyone ever gives

up...maybe we get so tired we can't go on, but then we "rest"....we don't quit...and if, during that rest, we are to come to the end of our earthly life, then so be it, our time has come.

Sue Tokuyama

Sue, 35, lives with her husband, Yoshi, and their two young children in Arizona, following a recent job transfer from New Jersey. She works as a database marketing director, and writes poetry and fiction.

In October 1994, Sue was diagnosed with Stage IIIB breast cancer, with thirteen of twenty-six lymph nodes positive. Following her mastectomy, she underwent induction chemotherapy with CAF for several months, followed by high-dose chemotherapy with thiotepa, Cytoxan and carboplatin, and a course in radiation to the chest wall. The following year, she underwent reconstructive surgery. Two years after her diagnosis, there is no evidence of disease.

> *As far as anyone can tell, the cancer is gone (there's always a little voice whispering, "yeah, no mets—yet"), but I know I won't die of breast cancer today, tomorrow, or next week. I love my work, and I'm strong enough to do it. My kids are amazing, and I love them very much. I'm closer to my parents than I was before. I see my marriage in a whole different light. Sometimes I feel a little bit like Scrooge, in* **A Christmas Carol.** *I've got my warning, and now I'm out to make sure that my eulogy, whenever it's read, is riveting!*

Chris Tribur (Candace)

Chris Tribur, 47, has twin sixteen-year-old daughters, lives in Colorado and is a partner in a commercial painting business. He and Candace, a journalist and copy editor, had been married over twenty years at the time of her death. Since then, Chris finds himself both comforted and challenged by his daughters. "My children have been my solace," Chris writes. "Parenting is the most all-consuming job and responsibility that any creature can have on this earth, and I think it has forced me to recoup fast and carry on."

Candace was diagnosed in 1991 with Stage IIB breast cancer, with six out of twelve lymph nodes positive for the spread of the disease. Following mastectomy, radiation and chemotherapy, her disease recurred a year later in the bones of her spine, leg and arm. High-dose chemotherapy with stem cell transplant failed to control the progression of the disease, which recurred less than six months later in her lung, bones and brain. Further treatment with Megace and Taxol were ineffective, and Candace died in July 1995.

> *Up until the last, I refused to acknowledge the inevitable.... To the best of my knowledge my wife did not wish to cease treatment and I certainly did not want to let her go. I think when the time comes, the choices narrow themselves and we do the best we can. These are extraordinarily difficult circumstances to find oneself in, but we do what we do and there is no value in second-guessing or beating oneself up after the fact.*

Gerry Wirth (Cindy)

Gerry and Cindy Wirth had been married for sixteen years, and had two young children, at the time of Cindy's death in early 1996. Gerry, 40, an electrical engineer, lives with his son and daughter in Illinois.

Cindy was 35 years old and was six months pregnant with their second child, when her breast cancer was diagnosed at Stage IIIB in 1991. Despite aggressive treatments, including Cytoxan, Adriamycin and 5-FU, the cancer spread to her supraclavicular nodes and lung. Two years after her original diagnosis, Cindy underwent high-dose chemotherapy with stem cell transplant, but the cancer recurred within a few months. Two years later, she developed metastases to her brain and liver, and further treatment was ineffective.

> *I miss Cindy very much. We were married for seventeen years and a major part of each other's life for twenty years. It is like a big part of the core of my being was removed. I know that I will heal—no, heal is not the right word because I will never be the same person I was before Cindy's death. I feel I am going through a metamorphosis. I will be different when it is over. I am trying to be sure I will become a butterfly, not a moth.*

Sandra Yandell

Sandra, 33, lives in Oregon with her boyfriend, Jim, with whom she took a romantic trip to Paris and London in the spring of 1997. She keeps a journal, loves writing and is organizing and planning a reunion of the Breast Cancer Discussion List in her home city of Portland in the fall of 1997.

Originally diagnosed in April 1991, Sandra was treated with lumpectomy and radiation. She found the lump that signaled a local recurrence two years later. A further recurrence to the chest wall in 1994 was treated with more radiation. Two years later, metastases to the spine were discovered and two thoracic vertebrae were replaced with titanium hardware in a fifteen-hour surgery. Since that time, metastases have spread to her pelvis, cervical spine and right shoulder. While they were treated with radiation, CMF and Navelbine, her bone mets are still showing progression. Currently, Sandra is not receiving treatment.

I remember hearing that 27-year-old women don't get breast cancer. But I did. I was too young to be considering my mortality. At 27 I was supposed to be thinking about buying a house, car payments, holding my marriage together, building a future. That future was supposed to be spread before me, a myriad of possibilities not including my death. Cancer was a blip on the screen, a traumatic episode to be "gotten over" so I could get on with my life. At 27, I had no clue that my life would be forever altered, and not all the scars would fade with time.

Resources

THIS APPENDIX IS ORGANIZED into eight main topics: General information, Financial and legal information and assistance, Emotional support, Research, Alternative and complementary treatment, Coping with treatment, pain and discomfort, Dying and hospice care, and Breast cancer advocacy. Within each category you will find organizations, books and other publications, and online resources.

Many resources overlap between topics; some appear in more than one. There is also some crossover between organizations, print and online resources. Many organizations have an online presence and offer reading material. Sometimes whole books are available online as well as in print. If you want to find every possible resource that is on the World Wide Web, you will want to look through the organizations and publications under the topic in which you are interested as well as the online resources. If you want to find everything in print, browse through the organizations and online resources as well as those listed under the Reading section.

Hopefully, the many resources listed here will offer you the support and information you seek.

General information

American Cancer Society
1599 Clifton Road N.E., Atlanta, GA 30329-4251
Hot line: (800) ACS-2345
http://www.cancer.org/

The American Cancer Society has a national network of both employees and volunteers who implement research, education and patient service programs to help cancer patients and their families cope with cancer:

- Through the Resources, Information, and Guidance program, ACS gives callers information about cancer. Community services and other resources meet the practical, social, psychological and other support needs of cancer patients and others coping with the burden of cancer.

- Reach to Recovery is a peer visitor program providing support and information for women who have had breast cancer surgery. Road to Recovery provides volunteer drivers to drive patients who have no other means of transportation to and from treatment.

- ACS may be able to arrange for durable medical equipment such as walkers, wheelchairs, hospital beds, etc., at no cost to the patient.

- Look Good...Feel Better helps women undergoing radiation or chemotherapy manage the temporary changes in appearance that their treatments can cause, such as skin problems and hair loss.

The Susan G. Komen Breast Cancer Foundation
(800) I'M AWARE or (800) 462-9273
http://www.komen.org/

The Komen Foundation was established in 1982 by Nancy Brinker in memory of her sister Susan, who died in 1980 after a three-year struggle with breast cancer. The primary mission of the Komen Foundation is to eradicate breast cancer as a life-threatening disease by advancing research, education, screening, and treatment. They are the sponsors of the annual Race for the Cure, run in cities around the country, and offer a helpline to callers needing information.

The Mautner Project for Lesbians with Cancer
1707 L Street N.W., Suite 1060, Washington, DC 20036
(202) 332-5536; Fax: (202) 265-6854
http://www.edisolwaynedotson.com/mautner/

Direct services to lesbians with cancer and their partners and caregivers. Offers education and information to the lesbian community about cancer, and education to the health care community about the special concerns of lesbians with cancer and their families. Active in advocacy on lesbian health issues in national and local arenas.

National Alliance of Breast Cancer Organizations (NABCO)
9 East 37th Street, 10th floor, New York, NY 10016
Toll Free: (888) 80-NABCO or (888) 806-2226
http://www.nabco.org/

The National Alliance of Breast Cancer Organizations (NABCO) is the leading non-profit central resource for information and education about breast cancer. In addition to information, they provide assistance and referrals to anyone with questions about breast cancer, and act as a voice for the interests and concerns of breast cancer survivors and women at risk. NABCO is a network of more than 375 breast cancer organizations providing detection, treatment and care to hundreds of thousands of American women. Information is available on its web site, by telephone and through the 1997/98 edition of the *NABCO Breast Cancer Resource List*. Other resources from NABCO include:

- NABCO Fact Sheets, for current information on risk, early detection, treatment, follow-up care and national statistics.

- NABCO News, a quarterly newsletter covering the latest developments in medicine, science, services and policy, including risk factors, early detection and treatment options.

- National Support Groups, a state-by-state listing of support groups, with contact numbers.

- Video: *"On with life: Practical information on living with metastatic breast cancer."*

- NABCO also will provide physicians with one free copy of the 1992, 30-minute video, *"Autologous Bone Marrow Transplantation: Facing the Challenge."*

National Cancer Institute (NCI)
Building 31, Room 10A16, 9000 Rockville Pike, Bethesda, MD 20892
Hot line: (800) 4-CANCER or (800) 422-6237
Fax: (301) 231-6941
CancerNet on the World Wide Web: *http://www.nci.nih.gov/*

The National Cancer Institute is the most comprehensive and up-to-date source of clinical and research information for cancer patients and for health care professionals. Detailed and extensive patient treatment information, reviewed and updated monthly, is available by a number of methods from NCI. A clinical trials finder that lists all NCI-sponsored clinical trials offers contact and other information. NCI publishes a variety of related materials, from supportive care guidelines to clinical updates, available free. More information about the various services offered by the NCI can be found in the "Research" section, later in this appendix.

National Coalition for Cancer Survivorship
323 Eighth Street S.W., Albuquerque, NM 87102
(505) 764-9956
http://www.access.digex.net/~mkragen/index.html

A national network of independent groups and individuals concerned with survivorship and support services for patients and families.

Sisters Network
8787 Woodway Drive, Suite 4207, Houston, TX 77063
(713) 781-0255
http://members.aol.com/SistersNet/sis.html

A national organization with seven affiliated chapters, founded in 1994. Support, education and advocacy for the African American community concerning breast cancer. Outreach, training and research. Newsletter, information and referrals, phone support, conferences. Assistance in starting new groups.

Y-Me National Breast Cancer Organization
212 W. Van Buren, 5th Floor, Chicago, Illinois 60607-3907
Hot line: (800) 221-2141 9:00 a.m. to 5:00 p.m. CST, Mon.-Fri.
Spanish hot line: (800) 986-9505
http://www.y-me.org/

For almost twenty years, Y-ME has served women with breast cancer and their families and friends—through a national hot line, open door groups, early detection workshops and many local chapters. They also offer peer support programs—breast cancer patients talking with survivors, and spouses of patients talking with spouses of survivors. Nineteen affiliated groups nationwide.

Local organizations

In addition to the national organizations listed above, there are many outstanding *local* organizations. Ask for referrals from one of the national organizations or your treatment center, or look in the telephone book under "Social Service Organizations." A few of the better-known ones are listed below.

Commonweal
P.O. Box 316, Bolinas, CA 94924
(415) 868-0970
http://www.commonwealhealth.org/

Commonweal is a health and environmental research institute located in Bolinas, California, run by Michael Lerner, author of *Choices in Healing*, and featured in Bill Moyers' PBS Series, *Healing and the Mind*. The Commonweal Cancer Help Program conducts weeklong support and learning programs for people with cancer. For information, please contact Asoka Thomas, Program Coordinator.

Community Breast Health Project
770 Welch Road, Suite 370, Palo Alto, CA 94304
(415) 725-1788; Fax: (415) 725-5474
http://www-med.stanford.edu/CBHP/

The Community Breast Health Project acts as a clearinghouse for information and support, providing volunteer opportunities for breast cancer survivors and friends dedicated to helping others with the disease, and serving as an educational resource and a community center for those concerned about breast cancer and breast health. Offers counseling, groups for metastatic and primary breast cancer patients, practical information and information on advocacy efforts.

SHARE: Self-Help for Women with Breast and Ovarian Cancer
19 West 44th Street, Suite 415, New York, NY 10036
(212) 719-0364
Hot line (English): (212) 382-2111
Hot line (Spanish): (212) 719-4454
Hot line (Chinese): (718) 296-7108

SHARE offers many support groups for women with breast and ovarian cancer, including groups in Spanish and Chinese. Operates a patient hot line (also multilingual) and presents an ongoing educational series on issues of interest to breast cancer patients. Particularly important for their extensive outreach programs to underserved communities in New York City.

General reading

Dollinger, Malin, Ernest Rosenbaum, and Greg Cable. *Everyone's Guide to Cancer Therapy,* 3rd Revised Edition. Kansas City, MO: Andrews & McMeel, 1998. Based on the PDQ database of the National Cancer Institute, this is a good resource on many types of cancer.

Hirshaut, Yashar and Peter Pressman. *Breast Cancer: The Complete Guide,* Second Edition. New York: Bantam, 1996. Another excellent basic "companion" book for breast cancer, with a chapter on metastatic disease.

Love, Susan, M.D. *Dr. Susan Love's Breast Book,* Second Edition. Boston: Addison-Wesley, 1995. Considered by many to be the primary breast cancer patient's "bible," the revised edition incorporates two chapters on metastatic disease.

Teamwork: The Cancer Patients' Guide to Talking with Your Doctor. National Coalition for Cancer Survivorship, 1010 Wayne Avenue, 5th Floor, Silver Spring, MD 20910. Online at: *http://www.access.digex.net/~mkragen/index.html*

When Cancer Recurs: Meeting the Challenge Again. #93-2709, 1992. A free pamphlet on recurrence, from the National Cancer Institute. Call (800) 4-CANCER. As a point of departure, this touches on many of the major issues metastatic breast cancer patients will face.

Zakarian, Beverly. *The Activist Cancer Patient.* New York, John Wiley & Sons, 1996. An well-organized, practical guide to becoming an "empowered patient," covering every aspect of taking charge of your treatment decisions, including researching state-of-the-art treatments, understanding how drug trials work, discovering what "experimental treatment" means, searching out relevant medical journals and accessing reliable databases, and enlisting the help of medical specialists and support groups.

General information online

BreastCancer.Net
http://www.breastcancer.net

An e-mail service that surveys popular Internet medical and health news sources for information, then e-mails it to you daily. Subscriptions to this newsletter are free.

Community Breast Health Project
http://www-med.stanford.edu/CBHP/

Among other resources, this web site contains the full text of Jenilu Schoolman's essay on living with metastatic breast cancer, *Within Measured Boundaries.*

Health News
http://www.healthdirect.com/usenew/news.shtml

Links to Reuters, AP and many other health news services online. All health topics, but most sites can be searched for disease-specific information.

NCI CancerNet
http://wwwicic.nci.nih.gov./

The NCI web site with the most updated information. See the Bonn and Oncolink web sites listed below for hyperlinked access to this information, so that references and abstracts appear when you click on the footnotes in the medical review articles.

NCI CancerNet Database Main Index
Redistributed by University of Bonn Medical Center
http://imsdd.meb.uni-bonn.de/cancernet/cancernet.html

This is a fully hyperlinked interface to all the NCI information, with links to PDQ Disease Topics; Supportive Care Topics; Search Clinical Trials Database at the NCI; News and NCI Publication Information including Full Text Publications; Cancer Information Service (800 4-CANCER); Journal of the NCI; CANCERLIT Citations and Abstracts; MEDLINE from PubMed; NCI Fact Sheets with Risk Factors, Prevention, Detection, Therapy, Rehabilitation, and Unconventional Methods; Search the CancerNet Files for Keywords (full-text retrieval).

Oncolink
http://www.oncolink.upenn.edu

The University of Pennsylvania Cancer Center Resource. The best single one-stop resource with information on all aspects of cancer, and pointers to other sites.

PDQ Physician Statement on Breast Cancer
http://imsdd.meb.uni-bonn.de/cancernet/100013.html
http://www.oncolink.upenn.edu/pdq_html/1/engl/100013.html

Although the NCI Statements can be obtained directly from the NCI, this excellent version hyperlinks references in the text to the article abstracts, a major convenience. It is also available in Spanish.

Scientific American
http://www.sciam.com/0996issue/0996currentissue.html

Selections from their excellent September 1996 single topic issue: "CANCER."

Financial and legal information and assistance

Affording Care
429 East 52nd Street, Suite 4G, New York, NY 10022-6431
(212) 371-4740
http://www.thebody.com/.../afford/affordix.html

Financial information for those with serious illness. Publishes a free newsletter, "The Affording Care Bulletin."

Barbara Anne Deboer Foundation
2069 S. Busse Road, Mount Prospect, IL 60056
(800) 895-8478 or (847) 981-0130; Fax: (847) 981-1575

A national non-profit organization to assist those in need of organ transplants and other life-saving procedures in obtaining resources specific to the individual needs. The Foundation is especially concerned with those life-saving procedures not covered by insurance, and provides outreach, support, and advocacy services to patients who are affected. The foundation responds to inquiries from both patients and professionals. They offer information on funding HDC through an individual fund-raising program. Help is available for planning a funding campaign, and managing the donations to insure full availability to you and full tax credit to those who donate.

Judges and Lawyers Breast Cancer Alert
Hot line for legal professionals: (212) 759-6630.

The National Insurance Consumer Helpline
Hot line: (800) 942-4242 8:00 a.m. to 8:00 p.m. EST, Mon.–Fri.

A general information source for all types of insurance-related issues, including life and health insurance.

Patient Advocate Foundation (PAF)
780 Pilot House Drive, Suite 100-C, Newport News, VA 23606
(800) 532-5274; Fax: (757) 873-8999
e-mail: *patient@pinn.net*
http://www.patientadvocate.org/paf/welcome.html

The purpose of PAF is to provide education and legal counseling to cancer patients concerning managed care, insurance and financial issues.

Pharmaceutical Reimbursement Assistance Programs
U.S. Senate, Department of Aging
Majority: 202-224-5364, Minority: 202- 224-1467
http://oncolink.upenn.edu/specialty/chemo/general/indigent_drugs.html.

Most pharmaceutical companies have programs for people who can't afford their medications to receive free drugs if they meet financial criteria. Copies of this list are available free of charge by calling the numbers above. Oncolink maintains a list of providers online. See also Appendix C, *Common Drugs in Use with Metastatic Breast Cancer*.

U.S. Social Security Administration
(800) 772-1213
http://www.ssa.gov/SSA_Home.html

If you have been or will be disabled for six months or longer, you may be entitled to disability benefits. Metastatic breast cancer is generally considered a qualifying disability. Pamphlets are available online at: *http://www.ssa.gov/pubs/englist.html*.

Organizations providing air transport

Air Care Alliance
The National Patient Air Transport Hot Line (NPATH)
Hot line: (800) 296-1217
http://www.wolf-aviation.org/aircare/

A "nationwide association of humanitarian flying organizations."

Airlifeline
(800)-446-1231
http://www.airlifeline.org/

Free, nationwide service that flies qualified patients to treatment sites within 500–700 miles.

Corporate Angel Network
Westchester County Airport, Building 1, White Plains, NY 10604
(914) 328-1313
http://www.corpangelnetwork.org/

Flies qualified patients to treatment sites, free, using empty seats on corporate flights.

Financial and legal information publications

Cancer Treatments Your Insurance Should Cover. March, 1991. The Association of Community Cancer Centers, 11600 Nebel Street, Suite 201, Rockville, MD 20852; (301) 984-9496. World Wide Web: *http://www.assoc-cancer-ctrs.org/*. Information for patients and their families sponsored by the Association of Community Cancer Centers, the Oncology Nursing Society, and the National Coalition for Cancer Survivorship.

Cancer—Your Job, Insurance and the Law. An informative pamphlet from the American Cancer Society; (800) ACS-2345.

Directory of Prescription Drug Patient Assistance Program. 1996. Pharmaceutical Research and Manufacturers of America, 1100 15th Street N.W. Washington, DC 20005; (800) PMA-INFA.

Free & Low Cost Prescription Drugs. Booklet #PD-360 from the Cost Containment Research Institute, 611 Pennsylvania Avenue S.E., Suite 1010, Washington, DC 20003-4303.

Health Care Bill of Rights/Standards. MacLean Center for Clinical Medical Ethics, at the University of Chicago. Online at: *http://ccme-mac4.bsd.uchicago.edu/CCMEPolicies/Laws/CBHC9602.*

Health Insurance Association of America (HIAA). A trade association that serves as the voice of health insurance. Publishes a number of consumer guides to various kinds of insurance, including: *The Consumer's Guide to Disability Insurance,* 1995; *The Consumer's Guide to Health Insurance,* 1995; *The Consumer's Guide to Long-Term Care Insurance,* 1995; and *The Consumer's Guide to Medicare Supplement Insurance,* 1995. Call (202) 824-1600. These are available online at: *http://www.hiaa.org/.*

The Managed Care Consumers' Bill of Rights. 1996. A Health Policy Guide for Consumer Advocates. Public Policy and Education Fund of New York, 94 Central Avenue, Albany, NY 12206.

Medical Records: Getting Yours. This booklet includes a summary of legal rights in each state and what to do if a request is denied or if the records are incorrect. Available from Public Citizen's Health Research Group, Washington, DC; (800) 289-3787 or (202) 588-1000 9:00 a.m. to 5:00 p.m., Mon.–Fri. Online at: *http://www.citizen.org.*

What Cancer Survivors Need To Know About Health Insurance. 1995. Available free from the National Coalition for Cancer Survivorship; (301) 650-8868. Provides a clear understanding of health insurance and how to receive maximum reimbursement on claims.

Financial information online

Needy Meds: The Place to Learn About Pharmaceutical Manufacturers' Drug Assistance Programs
http://www.needymeds.com/MainPage.html

Created and maintained by a family practice physician and a social worker, this excellent web site for those in financial need or with insurance coverage problems does just what it promises, giving contact information, guidelines on eligibility and enrollment, patient and provider responsibility and more for most drugs approved for cancer treatment.

Emotional support

Sometimes it is relatively easy to find a support group in which you feel comfortable; sometimes it takes a bit of looking around, maybe trying out a few until you find one that is a good fit for *you*. Below are some suggestions to help you get started, and several organizations that might also be helpful. If you are interested in joining an online support group, several are listed in the sections, "Listservs: Cancer mailing lists on the Internet" and "Other online support groups," that follow the reading lists.

How to find a support group

- Inquire at a local medical center or hospital. Check to see if there is a Breast Center, and if not, contact the social work or psychiatry department.

- Contact the American Cancer Society for a referral at (800) ACS-2345.

- Contact the National Alliance of Breast Cancer Organizations for a referral at (800) 719-9154.

- Contact Y-ME for a referral at (800) 221-2141.

- If there is no support group for metastatic patients nearby, call one in a neighboring community and ask for a referral to organizations or leaders who may help.

- If your local breast cancer support organization doesn't have a group for metastatic breast cancer patients, ask that one be started. Get together with other metastatic patients and let your needs be known.

- Look into starting a group yourself. A group of patients can get together to hire an experienced group leader—a social worker, psychologist or psychiatrist—who has experience in working with cancer patients and good group skills. You should be able to find a name of a good therapist from one of the above sources.

American Self-Help Clearinghouse
Northwest Covenant Medical Center, Denville, NJ 07834-2995
(201) 625-7101, (800) 367-6274 in NJ
TTY 625-9053 for hearing impaired
http://www.cmhc.com/selfhelp/

Referrals and suggestions for starting your own self-help group. Publishes the *Self-Help Sourcebook,* 1995. To order, write to the above address, Attn: Sourcebook. The Self-Help Sourcebook Online is a searchable database that includes information on approximately 700+ national and demonstrational model self-help support groups, ideas for starting groups, and opportunities to link with others to develop needed new national or international groups.

The National SelfHelp Clearinghouse
25 West 43rd Street, Room 620, New York, NY 10036
Hot line: (212) 354-8525
e-mail: *gar@cunyvmsl.gc.cuny.edu*

Provides information and referrals to self-help groups.

Buddy Program for Breast Cancer Clinical Trials
New England Research Institutes
9 Galen Street, Watertown, MA 02172
(800) 775-6374 x547; Fax: (617) 926-8246
e-mail: *AllisonM@neri.org*
http://www.gis.net/~allisonm/buddies.html

With the support of the NCI and the National Action Plan on Breast Cancer, researchers are pilot testing a Buddy Program for women with breast cancer who are eligible for a clinical trial. Trial candidates talk to a trained "buddy" —a breast cancer survivor who has been in a clinical trial and can tell about her experience. Contact Allison C. Morrill, Ph.D., for more information.

National Bone Marrow Transplant Link
29209 Northwestern Highway, #624, Southfield, MI 48034
(800) LINK-BMT

Clearinghouse and links to former patients. Volunteers will return your call.

The Wellness Community
10921 Reed Hartman Highway, Suite 215, Cincinnati, OH 45242
Toll-free: (888) 793-WELL or (888) 793-9355
e-mail: *wellnessnational@fuse.net*
http://www.brugold.com/wellness.html

The Wellness Community is a support program devoted to providing free psychological and emotional support to cancer patients and their families. The program is founded on the "Patient Active Concept," which combines the skill of the physician with the will of the patient. There are communities in many cities nationwide.

Emotional support reading

Benjamin, Harold H., Ph.D. *The Wellness Community Guide to Fighting for Recovery from Cancer.* Putnam, 1995. In this book, the founder of the Wellness Community, a nationwide cancer support organization with branches in a number of cities, offers strategies cancer patients can use to deal with the emotional and physical effects of cancer and treatments, including visualization, nutrition, exercise, and enhanced personal relationships.

Kneece, Judy C., R.N., O.C.N. *Helping Your Mate Face Breast Cancer.* Edu-Care Publishing, 1995. A book for support partners, designed to help them understand how to provide a caring, healthful environment while taking care of their own emotional needs during the crisis of breast cancer.

Sexuality and Cancer: For the Woman Who Has Cancer, and Her Partner. Free booklet gives information about cancer, sexuality and other areas of concern to the patient and her partner. Includes a resource list. American Cancer Society; (800) ACS-2345. 40 pages.

Spiegel, David, M.D. *Living Beyond Limits.* New York: Random House, 1993. This excellent book on coping with metastatic illness is by the Stanford University psychiatrist responsible for the groundbreaking study suggesting that support groups for metastatic breast cancer patients extend both quality and quantity of life. Very strong chapters on psychosocial support and on the use of hypnosis and relaxation for controlling pain and other symptoms, with an outstanding bibliography. *Chapter Six: Detoxifying Dying* can be found online at: *http://www-med.stanford.edu/school/Psychiatry/PSTreatLab/lbltext.html*

Taking Time: Support for People with Cancer and the People Who Care About Them. NCI publication #93-2059, 1993. Free booklet from NCI; (800) 4-CANCER. This sensitively written booklet for persons with cancer and their families addresses the feelings and concerns of others in similar situations and how they have coped. 68 pages. Available online at *http://wwwicic.nci.nih.gov/taking_time/timeintro.html.*

Personal stories

Butler, Sandra, and Barbara Rosenblum. *Cancer in Two Voices.* Spinsters Book Company, 1991. (Also 16mm/video, Women Make Movies, New York.) A moving journal of illness, written by Rosenblum and her partner.

Ireland, Jill. *Life Lines* and *Life Wish.* Jove Publications, 1988. The actress's two memoirs provide affecting portraits of celebrity in the shadow of cancer.

Lorde, Audre. *The Cancer Journals.* San Francisco: Aunt Lute Books, 1980. Paperback. Reflections on her breast cancer experience by a well-known poet and feminist.

Lorde, Audre. *A Burst of Light.* Firebrand Books, 1988. A second essay collection, this one about Lorde's recurrence and subsequent treatment.

Middlebrook, Christina. *Seeing the Crab: A Memoir of Dying*. Basic Books, 1996. A vivid and honest account by a Jungian analyst of her experience with high-dose chemotherapy and metastatic disease.

Photopulos, Georgia, and Bud Photopulos. *Of Tears and Triumphs: One Family's Courageous Fight Against Cancer*. Contemporary Books, 1991. An account of how a political figure and his wife dealt with her metastatic breast cancer. Out of print, but available in libraries.

Richards, Eugene, and Dorothy Lynch. *Exploding into Life*. Aperture, 1986. A compelling and unsparing journal in photographs and words by a metastatic breast cancer patient and her partner. Out of print, but available in libraries.

Wilber, Ken. *Grace and Grit: Spirituality and Healing in the Life and Death of Treya Killam Wilber*. Boston: Shambala Publications, 1993. This book interweaves the physical and spiritual journeys of a woman with metastatic breast cancer, using her own journals and the words of her husband.

Helping children deal with a parent's cancer

Brack, Pat, with Ben Brack. *Moms Don't Get Sick*. Pierre, SD: Melius Publishing, 1990. (800) 882-5171.

Harpham, Wendy Schlessel. *Becky and the Worry Cup: A Children's Book About a Parent's Cancer*. HarperPerennial Library, 1997.

Harpham, Wendy Schlessel. *When a Parent Has Cancer: A Guide to Caring for Your Children*. HarperCollins Publishers, 1997.

Kohlenberg, Sherry. *Sammy's Mommy Has Cancer*. Magination Press, 1993. (800) 825-3089 or (212) 924-3344.

McCue, Kathleen. *How to Help Children Through a Parent's Serious Illness*. St. Martin's Press, 1994.

Parkinson, Carolyn Stearns. *My Mommy Has Cancer*. Solace Publications, 1991.

Helping children deal with a parent's death

Grollman, Earl. *Talking About Death: A Dialogue Between Parent and Child*. Boston: Beacon Press, 1990. An excellent book for helping children cope with grief. In comforting language, it teaches parents how to explain death, understand how children feel and know when to seek professional help.

Grollman, Earl. *Straight Talk About Death for Teenagers: How to Cope with Losing Someone You Love*. Boston: Beacon Press, 1993. Wonderful book that talks to teens, not at them. Discusses denial, pain, anger, sadness, physical symptoms, and depression, and offers techniques for working through feelings.

Jarratt, Claudia Jewett. *Helping Children Cope with Separation and Loss,* revised edition. Cambridge, MA: Harvard Common Press, 1994. Written by a child and family therapist, this book covers many kinds of loss, and describes simple techniques that adults can use to help children through grief.

Mellonie, Bryan, and Robert Ingpen. *Lifetimes: The Beautiful Way to Explain Death to Children.* New York: Bantam Books, 1983. Paintings and simple text explain that dying is as much a part of life as being born.

White, E. B. *Charlotte's Web.* New York: Harper, 1952. The classic tale of friendship and death as a part of life.

Listservs: Cancer mailing lists on the Internet

As of July 1998, there are eight Internet mailing lists that may be of interest to metastatic breast cancer patients and their families. Most of the quotes in this book came from people on the Breast cancer discussion list. To join, you only need to have a computer with a modem, a subscription to an Internet server, and an e-mail account. Access to the World Wide Web is not necessary. Instructions on how to subscribe are below, but if you do have WWW access, you can also use the "interact" option at Medinfo, listed below.

Medinfo.Org
http://www.medinfo.org/listserv.html

The MedInfo web site maintains the searchable archives of all the oncology listservs, and provides a convenient interface for subscribing, searching, browsing and other functions.

BMT-TALK
Subscription address: *bmt-talk-request@ai.mit.edu*
Address to post: *bmt-talk@ai.mit.edu*

A moderated mailing list for the discussion of bone marrow transplants. To subscribe, leave subject blank; in body of message, write only: subscribe BMT-TALK YourFirstName YourLastName.

BREAST-CANCER
Subscription address: *listserv@morgan.ucs.mun.ca*
Address to post: *breast-cancer@morgan.ucs.mun.ca*

The breast cancer discussion list. To subscribe, leave subject blank; in body of message, write only: subscribe BREAST-CANCER YourFirstName Your-LastName.

CANCER-L
Subscription address: *listserv@wvnvm.wvnet.edu*
Address to post: *cancer-l@wvnvm.wvnet.edu*

The general cancer support group. To subscribe, leave subject blank; in body of message, write only: subscribe CANCER-L YourFirstName YourLastName.

FACING-AHEAD
Subscription address: *listserv@maelstrom.stjohns.edu*
Address to post: *facing-ahead@maelstrom.stjohns.edu*

Helping to face the death of a loved one and its aftermath. To subscribe, leave subject blank; in body of message, write only: subscribe FACING-AHEAD YourFirstName YourLastName.

IBC
Subscription address: *ibc-request@bestiary.com*

Inflammatory breast cancer mailing list. To subscribe, leave subject blank; in body of message, write only: subscribe IBC YourFirstName YourLastName. Also see the Inflammatory Breast Cancer help page at: *http://www.bestiary.com/ibc/*.

LYMPHEDEMA
Subscription address: *listserv@acor.org*
Address to post: *lymphedema@acor.org*

The lymphedema e-support group. To subscribe, leave subject blank; in body of message, write only: subscribe LYMPHEDEMA YourFirstName Your-LastName.

MALEBC
Subscription address: *listserv@maelstrom.stjohns.edu*
Address to post: *malebc@maelstrom.stjohns.edu*

A male breast cancer discussion list. To subscribe, leave subject blank; in body of message, write only: subscribe MALEBC YourFirstName YourLast-Name.

Other online support groups

AOL Cancer Board

Go to The New Better & Medical Cancer Forum, then Glenna's Garden, and you arrive at dozens of Cancer Message Boards.

Compuserve Cancer Forum

At main menu: GO CANCER. Has Library, Message Boards, and a link to CancerNet.

Research

National Cancer Institute (NCI)
Building 31, Room 10A16, 9000 Rockville Pike, Bethesda, MD 20892
Hot line: (800) 4-CANCER or (800) 422-6237
Fax: (301) 231-6941
CancerNet on the World Wide Web: *http://www.nci.nih.gov/*

The National Cancer Institute is the most comprehensive and up-to-date source of clinical and research information for cancer patients and for health care professionals. Detailed and extensive patient treatment information, reviewed and updated monthly, is available by a number of methods from NCI. A clinical trials finder that lists all NCI-sponsored clinical trials offers contact and other information. NCI publishes a variety of related materials, from supportive care guidelines to clinical updates, available free. Following is more specific information about each of several services provided by NCI:

- Cancer Information Service: (800) 4-CANCER or (800) 422-6237

Callers are automatically connected to the office serving their region. Provides education and support. Performs PDQ (Physician Data Query) searches to provide up-to-date information on latest treatments, research and clinical trials. Offers free publications or the opportunity to speak directly with a cancer specialist, who is not a physician, but who is trained to provide accurate information on treatment and prevention of cancer and to make appropriate referrals. Informational materials are available on a huge variety of cancer-related topics.

- PDQ Search Service: (800) 345-3300

Access to Physicians Data Query database. PDQ, NCI's comprehensive cancer database, contains peer-reviewed statements on treatment, supportive care, screening, and prevention; a registry of clinical trials from around the world; and directories of physicians and organizations that provide cancer care.

- CANCERFAX: (301) 402-5874

Provides treatment guidelines, with current data on prognosis, staging, and histologic classifications. To use CANCERFAX, you need a fax machine with a telephone set to touch-tone dialing. You do not need to send anything. Pick up the receiver and enter the CANCERFAX number. A recording will come on to guide you. All documents are also available by mail.

- CancerNet: *http://wwwicic.nci.nih.gov/* or *http://pdqsearch@icicc.nci.nih.gov/*

Online access to the entire PDQ database system, including:

> Treatment information.
> Screening, prevention and genetics.
> Supportive care and advocacy issues.
> Clinical trial information.
> CANCERLIT topic searches.
> Cancer statistics.
> Journal of the National Cancer Institute.
> PDQ supportive care information.
> Managing side effects.

- CancerNet by e-mail: *cancernet@icicc.nci.nih.gov*

You don't need World Wide Web access to access CancerNet. You can send e-mail to the address above with a blank subject and the single word "help" in the message field to obtain the file of available e-mail resources.

Research and reference publications

Altman, Roberta and Michael J. Sarg, M.D. *The Cancer Dictionary.* New York: Facts on File, 1992. A valuable resource which combines cancer-related terms with simple definitions. Includes acronyms for chemotherapy protocols and some illustrations. Order from Facts on File; (800) 322-8755, or online at *http://www.factsonfile.com/*.

Baldwin, Fred D., and Suzanne McInerney. *INFOMEDICINE: A Consumer's Guide to Finding the Latest Medical Research.* Little, Brown and Company, 1996. A good layperson's guide to the benefits of researching and gathering medical information. Includes basic information on Medline searches, clinical trials, as well as a sound rationale on why information-seeking can be so important. Like any print resource, it is slightly outdated with regard to online resources.

The Bantam Medical Dictionary, revised. Bantam Books, 1990. An inexpensive paperback book that gives brief definitions of medical terms and concepts.

The Merck Manual of Diagnosis and Therapy, Sixteenth Edition. Merck & Co., Inc., 1992. The most widely used medical text in the world. While the *Manual* has grown from only 263 pages nearly 100 years ago to about 2,800 pages today, its primary purpose remains the same—to provide useful clinical information to practicing physicians, medical students, interns, residents, and other health care professionals. Gives overall, concise diagnostic and treatment information for all but the most obscure diseases. World Wide Web: *http://www.merck.com/!!quLzx2cATquOnv2W4I/pubs/mmanual/.*

Physicians' Desk Reference. Oradell, NJ: Medical Economics Data, 1997. Reference issued yearly lists authoritative information on all FDA approved drugs in technical language.

Rosenfelt, Isadore, M.D. *Second Opinion: Your Comprehensive Guide to Treatment Alternatives.* New York: Simon & Schuster, 1981. Basic information from a physician about the importance of second opinions.

Thomas, Clayton L., editor. *Taber's Cyclopedic Medical Dictionary,* seventeenth illustrated edition. F. A. Davis Company, 1993. A comprehensive resource with illustrations intended for "nurses and allied health professionals."

Research online

CancerGuide
http://cancerguide.org/index.html

Steve Dunn's cancer information page. One of the best resources on how to go about researching particular diagnoses, as well as a thoughtful collection of materials on pitfalls and benefits of seeking information, including "The Median Isn't the Message," an essay by evolutionary biologist and cancer patient Stephen Jay Gould. Steve Dunn calls it, "The wisest, most humane thing ever written about cancer and statistics."

CancerGuide: How to Research the Medical Literature
http://cancerguide.org/research.html

Steve Dunn has written the best online step-by-step thorough introduction to researching your own disease and treatments. A must-read.

CANCERLIT
http://www.healthgate.com/HealthGate/MEDLINE/search.shtml

A database in the MEDLARS group, CANCERLIT contains over a million citations, including some government reports, meeting abstracts, monographs and some foreign language journals not included in MEDLINE.

EMBASE
http://www.healthgate.com/HealthGate/price/embase.html

EMBASE is a giant database located in Holland. With more depth on drugs and the international pharmaceutical industry, it can be a source for information about drugs not yet approved in the United States. If you wish to access this database, you will be asked to pay a fee.

In Vitro Chemosensitivity Testing/Cell Culture Drug Resistance Testing (CCDRT)
http://www-med.stanford.edu/CBHP/Medical/Chemotherapy/
Chemosensitivity/TofC.html
http://www.oncolink.upenn.edu/specialty/chemo/general/chemosens_1.html

Note: This procedure is not yet widely accepted among oncologists.

From *Cell Culture Drug Resistance Testing (CCDRT)* by Larry M. Weisenthal, M.D., Ph.D.: "Cell culture drug resistance testing (CCDRT) refers to testing a patient's own cancer cells in the laboratory to drugs that may be used to treat the patient's cancer. The idea is to identify which drugs are more likely to work and which drugs are less likely to work. By avoiding the latter and choosing from among the former, the patient's probability of benefiting from the chemotherapy may be improved."

Weisenthal's extensive material on this controversial test can be found at the above URL. You may also send e-mail to Larry Weisenthal at *72203.2235@compuserve.com*, or phone: (714) 894-0011; Fax: (714) 893-3658.

Another source is Rational Therapeutics Cancer Laboratories, where the test is called the Ex Vivo Apoptotic Assay (EVA). Web site: *http://www.rational-t.com/*. Send e-mail to *RationalT@aol.com*. Phone: (562) 989-8128; Fax: (562) 989-8160.

Medical News and Alerts Doctor's Guide to the Internet (P\S\L Consulting Group Inc.)
http://www.pslgroup.com/breastcancer.htm#News

A list of press releases on new findings, treatments and drugs related to breast cancer.

MEDLINE
http://www.ncbi.nlm.nih.gov/PubMed/

MEDLINE is the single most important resource for researching the published medical literature. It contains nearly nine million medical journal citations and abstracts in every field of medicine from thousands of journals, back to 1966. It is the online version of the *Index Medicus*, indexed by medical subject headings (MeSH) to enable effective searches. MEDLINE is now available free, from the NIH at PubMed.

NCCS Guide to Cancer Resources: Cansearch
http://www.access.digex.net/~mkragen/index.html

Marshall Kragen, the Internet Liaison for the National Coalition for Cancer Survivorship, walks you through the process. Look in the "Basic Research" section. Also gathers links to clinical trials, mailing lists and other support online.

The Online Medical Dictionary
http://www.graylab.ac.uk/omd/index.html

CancerWEB's comprehensive online dictionary gives convenient definitions and derivations for medical terms and concepts.

PDQ Physician Statement on Breast Cancer
http://imsdd.meb.uni-bonn.de/cancernet/100013.html
http://www.oncolink.upenn.edu/pdq_html/1/engl/100013.html

Although the NCI Statements can be obtained directly from the NCI, this excellent version hyperlinks references in the text to the article abstracts, a major convenience. It is also available in Spanish at: *http://www.oncolink.upenn.edu/pdq_html/1/span/100013.html.*

Drug information online

Clinical Pharmacology Online
http://www.cponline.gsm.com/

A good source for comprehensive pharmacology monographs.

PharmInfo DrugDB
http://pharminfo.com/drugdb/db_mnu.html

This database provides access to the drug information resources on PharmInfoNet and elsewhere on the Internet. The database, listed by generic or trade name, has links to published articles on listed drugs.

RxMed
http://www.rxmed.com/prescribe.html

RxMed is a web site for family physicians that has an excellent "prescribing information" section, which includes most of the materials found in the *1996* [or later edition] *Physicians' Desk Reference,* published by Medical Economics Data.

University of Maryland at College Park Libraries, Drug and Toxicology Information
http://www.lib.umd.edu/UMCP/MCK/GUIDES/drug.html

A comprehensive review of existing sources for drug information.

Clinical trials information online

What Are Clinical Trials All About?
http://cancernet.nci.nih.gov/clinical_trials/trialintro.html

NCI Pamphlet #90-2706. This booklet is designed for patients who are considering taking part in research for new cancer treatments. It explains clinical trials to patients in easy-to-understand terms and gives them information that will help them decide about participating. Available in print by calling (800) 4-CANCER. 24 pages.

CenterWatch Clinical Trials Listing Service
http://www.centerwatch.com/

An international listing of clinical research trials. Here you'll also find profiles of centers conducting clinical research and listings of newly approved drug therapies.

NABCO's "Participate in Clinical Trials" Web page
http://www.nabco.org/trials/

In an effort to increase awareness of clinical trials, NABCO is collaborating with the National Cancer Institute in offering a new web page for breast cancer clinical trials listing. Includes: "Joining a Clinical Trial," "Clinical Trial Basics" and "Breast Cancer Trial Directory."

NCCS Guide to Cancer Resources: Cansearch
http://www.access.digex.net/~mkragen/index.html

This is a general orientation to clinical trials, with links to helpful sites.

NCI Patient Clinical Trials
http://wwwicic.nci.nih.gov/trials/p_clinic.htm

NCI Selected High Priority Breast Cancer Treatment and Prevention Trials
http://wwwicic.nci.nih.gov/proto/breast.html

Oncolink Clinical Trials Information
http://oncolink.upenn.edu/clinical_trials/

A web page devoted to links that provide information on clinical trials.

PDQ Clinical Trial Search Form for Patients
http://wwwicic.nci.nih.gov/prot/patsrch.shtml

Bone marrow transplantation/high-dose chemotherapy information online and in print

Blood and Marrow Transplant Newsletter
http://www.oncolink.upenn.edu/specialty/chemo/bmt/newsletter/

Edited by the List owner of the BMT-Talk listserv on the Internet, the *Blood and Marrow Transplant Newsletter* (formerly *BMT Newsletter*) has reviewed the major issues surrounding allogenic and autologous high-dose chemotherapy with stem cell or bone marrow transplant for all types of cancer. Issues from 1992 to the present are available online. You can also get free print copies from the *Blood and Marrow Transplant Newsletter*, 1985 Spruce Avenue, Highland Park, IL 60035; (708) 831-1913, Fax: (708) 836-1943.

ECRI Patient Reference Guide: *High-Dose Chemotherapy with BMT for Metastatic Breast Cancer*
http://www.hslc.org/emb/bctoc.html

This meta-analysis of clinical studies of HDC reviews all the available scientific and medical literature as of 1995. A must-read for anyone considering HDC. ECRI, 5200 Butler Pike, Plymouth Meeting, PA 19462-1298; (610) 825-6000.

Bone Marrow Transplants: A Book of Basics for Patients
http://www.oncolink.upenn.edu/specialty/chemo/bmt/contents.html

Written by Susan K. Stewart, this is an excellent handbook for patients about what to expect from this treatment, covering medical, emotional and insurance issues. Technically accurate, yet easy to read. For a print copy, write or call the *Blood and Marrow Transplant Newsletter*, 1985 Spruce Avenue, Highland Park, IL 60035; (708) 831-1913, Fax: (708) 836-1943.

Alternative and complementary treatment

The National Institutes of Health Office of Alternative Medicine
OAM Clearinghouse
P.O. Box 8218, Silver Spring, Maryland 20907-8218
Toll Free: (888) 644-6226; Fax: 301-495-4957
http://altmed.od.nih.gov/

The National Institutes of Health (NIH) Office of Alternative Medicine (OAM) identifies and evaluates unconventional health care practices. The OAM supports and conducts research and research training on these practices and disseminates information.

Stress Reduction Clinic
University of Massachusetts Medical Center
Worcester, MA 01655
(508) 856-2656, Fax: (508) 856-1977

Offers an eight-week non-residential meditation-based program for medical patients. Also featured in Moyers' series, above. Director Jon Kabat-Zinn describes the program as "an eight-week-long course designed to teach people with a wide range of chronic medical diagnoses and varying degrees of chronic stress, pain, and illness how to take care of themselves as a complement to the care and treatment they are receiving through more traditional routes. The core of the program is a relatively intensive training in mindfulness meditation and its application in daily living to coping with stress and pain." This program has been widely taught to health care professionals around the country, and is offered in other settings.

Alternative and complementary treatment reading

Audiotapes: Miller, Emmett, M.D., and Steven Halpern, Ph.D. P.O. Box W, Stanford, CA 94309; (800) 52-TAPES. One example: *An Answer to Cancer, Side 1: The Healing Image; Side 2: Targeting your Treatment.* These beautifully made audiotapes offer soothing music with meditation, visualization, self-healing and pain control. Call or write for a list of offerings.

Boik, John. *Cancer and Natural Medicine: A Textbook of Basic Science and Clinical Research.* Oregon Medical Press, 1996. A thorough review of the published scientific evidence for a wide range of therapies, including herbs, vitamins and minerals, dietary factors, electrotherapy, psychological approaches, and a grab bag of other interesting substances. From the author: "Since the clinical efficacies of the natural therapies discussed in the book are still largely unknown, this book is not written as a treatment guide. Rather, it presents the current state of research, and points to promising therapies and research needs."

Cousins, Norman. *Head First: The Biology of Hope and the Healing Power of the Human Spirit.* New York: E. P. Dutton, 1989. Reviews some of the evidence on the influence of attitudes and beliefs on illness, and has excellent material on the doctor-patient relationship.

Goleman, Daniel and J. Gurin, editors. *Mind/Body Medicine: How to Use Your Mind for Better Health*. Yonkers, NY: Consumer Reports Books, 1993. This collection of articles by top health professionals looks at the relationship between mind and body, and how it can be influenced. Describes mind-body techniques such as hypnosis, meditation, imagery, support groups and psychotherapy, with a good list of resources.

Holland, Jimmie C., and S. Lewis. "Emotions and Cancer: What Do We Really Know?" in *Mind Body Medicine: How to Use Your Mind for Better Health*. Daniel Goleman and Joel Gurin, editors. Yonkers, NY: Consumer Reports Books, 1993. This review of a controversial topic looks past popular approaches to take a thoughtful look at what the research has actually shown.

"Information Packages" on selected unconventional therapies. Published by the Canadian Breast Cancer Research Initiative. Available from the Canadian Cancer Society/National Cancer Institute of Canada by calling the Cancer Information Service (in Canada) at (888) 939-3333; or outside Canada at (416) 961-7223 x372; Fax: (416) 961-4189.

Kabat-Zinn, Jon. *Full Catastrophe Living: Using the Wisdom of Your Body and Mind to Face Stress, Pain, and Illness*. New York: Delacorte Press, 1990. From the pioneering work done in the Stress Reduction Clinic of the University of Massachusetts Medical Center, this innovative and comprehensive book is about using mindfulness, meditation and yoga to cope with pain and illness. These easy-to-learn techniques have been taught to many thousands of medical patients, referred by their physicians. Also, try the companion set of *Stress Reduction Tapes*, available from P.O. Box 547, Lexington, MA 02173. These are simple, easy-to-do yoga, relaxation and meditation tapes that are used in the clinic.

Lerner, Michael. *Choices in Healing: Integrating the Best of Conventional and Complementary Approaches to Cancer*. Cambridge, MA: MIT Press, 1994. Lerner, Director of Commonweal, a California retreat center for cancer patients, gives a lucid, unbiased, thorough and thoughtful presentation of this complex and confusing topic. The entire book is now available online in searchable format at the Commonweal web site: *http://www.commonweal-health.org/choicescontents.html*.

Moss, Ralph, Ph.D. *Cancer Therapy: The Independent Consumer's Guide to Non-Toxic Treatment and Prevention*. Equinox Press, 1992. A widely respected review of 100 nontoxic or relatively nontoxic treatment options. Of particular interest is his review of the evidence that some of these substances can enhance conventional therapy or reduce its side effects. Moss's web site is at: *http://www.ralphmoss.com/*.

Ontario Breast Cancer Information Exchange Project. *A Guide to Unconventional Cancer Therapies.* 1994. To order, write, call or fax R & R Bookbar, 14800 Yonge Street, Unit 106, Aurora, Ontario, Canada L4G 1N3; (905) 727-3300; Fax: (905) 727-2620. This book is also online at: *http:// aorta.library.mun.ca/bc/uct/accept.htm.*

Walters, Richard. *Options: The Alternative Cancer Therapy Book.* Garden City Park, NY: Avery Publishing Group Inc., 1993. Less thorough-going and research-based than the above listed guides by John Boik and Ralph Moss, but according to Steve Dunn of CancerGuide: "It includes extensive references to both the popular and alternative therapy literature, with some references to the scientific literature. In my opinion, this book sometimes puts too much credence in marginal therapies for which evidence is lacking, but it is still useful."

Alternative and complementary treatment information online

Quackwatch: Your Guide to Health Fraud, Quackery, and Intelligent Decision-making
http://www.quackwatch.com/

Quackwatch, Inc., is a nonprofit corporation whose purpose is to combat health-related frauds, myths, fads, and fallacies. Dr. Stephen Barrett, a retired psychiatrist, is on the board of the National Council Against Health Fraud, and is a scientific advisor to the American Council on Science and Health. He has written a number of books exposing and debunking fraudulent health scams. His ambitious goals include investigating questionable claims, distributing reliable publications, reporting illegal marketing, and improving the quality of health information on the Internet. Of particular interest is "A Special Message for Cancer Patients Seeking 'Alternative' Treatments."

The WellnessWeb
http://wellweb.com/altern/index.htm

WellnessWeb is a collaboration of patients, health care professionals, and other caregivers, to help people find the best and most appropriate medical information and support available. Information about clinical trials, community health, drug dosages and compliance, treatment options and research, how to select a health care provider, reports on dozens of illnesses and conditions, tips about healthy lifestyles, complementary treatment alternatives and options, and many more topics.

Coping with treatment, pain and discomfort

American Hair Loss Council
(800) 274-8717
http://www.ahlc.org/

The American Hair Loss Council (AHLC) is a non-profit organization designed to provide the public with non-biased information on treatments and options for men, women and children experiencing hair loss. The Web site has extensive links.

American Pain Society (APS)
4700 West Lake Avenue, Glenview, IL 60025
(847) 375-4715; Fax: (847) 375-4777
e-mail: *info@ampainsoc.org*
http://www.ampainsoc.org/

APS is a multidisciplinary educational and scientific organization dedicated to serving people in pain. They offer help and resources to patients and professionals.

Cancer Care
1180 Avenue of the Americas, New York, NY 10036
(212) 221-3300
Free counseling hot line: (800) 813-HOPE or (800) 813-4673
http://www.cancercareinc.org/

A social service agency dedicated to helping patients and families cope with the emotional impact of cancer. Provides services in the New York area, and referrals elsewhere. Ask for Cancer Care's Pain Resource Center. Educational teleconferences in Real Audio format are available for listening at: *http://www.cancercareinc.org/audio/teleconferences.htm*.

Chemocare
Hot line: (800) 55-CHEMO or (908) 233-1103 in New Jersey

Chemocare is a non-profit, voluntary program whose chief goal is to encourage people undergoing treatment for cancer to continue despite adverse side effects. Support is given by people who have survived a similar experience and have resumed living normal lives.

Encore
YWCA of the USA, Office of the Women's Health Initiative
624 9th Street, 3rd Floor, Washington, DC 20001-5394
(202) 628-3636

Encore is a program of peer support and exercise for women who have had breast cancer surgery. Operated through local YWCA member associates.

Look Good...Feel Better
(800) 395-LOOK or (800) ACS-2345
http://nysernet.org/bcic/numbers/look-good.html

A collaboration of the American Cancer Society, the Cosmetic, Toiletry and Fragrance Association, and the National Cosmetology Association, the "Look Good...Feel Better" program is a community-based, free national service which teaches female cancer patients beauty techniques to help enhance their appearance and self-image during chemotherapy and radiation treatments.

National Lymphedema Network
2211 Post Street, Suite 404, San Francisco, CA 94115
Toll-free support hot line: (800) 541-3259
http://www.wenet.net/users/lymphnet/

Provides patients and professionals with information about prevention and treatment of this complication of lymph node surgery. Offers guidelines and referrals for medical treatment, physical therapy, and support. Publishes a quarterly newsletter and sponsors national conferences. They will send out an information packet.

Coping with treatment: Reading and video

Bruning, Nancy. *Coping with Chemotherapy.* Ballantine Books, 1993. Paperback. Very good book on all aspects of coping with treatment, both practical and emotional, from a breast cancer survivor.

Dodd, Marylin J., R.N., Ph.D. *Chemotherapy and Radiation Therapy for Patients and their Families*, third edition. UCSF Nursing Press, 1996. Offers detailed coping strategies and information. May be available online from Sapient Health Network at: *http://www.shn.net/.*

Holland, Jimmie C., and Julia H. Rowland, editors. *Handbook of Psychooncology: Psychological Care of the Patient with Cancer.* Oxford University Press, 1989. Written for professionals working with cancer patients, this anthology of scholarly articles concerns all aspects of emotional and psychological care for persons coping with cancer. Particularly useful for its review of the literature of psychooncology, an emerging discipline.

Home Care Guide for Cancer: How to Care for Family and Friends at Home. Published by the American College of Physicians. Softcover, 276 pages. To purchase, contact the ACP Customer Service at (800) 523-1546, extension 2600, or (215) 351-2600. View a sample article on fatigue at the Cancer Care web site at: *http://www.cancercareinc.org/campaigns/fatigue1.htm.*

Lang, Susan S., and Richard B. Patt, M.D. *You Don't Have to Suffer: A Complete Guide to Relieving Cancer Pain for Patients and Their Families.* Oxford University Press, 1994. This easy-to-read handbook looks at the needless pain that results from undertreatment and from unfounded fears of addiction, and offers helpful information about specific pain medications, side effects, and emotional concerns.

McKay, Judith, R.N., Nancee Hirano, R.N., and Miles Lampenfeld. *The Chemotherapy and Radiation Therapy Survival Guide, second edition.* Oakland, CA: New Harbinger Publications, 1998. A basic guide to understanding and coping with treatment.

Morra, Marion, and Eve Potts. *Choices,* third edition. Avon Books, 1994. A classic in the field, this well-thought-out basic compendium of treatment and resources, written in a clearly understandable format, is for all cancer patients. Sections on basic understanding of cancer and its treatments are particularly useful.

Questions and Answers About Pain Control: A Guide for People with Cancer and Their Families. American Cancer Society #4518-PS, 1992. ACS, (800) ACS-2345; NCI, (800) 4-CANCER. A good basic introduction on pain and pain control. Available online at: *http://cancernet.nci.nih.gov/pain_control/paincont.html.*

Videotape: *The Beauty of Control.* Created by Laurie Feldman, a member of the breast cancer discussion list until her death in 1996. Narrated by Jill Eikenberry. This 17-minute videotape helps patients emotionally during treatment through advice on improving physical appearance with cosmetics and other aids. Medical Video Productions, 450 North New Ballas Road, Suite 266, St. Louis, MO 63141. (800) 822-3100 or (314) 991-5510.

Coping with treatment information online

Chemotherapy and You: A Guide To Self-Help During Treatment
http://cancernet.nci.nih.gov/chemotherapy/chemoint.html

NCI publication #94-1136, 1993. Gives basic principles for handling side effects of treatment, in an easy-to-follow format. Available in print by calling (800) 4-CANCER.

Managing Cancer Pain
http://www.ahcpr.gov/clinic/

These extensive guidelines, written for physicians, can be accessed from the web page by following the link "Clinical Practice Guidelines Online" and clicking on the documents for managing cancer pain. Published by the U.S. Government's Agency for Health Care Policy and Research, 1994, a free print version can be ordered from AHCPR Publications Clearinghouse, P.O. Box 8547, Silver Spring, MD 20907-8547; (800) 358-9295.

National Cancer Institute PDQ Physician Statement: Pain
http://www.oncolink.upenn.edu/pdq_html/3/engl/304470.html

Intended for physicians, this Quick Reference Guide focuses on pharmacologic, physical and psychosocial ways to manage cancer pain, and is adapted from the more extensive "Clinical Practice Guidelines" (see the previous resource, *Managing Cancer Pain*).

Pharmacologic Treatment of Cancer Pain: A Nursing Continuing Education Program
http://www.powerpak.com/CE/CancerPain/lesson.htm

A good, medically oriented online tutorial on pain management by Bridget Bernstein, Pharm.D.

Radiation Therapy and You: A Guide to Self-Help During Treatment
http://wwwicic.nci.nih.gov/Radiation/radintro.html

NCI publication #94-2227, 1993. A basic introduction to the topic of radiation treatment, how and why it is done, and coping with the side effects. Print version available from NCI, (800) 4-CANCER.

Roxane Pain Institute
http://pain.roxane.com/index.html

Talarian Index
http://www.stat.washington.edu/TALARIA/index.html

Dying and hospice care

Choice in Dying, Inc.
200 Varick Street, New York, NY 10014
(212) 366-5540
http://www.choices.org/

Dedicated to fostering communication about complex end-of-life decisions. The nonprofit organization provides advance directives, counsels patients and families, trains professionals, advocates for imporoved laws, and offers a range of publications and services. Free information and forms on living wills, advance directives and health care proxies, as applicable in each state.

Foundation for Hospice and Home Care
519 C Street N.E., Washington, DC 20002
(202) 547-7424

Information and referrals.

HOSPICELINK
Hospice Education Institute Suite 3-B, P.O. Box 7135
Essex Square, Essex, CT 06426-0713
(800) 331-1620, (203) 767-1620 in Alaska and Connecticut

HOSPICELINK maintains a computerized and continually updated direc-tory of hospice programs in the United States, and operates a toll-free tele-phone number to refer callers to local hospice and palliative care programs. HOSPICELINK also provides general information about the principles and practice of hospice care. Staff members will listen sympathetically and give limited, informal support to callers who wish to discuss immediate personal problems relating to terminal illness and bereavement. (HOSPICELINK does not offer medical advice or provide psychological counseling.) There is no charge for any HOSPICELINK service.

National Hospice Organization
1901 North Moore Street, Suite 901, Arlington, VA 22209
(800) 658-8898
http://nho.org/

Information, free publications and referrals regarding hospice care.

Grief Recovery Institute
8306 Wilshire Blvd., #21A, Beverly Hills, CA 90211
(800) 334-7606, (213) 650-1234

Organization that sponsors workshops, supports people who are grieving, and provides publications on recovery.

Grief Recovery Helpline
(800) 445-4808

Free service staffed by trained personnel to help anyone who is grieving.

Dying and hospice care reading

Buckingham, Robert W. *The Handbook of Hospice Care.* Prometheus Books, 1996. An introduction and explanation of hospice, and how it can help.

Caring for the Patient with Cancer at Home: A Guide for Patients and Families. A guidebook that provides detailed, helpful information on how to care for the patient at home. American Cancer Society; (800) ACS-2345.

Harwell, Amy. *Ready to Live, Prepared to Die: A Provocative Guide to the Rest of Your Life.* Harold Shaw, 1995. Written from a Christian perspective by a cancer patient, this well-organized book deals with such practicalities as health-care directives, legal documents, and funeral arrangements, as well as the emotional realities of saying good-bye.

Home Care Guide for Advanced Cancer. Published by the American College of Physicians. "For family, friends, and hospice workers caring for persons with advanced cancer at home, when quality of life is the primary goal." Contact the ACP Customer Service at (800) 523-1546, extension 2600, or write to: American College of Physicians, Customer Service Center, Independence Mall West, Sixth Street and Race, Philadelphia, PA 19106-1572. Available free online at the ACP web site: *http://www.acponline.org/public/homecare/index.html.*

Kubler-Ross, Elisabeth, M.D. *On Death and Dying.* New York: Macmillan, 1969. A classic in this field. Kubler-Ross discusses attitudes toward death, emotional stages of dying (anger, bargaining, depression, acceptance, hope), family reactions and therapy.

Levine, Stephen. *Who Dies?* Garden City: Anchor Press, 1982. Also, *Meetings at the Edge: Dialogues with the Grieving and Dying,* Garden City: Anchor Press, 1984; and *Healing into Life and Death,* Garden City: Doubleday, 1987. A meditation teacher and counselor of the terminally ill, Levine's focus is on learning to live fully in the moment. Excellent resources on the process and practice of mindfulness meditation, these inspirational books also include sections on relaxation and guided imagery.

Nuland, Sherwin B., M.D. *How We Die: Reflections on Life's Final Chapter.* New York: Alfred A. Knopf, 1994. A Yale professor demystifies the dying process in this beautifully written, insightful book on the way different diseases lead to death. Touches on end-of-life decision-making and other issues connected with preserving the human side of dying.

Rando, Therese, Ph.D. *Grieving: How to Go On Living When Someone You Love Dies.* Lexington, MA: Lexington Books, 1988. Written by a grief counselor, this is a comprehensive and compassionate book.

Ray, M. Catherine. *I'm With You Now: A Guide Through Incurable Illness for Patients, Families, and Friends.* Bantam Books, 1997. An experienced hospice worker gives useful guidelines for end-of-life care and for facing difficult discussions and topics.

Helping children deal with a parent's death

Grollman, Earl. *Talking About Death: A Dialogue Between Parent and Child.* Boston: Beacon Press, 1990. An excellent book for helping children cope with grief. In comforting language, it teaches parents how to explain death, understand how children feel and know when to seek professional help.

Grollman, Earl. *Straight Talk About Death for Teenagers: How to Cope with Losing Someone You Love.* Boston: Beacon Press, 1993. Wonderful book that talks to teens, not at them. Discusses denial, pain, anger, sadness, physical symptoms, and depression, and offers techniques for working through feelings.

Jarratt, Claudia Jewett. *Helping Children Cope with Separation and Loss,* revised edition. Cambridge, MA: Harvard Common Press, 1994. Written by a child and family therapist, this book covers many kinds of loss, and describes simple techniques that adults can use to help children through grief.

Mellonie, Bryan, and Robert Ingpen. *Lifetimes: The Beautiful Way to Explain Death to Children.* New York: Bantam Books, 1983. Paintings and simple text explain that dying is as much a part of life as being born.

White, E. B. *Charlotte's Web.* New York: Harper, 1952. The classic tale of friendship and death as a part of life.

Dying and hospice care online

Hospice Hands
http://hospice-cares.com/hlinks.html

Online links.

Hospice Web
http://www.teleport.com/~hospice/links.htm

Online links.

FACING-AHEAD
Subscription address: *listserv@maelstrom.stjohns.edu*
Address to post: *facing-ahead@maelstrom.stjohns.edu*

Helping to face the death of a loved one and its aftermath. To subscribe, leave subject blank; in body of message, write only: subscribe FACING-AHEAD YourFirstName YourLastName.

GriefNet
http://www.rivendell.org/

A collection of resources of value to those who are experiencing loss and grief.

Breast cancer advocacy

Breast Cancer Fund
282 Second Street, 3rd Floor, San Francisco, CA 94105
(800) 487-0492 or (415) 543-2979; Fax: (415) 543-2975
http://www.letlive.com/text/bcfund.htm

Cancer Prevention Coalition
520 North Michigan Avenue, Suite 410, Chicago, IL 60611
(312) 467-0600

National Action Plan on Breast Cancer
http://www.napbc.org/napbc/index.htm

The NAPBC, a public/private partnership of many member organizations in government and the private section, is coordinated by the Public Health Service's Office on Women's Health, Department of Health and Human Services. The mission of the NAPBC is to speed progress toward eradicating breast cancer. Has good links to a variety of organizations and background information.

The National Breast Cancer Coalition
1707 L Street, N.W., Suite 1060, Washington, DC 20036
(202) 296-7477; Fax: (202) 265-6854
World Wide Web: *http://www.natlbcc.org/*

The National Breast Cancer Coalition is a grassroots effort in the fight against breast cancer, composed of a network of activists across the country—350 organizations and 41,000 individuals in 1997. In five years, NBCC has increased U.S. federal government funding for breast cancer research nearly sixfold—from $90 million to more than $500 million. Its goals are: research—increasing appropriations for high quality, peer-reviewed research and working within the scientific community to focus research on prevention and finding a cure; access—increasing access for all women to high quality treatment and care and to breast cancer clinical trials; influence—increasing the influence of women living with breast cancer and other breast cancer activists in the decision-making that impacts all issues surrounding breast cancer.

Project LEAD is a science program for breast cancer advocates developed by NBCC. The goal is to empower activists to fully participate everywhere that breast cancer research decisions are being made. After an intensive four-day science course, graduates go on to utilize their newly acquired skills by serving on influential research boards and committees.

In 1992, the National Breast Cancer Coalition created a memorial exhibit called "The Face of Breast Cancer," a photographic essay to humanize the overwhelming statistics of breast cancer. Photographs of 84 women, with sentiments contributed by their family members and friends, make real the personal stories behind the staggering statistics of breast cancer.

Women's Environment and Development Organization (WEDO)
355 Lexington Avenue, 3rd Floor, New York, NY 10017
(212) 973-0325
e-mail: *wedo@igc.apc.org*
World Wide Web: *http://www.wedo.org*

Co-sponsor of the 1997 World Breast Cancer Conference in Kingston, Ontario, this organization has a focus on prevention of breast cancer through education and action. Ask for their "Action for Prevention: Breast Cancer and the Environment" program.

Local advocacy organizations

There are local breast cancer advocacy organizations in almost every state and in many major cities in the U.S. and Canada. Contact the National Breast Cancer Coalition (NBCC) listed above for one in your area. Many publish informative newsletters, offer informational programs to members and the public, and lobby to influence local and national legislation. Following are two examples among many—one American and one Canadian:

Breast Cancer Action
55 New Montgomery, Suite 624, San Francisco, CA 94105
(415) 243-9301; Fax: (415) 243-3996
http://www-med.stanford.edu/bca/index.html

Breast Cancer Action, Ottawa
Billings Bridge Plaza, P.O. Box 39041
Ottawa, ON Canada K1H 1A1
(613) 736-5921, Fax: (613) 736 8422
e-mail: *bcanet@magi.com*
http://infoweb.magi.com/~bcanet/

Advocacy reading and videotape

Altman, Roberta. *Waking Up/Fighting Back: The Politics of Breast Cancer.* New York: Little, Brown & Company, 1996. A detailed, thorough and accessible examination of the important issues related to breast cancer causation, diagnosis and treatment, examined historically from the social perspective of the women's health movement.

Batt, Sharon. *Patient No More: The Politics of Breast Cancer.* Gynergy Books/Ragweed Press, 1994. This outspoken book exposes the "fear and cheer" filter, as the author terms the unrealistically optimistic assessments of various treatments on the part of the medical community, insurance companies, pharmaceutical companies, government researchers and regulators, the media and various purveyors of popular culture, as well as cancer charities.

"Breast Cancer Bulletin: News from the Canadian Breast Cancer Research Initiative." Canadian Cancer Society and the National Cancer Institute of Canada, 19 Alcorn Avenue, Suite 200, Toronto, Ontario M4V 3B1. This free newsletter contains information about research on breast cancer and the environment.

Carson, Rachel. *Silent Spring.* New York: Houghton-Mifflin, 1962. The book that inspired the environmental movement. Two years after its publication, Carson died of breast cancer.

Stabiner, Karen. *To Dance with the Devil: The New War on Breast Cancer.* New York: Delacorte Press, 1997. A journalist's intriguing view of one year in the breast cancer advocacy movement and the current state of breast cancer treatment and research, told through the filter of a detailed portrait of Dr. Susan Love and a number of her patients at the UCLA Breast Center.

Steingraber, Sandra. *Living Downstream: An Ecologist Looks at Cancer and the Environment.* New York: Addison Wesley, 1997. An eye-opening review of the research to date on environmental links to cancer, from a biologist and cancer survivor. Consider this book a very readable jumping-off place for further investigation of the role that environmental pollution of all kinds may play as a cause of breast and other cancers.

Videotape: *Exposure: Environmental Links to Breast Cancer.* Women's Network on Health & Environment, 736 Bathurst Street, Toronto, ON Canada M5S 2R4; (416) 516-2600. This hour-long video raises awareness about the role that pesticides, chlorine, plastics, radiation, electromagnetic fields and air quality may play in causing breast cancer.

Common Drugs in Use with Metastatic Breast Cancer

ALKYLATING AGENTS (AND RELATED COMPOUNDS)

Generic Name	Brand Name	Manufacturer
Busulfan	Myleran®	Glaxo Wellcome
Carboplatin	Paraplatin®	Bristol-Myers Squibb Oncology Division
Carmustine, (BCNU)	BiCNU®, Gliadel®	Bristol-Myers Squibb Oncology Division
Chlorambucil	Leukeran®	Glaxo Wellcome
Cisplatin	Platinol®	Bristol-Myers Squibb Oncology Division
Cyclophosphamide	Cytoxan®	Bristol-Myers Squibb Oncology Division
Ifosfamide	Ifex®	Bristol-Myers Squibb Oncology Division
Melphalan, (L-PAM)	Alkeran®	Glaxo Wellcome
Thiotepa	Thioplex®	Immunex Corporation

TAXANES

Generic Name	Brand Name	Manufacturer
Docetaxel	Taxotere®	Rhône-Poulenc Rorer
Paclitaxel	Taxol®	Bristol-Myers Squibb Oncology Division

ANTHRACYCLINES (AND RELATED COMPOUNDS)

Generic Name	Brand Name	Manufacturer
Doxorubicin, (DOX)	Adriamycin® Doxil® Doxorubicin HCl Rubex®	Pharmacia & Upjohn Sequus Pharmaceuticals Ben Venue Bristol-Myers Squibb Oncology Division
Etoposide, (VP-16)	Etopophos® Toposar® VePesid®	Immunex Pharmacia & Upjohn Bristol-Myers Squibb Oncology Division
Idarubicin	Idamycin®	Pharmacia & Upjohn
Liposomal Doxorubicin	Doxil®	Sequus Pharmaceuticals

VINCA ALKALOIDS

Generic Name	Brand Name	Manufacturer
Vinblastine, (VBL)	Velban® Vinblastine	Eli Lilly and Company Schein
Vincristine	Oncovin®	Eli Lilly and Company
Vinorelbine, (VNB)	Navelbine®	Glaxo Wellcome

ANTIMETABOLITES

Generic Name	Brand Name	Manufacturer
Capecitabine	Xeloda®	Hoffmann-La Roche
Fluorouracil, (5-FU)	Adrucil® Efudex® Fluoroplex® Fluorouracil IV	Adria Roche Laboratories Allergan Inc. Solopak
Methotrexate	Methotrexate Methotrexate	Lederle Laboratories Mylan
Mitoxantrone	Novantrone	Immunex

HORMONAL DRUGS

Generic Name	Brand Name	Manufacturer
Anastrozole (a nonsteroidal aromatase inhibitor)	Arimidex®	Zeneca Pharmaceuticals
Goserelin, (FZ)	Zoladex®	Zeneca Pharmaceuticals
Letrozole	Femara®	Novartis

HORMONAL DRUGS (continued)

Generic Name	Brand Name	Manufacturer
Megestrol	Megestrol Acetate Megace®	Par Bristol-Myers Squibb Oncology Division
Tamoxifen	Nolvadex®	Zeneca Pharmaceuticals
Toremifene	Fareston®	Orion/Schering

DRUGS TO DEAL WITH CHEMOTHERAPY SIDE EFFECTS and QUALITY OF LIFE ISSUES (Does not include pain medications)

Generic Name	Brand Name	Manufacturer	Use
Clodronate	Bonefos®	Rhône-Poulenc Rorer	Bone metabolism regulator, antihyper-calcemic agent.
Dexamethasone (closely related to Prednisone)	Decadron		A commonly pre-scribed oral corticos-teroid, sometimes used with chemother-apy for anti-inflamma-tory and antiemetic properties.
Dexrazoxane	Zinecard®	Pharmacia & Upjohn	Reduces the cardiac side effects of doxo-rubicin.
Dolasetron	Anzamet®	Hoechst Marion Roussel	5HT3 antagonist for prevention of chemo-therapy-induced nau-sea and vomiting.
Erythropoietin	Epogen® Procrit®	Amgen Ortho Biotech	Stimulates red cell production.
Filgrastim, G-CSF	Neupogen®	Amgen	Granulocyte colony-stimulating factor, used in chemother-apy-related febrile neutropenia.
Granisetron	Kytril®	SmithKline Beecham Pharmaceuticals	One of the newer, highly effective anti-emetics that helps nausea and vomiting.
Leucovorin	Wellcovorin® Leucovorin® Leucovorin IM/IV®	Glaxo Wellcome Barr Labs Lederle	Offsets the hemato-logic toxicity of folic acid antagonists like methotrexate.

DRUGS TO DEAL WITH CHEMOTHERAPY SIDE EFFECTS and QUALITY OF LIFE
ISSUES (Does not include pain medications) (continued)

Generic Name	Brand Name	Manufacturer	Use
Ondansetron	Zofran®	Cerenex Pharmaceuticals	Another of the newer, highly effective anti-emetics that helps nausea and vomiting.
Pamidronate	Aredia®	CibaGeneva Pharmaceuticals	Decreases the extent of accelerated bone resorption with osteolytic bone metastases, decreasing fractures and hypercalcemia.
Prednisone (closely related to Dexamethasone)	Deltasone® Orasone® Prednisone	Pharmacia & Upjohn	A commonly prescribed oral corticosteroid, sometimes used with chemotherapy for anti-inflammatory and antiemetic properties.

Financial assistance

Many pharmaceutical companies have patient assistance programs to aid patients who cannot afford the cost of the drugs their physicians prescribe for them. The following table lists the names of some of these companies and the numbers you can call to ask for an application. Your physician will need to send the application back, along with a prescription for the requested drugs. The drugs will be sent to your physician's office, where you can pick them up. Programs may vary from one company to the next, so be sure to ask for the details of the program for each company you call. Additional programs can be found by contacting the Pharmaceutical Manufacturers Association. Information about this organization is listed after the table.

CONTACT NUMBERS FOR DRUG COMPANY PATIENT ASSISTANCE PROGRAMS

Company Name	Telephone Number
Amgen	(800) 272-9376
Bristol Myers Oncology	(800) 272-4878
Burroughs Wellcome	(800) 722-9294
Glaxo	(800) 745-2967
Immunex	(800) 466-8639
Janssen	(800) 544-2987
Lederle Oncology	(800) 533-2273

Company Name	Telephone Number
Ortho Biotech	(800) 553-3851
Pharmacia & Upjohn	(800) 366-5570
Purdue Frederick	(203) 853-0123
Roxane	(800) 274-8651
Sandoz	(800) 447-6673
Schering Oncology	(800) 521-7157
Tap	(800) 453-8438
Zeneca	(800) 424-3727

Pharmaceutical Manufacturers Association
1100 Fifteenth Street NW
Washington, DC 20005
(800) 762-4636

This organization publishes the *Directory of Prescription Drug Indigent Programs* from information provided by member companies. Request for a free copy must be on the letterhead of a health-care professional.

Investigational drugs

New drugs are being investigated all the time. When this book went to press, there were many new drugs being tested in clinical trials. Consult Appendix B, *Resources*, for sources to help you research drugs being tested at the time you read this, as well as those which may have come into standard use since this writing. The organization listed below might be able to help you gain access to investigational drugs before they are approved for standard use.

Emergency Investigational New Drug Program
Food and Drug Administration
HF-12 Parklawn Building Room 12A40
5600 Fishers Lane
Rockville, MD 20857
(301) 443-0104

Patients not eligible for clinical trials and in a medical crisis may be able to receive drugs not yet approved by the FDA by having their doctor apply to the FDA for an Emergency IND. The physician should call for additional application information. The FDA usually responds to an application within 24 to 48 hours.

Notes

Preface

1. From Ann Landers's column.
2. Mayer, Musa, *Examining Myself: One Woman's Story of Breast Cancer Treatment and Recovery* (Faber & Faber, 1993).
3. Kleinman, Arthur, *The Illness Narratives: Suffering, Healing, and the Human Condition* (New York: Basic Books, 1988), i

Chapter One

1. Brenner, Barbara, "Let them lick stamps," *Breast Cancer Action Newsletter* #37, August/September 1996, p. 2.
2. Sontag, Susan, *Illness As Metaphor and AIDS and Its Metaphor* (New York: Doubleday, 1990), p. 3.
3. Taylor, Shelley, *Positive Illusions: Creative Self-Deception and the Healthy Mind* (New York: Basic Books, 1989).
4. Goleman, Daniel, "Insights into Self-Deception," *The New York Times Magazine*, May 12, 1985, p. 36.
5. Slater, Philip, *The Pursuit of Loneliness: American Culture at the Breaking Point* (Boston: Beacon Press, 1976), p. 19.
6. Frank, Arthur, *At the Will of the Body: Reflections on Illness* (New York: Houghton Mifflin, 1991), p. 13.
7. "NABCO Survey Challenges Public Perception About Metastatic Breast Cancer," PR Newswire, October 19, 1995.
8. *Breast Cancer Resource List: 1996/97 Edition*, p. 16. National Alliance of Breast Cancer Organizations (NABCO), 9 East 37th Street, 10th Floor, New York, NY 10016, (212) 719-0154. Single copies $3.00.
9. "When Cancer Recurs: Meeting the Challenge Again," National Cancer Institute, 1992, publication 93-2709.
10. American Cancer Society website, at *http://www.cancer.org*.

Chapter Two

1. *SEER Cancer Statistics Review* (CSR). The SEER (Surveillance, Epidemiology, and End Results) Program of the National Cancer Institute collects and publishes cancer incidence and survival data from popula-

tion-based cancer registries. Breast Cancer Statistics on Incidence and Survival can be found at *http://www-seer.ims.nci.nih.gov/Publications/ CSR7393/index.html.*

2. Charmaz, Kathy, *Good Days, Bad Days: The Self in Chronic Illness and Time* (New Jersey: Rutgers University Press, 1991), p. 2.
3. *Ibid.,* p. 12.
4. Wortman, CB, and Dunkel-Schetter, C., "Interpersonal Relationships and Cancer," *Journal of Social Issues*, 35: 120–155, Winter, 1979.
5. Videka, LM, "Psychosocial Adaptations in a Medical Self-Help Group," in *Self-Help Groups for Coping with Crisis,* ML Leiberman, LD Borman, and Associates, eds. (San Francisco: Jossey-Bass, 1979).
6. Benjamin, Harold, *From Victim to Victor* (Los Angeles: Tarcher Books, 1987), p. 80.
7. *Ibid.,* p. 81.
8. Love, Susan, *Dr. Susan Love's Breast Book, Second Edition,* with Karen Lindsey (Reading, MA: Addison-Wesley, 1995), p. 476.
9. Hirshaut, Yashar, and Pressman, Peter, *Breast Cancer: The Complete Guide* (New York: Bantam, 1992), p. 219.
10. Love, Susan, *Op. Cit.,* p. 475.
11. Spiegel, David, *Living Beyond Limits: New Hope and Help for Facing Life-Threatening Illness* (New York: Times Books, 1993), p. 4.
12. Greer, S., Morris, T., and Pettingale, K.W., "Psychological response to breast cancer: Effect on outcome," *Lancet* 2:785–87, 1979.
13. Spiegel, D., Bloom, JR, Kraemer, HC, and Gottheil, E., "Effect of psycho-social treatment on survival of patients with metastatic breast cancer," *Lancet* ii: 888–91, 1989.
14. Spiegel, David, Personal communication with the author, May 1, 1997.

Chapter Three

1. Ellis, Lee N., and Fidler, Isaiah J., "Angiogenesis and breast cancer metastasis," *Lancet*, Vol. 346, p. 388, August 12, 1995.
2. Buhle, Loren, Personal communication, August 3, 1996.
3. Aaron, Alan D., "The management of cancer metastatic to bone," *JAMA, the Journal of the American Medical Association*, Vol. 272, p. 1206. October 19, 1994.
4. Ruoslahti, Erkki, "How Cancer Spreads," *Scientific American*, September, 1996.
5. Hurd, DD, and Peters, WP, "Randomized, comparative study of high-dose (with autologous bone marrow support) versus low-dose cyclophosphamide, cisplatin, and carmustine as consolidation to adjuvant cyclophosphamide, doxorubicin, and fluorouracil for patients with operable stage II or III breast cancer involving 10 or more axillary lymph nodes" (CALGB Protocol 9082). Cancer and Leukemia Group B. *J Natl Cancer Inst Monogr* 19: 41–44, 1995.
   Schwartzberg, L., Birch, R., Weaver, C., Palmer, P., Tauer, K., McAneny,

B., Kalman, L., and West, W., "Prognostic factors after high-dose chemotherapy (HDC) for high-risk stage II and III breast cancer," *Proc
Annu Meet Am Soc Clin Oncol* 14: A114, 1995.

Huelskamp, AM, Abeloff, MD, Armstrong, DK, Fetting, JH, Gordon, G.,
Davidson, NE, and Kennedy, MJ, "High-dose consolidation chemotherapy for stage IIIB breast cancer in remission: intermediate follow-up and
comparison with intensively treated historical controls," *Proc Annu Meet
Am Soc Clin Oncol* 14: A93, 1995.

6. Clark, GM, Sledge, GW, Jr., Osborne, CK, and McGuire, WL, "Survival
   from first recurrence: relative importance of prognostic factors in 1,015
   breast cancer patients," *J Clin Oncol* 5 (1): 55–61, Jan 1987.

7. Lichter, AS, Lippman, ME, Danforth, DN, et al., "Mastectomy versus
   breast-conserving therapy in the treatment of Stage I and II carcinoma
   of the breast: a randomized trial at the National Cancer Institute," *J Clin
   Oncol* 10 (6): p. 976–983, 1992.

8. Scanlon, Edward F. and Murthy, Satya, "The process of metastasis," *Ca,
   the Journal of the American Cancer Society*, Vol. 41, No. 5, p. 301, September, 1991.

9. "Recurrent breast cancer," PDQ database, CancerNet, *http://wwwicic.
   nci.nih.gov/*.

10. Scanlon, Edward, *Op. Cit.*, p. 476.

11. Leonard, RCF, Rodger, A., and Dixon, JM, "Metastatic Breast Cancer;
    ABC of Breast Diseases," *British Medical Journal*, Vol. 309, p. 1501, De-
    cember 3, 1994.

12. Aaron, Alan D., *Op. Cit.*, p. 1206.

13. *Ibid.*, p. 1206.

14. Love, Susan, *Op. Cit.*, p. 477.

15. *Ibid.*, p. 478.

Chapter Four

1. Backman, Margaret E., *The Psychology of the Physically Ill Patient: A Clinician's Guide* (New York: Plenum Press, 1989), p. 8.

2. *Ibid.*, p. 8.

3. Worden, William J., "The experience of recurrent cancer," *Ca*, Vol. 39,
   No. 5, p. 305, September, 1989.

4. *Ibid.*, p. 305.

5. Lazarus, RS, and Folkman, S., *Stress Appraisal and Coping* (New York:
   Springer-Verlag, 1984).

Chapter Five

1. Novack, DH, et al., "Changes in physicians' attitudes toward telling the
   cancer patient," *Journal of the American Medical Association*, 241 (9):
   897–900, March 2, 1979.

2. Cassileth, BR, et al., "Information and participation preferences among cancer patients," *Annals of Internal Medicine*, 92 (6): 832–6, June 1980.
3. Annas, George J., "Informed Consent, Cancer, and Truth in Prognosis," *New England Journal of Medicine*, 330: 223–225, January 20, 1994.
4. Annas, George J., *Op. Cit.*
5. Roan, Shari, "What to do when the news is bad," *Los Angeles Times*, October 7, 1993.
6. Reiser, SJ, "Words as Scalpels: transmitting evidence in the clinical dialogue," *Annals of Internal Medicine*, 92 (6): 837–42, June 1980.
7. Tversky, A., and Kahneman, D., "The framing of decisions and the psychology of choice," *Science*, 211:453–458, 1981.
8. Cousins, Norman, "Tapping Human Potential: an Interview," *Second Opinion,* 14: p. 56, July 1990.
9. Roan, Shari, *Op. Cit.*, p. 1.
10. *Ibid.*, p. 1.
11. Gould, Stephen Jay, "The Median Isn't the Message." For the entire article, see Steve Dunn's Cancer Guide at *http://cancerguide.org/median_not_msg.html*.
12. Dunn, Steve, *CancerGuide: Steve Dunn's Cancer Information Page*, *http://cancerguide.org/*.
13. Macklin, Ruth, *Mortal Choices: Ethical Dilemmas in Modern Medicine* (Boston: Houghton Mifflin, 1987), pp. 35–36.
14. Hirshaut, Yashar, and Pressman, Peter, *Breast Cancer: The Complete Guide, Revised Edition* (New York: Bantam Books, 1996), p. 223.
15. Franks, Arthur, *Op. Cit.*, p. 14.

Chapter Six

1. Winer, Dr. Eric P., "Treatment Options for Patients with Refractory Breast Cancer," *Oncology*, Vol. 10/6, p. 16.
2. *PDQ—NCI's Comprehensive Cancer Database*, description from the NCI website at *http://wwwicic.nci.nih.gov/pdq.htm*.
3. Love, Susan, *Dr. Susan Love's Breast Book, Second Edition,* with Karen Lindsey (Reading, MA: Addison-Wesley, 1995), Chapter 31, "When Cancer Comes Back," pp. 468–485, and Chapter 32, "Metastatic Disease: Treatments," pp. 486–501.
4. Hirshaut, Yashar, and Pressman, Peter, *Breast Cancer: The Complete Guide, Revised Edition* (New York: Bantam Books, 1996), Chapter 13: "Recurrence," pp. 221–240.
5. Zakarian, Beverly, *The Activist Cancer Patient: How to Take Charge of Your Treatment* (New York: John Wiley and Sons, 1996), p. 71.
6. Love, Susan, *Op. Cit.*, p. 490–91.
7. *Joining a Clinical Trial*, from the National Alliance of Breast Cancer Organizations (NABCO) website at *http://www.nabco.org/trials*.
8. Zakarian, Beverly, *Op. Cit.*, p. 120.

9. NCI CancerNet Clinical Trials information is at *http://wwwicic. nci.nih.gov/trials/h_clinic.htm* and Centerwatch Clinical Trials Listing Service is at *http://www.centerwatch.com/*.

10. Newsmith, Jeff, "Can Those New Cancer Drugs Win FDA Approval?" Cox News Service at *http://www.coxnews.com*.

11. Boyd, Robert S., "Sharpening the Attack on Cancer," *The Philadelphia Enquirer*, May 9, 1998.

12. Horowitz, Craig, "The Cancer Killer," *New York Magazine*, Vol. 31, No. 20, p. 68, May 25, 1998.

13. Wallis, Claudia, "Molecular Revolution," *Time*, Vol. 151, No. 19, May 18, 1998.

14. Tannock, Ian F., "Conventional Cancer Therapy: Promise Broken or Promise Delayed?" *Lancet*, 351 (suppl II), pp. 9-16, 1998.

15. Lane, David, "The Promise of Molecular Biology," *Lancet*, (suppl II), pp. 17-20, 1998.

16. Brownlee, Shannon, and Shute, Nancy, "Killing Cancer," *U.S. News*, May 18, 1998.

17. Norton, Larry, "Evolving Concepts in the Systemic Drug Therapy of Breast Cancer," *Seminars in Oncology*, Vol. 24, No. 4 (Suppl 10), August, 1997.

18. Oliff, Allen, Gibbs, Jackson B., and McCormick, Frank, "New Molecular Targets for Cancer Therapy," *Scientific American*, September, 1996.

19. Haber, Daniel A., and Fearon, Eric R., "The Promise of Cancer Genetics," *Lancet*, 351 (suppl II) pp. 1-8, 1998.

20. Oliff, Allen, Gibbs, Jackson B., and McCormick, Frank, *Op. Cit.*

21. Boyd, Robert S., "Sharpening the Attack on Cancer," *The Philadelphia Enquirer*, May 9, 1998.

22. Old, Lloyd J., "Immunotherapy for Cancer," *Scientific American*, September, 1996.

23. Folkman, Judah, "Fighting Cancer by Attacking Its Blood Supply," *Scientific American*, September, 1996.

24. NCI CancerNet Clinical Trials information is at *http://wwwicic.nci.nih. gov/trials/h_clinic.htm* and Centerwatch Clinical Trials Listing Service is at *http://www.centerwatch.com/*.

25. Belkora, Jeff, *Top ten decision lessons from CHBP Open Houses, http:// www-med.Stanford.EDU:80/CBHP/Practical/Belkora.html.*

26. "High-Dose Chemotherapy with Stem Cell Transplant as Breast Cancer Treatment," from *Cancer Facts* National Cancer Institute, National Institutes of Health.

27. Antman, Karen H., et al., "High-Dose Chemotherapy with Autologous Hematopoietic Stem-Cell Support for Breast Cancer in North America," *Journal of Clinical Oncology*, Vol. 15, pp. 1870–79, 1997.

28. Zujewski, JoAnne, Nelson, Anita, and Abrams, Jeffrey, "Much Ado About Not. . .Enough Data: High-Dose Chemotherapy with Autologous

Stem Cell Rescue for Breast Cancer," *Journal of the National Cancer Institute*, Vol. 90, pp. 200-209, February 4, 1998.

29. Zones, Jane, "Autologous bone marrow transplant: what is the price of hope?" *The Network News*, Vol. 20; No. 6; p. 6. National Women's Health Network, November, 1995.

30. Antman, Karen, et al., *Op. Cit.*

31. *Ibid.*

32. "Breast Cancer (Therapy) Chemotherapy with Autologous Bone-Marrow Transplant Re-Evaluated," *Cancer Biotechnology Weekly*, March 18, 1996.

33. Burrus, William M., "Current treatment of advanced breast cancer," *OT*, p. 31, January 25.

34. Hortobagyi, Gabriel N., "Management of breast cancer: Status and future trends," *Seminars on Oncology*, Vol. 22, No. 5, Suppl 12, p. 103, October 1995.

35. Greenberg, PA, Hortobagyi, GN, et al., "Ten-Year Results of FAC Adjuvant Chemotherapy Trial in breast Cancer," *Journal of Clinical Oncology*, Vol. 14, pp. 2197-2205, 1996.

36. Hirshaut, Yashar, and Pressman, Peter, *Breast Cancer: The Complete Guide* (New York: Bantam, 1996), p. 239.

37. Bezwoda, WR, "High-dose chemotherapy with hematopoietic rescue as a primary treatment for metastatic breast cancer: a randomized trial," *The Journal of Clinical Oncology*, pp. 2483–89, October 1995.

38. Bearman, SI, "High-dose chemotherapy for metastatic and primary breast cancer," *Perspectives in Breast Cancer*, pp. 28–9, September 29–30, 1995, Phoenix, Arizona.

39. *High-Dose Chemotherapy with Bone Marrow Transplant for Metastatic Breast Cancer: ECRI Patient Reference Guide*, Second Edition, March 1996, available at *http://www.hslc.org/emb/bc1.html*.

40. Hortobagyi, GN, *Is High-dose Chemotherapy an Established Treatment for Breast Cancer?* ASCO Educational Book, 1995, pp. 341-346.

41. Zujewski, JoAnne, et al., *Op. Cit.*

42. Rodenhuis, S., et al., "Randomized trial of high-dose chemotherapy and haemopoietic progenitor-cell support in operable breast cancer with extensive axillary lymph-node involvement," *Lancet*, 352, pp. 515-21, 1998.

43. Slevin, ML, Stubbs, L., Plant, HJ, Wilson, P., Gregory, WM, Armes, PJ, and Downer, SM, "Attitudes to chemotherapy: comparing views of patients with cancer with those of doctors, nurses, and general public," *British Medical Journal*, 300 (6737): pp. 1458–60, 1990 Jun 2.

44. "Most patients seek aggressive therapy," *The Press-Enterprise* p. D01, March 5, 1996, Riverside, CA.

45. Lerner, Michael, *Choices in Healing* (Cambridge, MA: MIT Press, 1994).

Chapter Seven

1. Brody, Jane, "Alternative medicine has its place. But be careful," *The New York Times*, November 13, 1996, p. C13.

2. Brigden, Malcolm L., "Unproven questionable cancer therapies," *The Western Journal of Medicine*, 163: p. 463, 1995.

3. Callahan, Daniel, *The Troubled Dream of Life: In Search of a Peaceful Death* (New York: Simon & Shuster, 1993).

4. As quoted in Brody, Jane, *Op. Cit.*

5. Elizabeth J. Clark, Ph.D., "Words That Heal, Words That Harm," The National Coalition for Cancer Survivorship (NCCS) at *http://www.access.digex.net/~mkragen/healharm.html*.

6. Spiegel, David, "Compassion Is the Best Medicine," *The New York Times*, June 12, 1994, Section 4A, p. 3.

7. Gordon, James S., "Healing With Feeling; Bringing Holistic Medicine in From the Therapeutic Fringe," *The Washington Post*, August 29, 1993, p. C3.

8. Lerner, Michael, "Hedging The Bet Against Cancer," *The New York Times*, October 2, 1994, Section 6, p. 65.

9. Taylor, SE, Lichtman, RR, and Wood, JV, "Attributions, beliefs about control and adjustment to breast cancer," *Journal of Perspectives on Sociology and Psychology*, 46: p. 489, 1984.

10. Sontag, Susan, *Illness as Metaphor* (New York: Vintage Books, 1977).

11. Klass, Perri, "Life without euphemisms," *The New York Times*, April 27, 1986, Section 7, p. 21.

12. Frank, Arthur, *Op. Cit.*, p. 8.

13. Massie, Mary Jane, "Depression and Anxiety, Panic and Phobias," in *Handbook of Psychooncology: Psychological Care of the Patient with Cancer*, Holland and Towland, editors (New York: Oxford University Press, 1990), pp. 283–84.

14. *Ibid.*, pp. 300–303.

15. Mastrovito, Rene, "Behavioral Techniques: Progressive Relaxation and Self-Regulatory Therapies," In *Handbook of Psychooncology*, *Op. Cit.*, pp. 492–500.

16. Kabat-Zinn, Jon, *Full Catastrophe Living: Using the Wisdom of Your Body and Mind to Face Stress, Pain, and Illness* (New York: Bantam, 1990), pp. 5–6.

17. Spiegel, David, "How do you feel about cancer now?—survival and psychosocial support," *Public Health Reports,* Vol. 110, No. 3, p. 298, May 1995.

18. Classen, C., Diamond, S., Soleman, A., Fobair, P., Spira, J., and Spiegel, D., *Brief Supportive-Expressive Group Therapy for Women with Primary Breast Cancer: A Treatment Manual* (Stanford University, 1993). *http://www-med.stanford.edu/school/Psychiatry/PSTreatLab/*.

19. Lerner, Michael, "Hedging The Bet Against Cancer," *The New York Times*, Sunday, October 2, 1994, Section 6, p. 65.

Chapter Eight

1. Harpham, as quoted in Jane Brody, "Fighting Fatigue That Accompanies Cancer," *The New York Times*, Personal Health, April 2, 1997.
2. Bukberg, J., Penman, D., and Holland, JC, "Depression in hospitalized cancer patients," *Psychosomatic Medicine*, 46: 999–1004, 1980.
3. Scheiner, Ellen, "Health Care Professionals with Cancer: A Physician's Perspective," Presented at the Third Annual Psycho-Oncology Congress, New York, New York, October 4, 1996.
4. Melzack, Ronald, "Pain relief won't create addicts; children and the elderly suffer most when physicians underprescribe narcotics." *Medical World News*, Vol. 31/No. 13, p. 67, July 1990.
5. Hermann, Joan F., A.C.S.W., Wojtkowiak, Sandra L., R.N., M.S.N., Houts, Peter S., Ph.D., and Kahn, S. Benham, M.D., "Helping People Cope, Introduction: How Can This Guide Help You?" from Oncolink: The University of Pennsylvania Cancer Center Resource at *http://www.oncolink.upenn.edu/*.
6. Cherny, Nathan I., and Portenoy, Russell K., "The Management of Cancer Pain," *CA: A Cancer Journal for Clinicians*, Vol. 44, No. 5, Sept/Oct 1994.
7. Spiegel, David, *Op. Cit.*, p. 242.

Chapter Nine

1. Rait, Douglas, and Lederberg, Marguerite, "The Family of the Cancer Patient," in *Handbook of Psychooncology*, *Op. Cit.*, pp. 585–589.
2. *Ibid.*
3. *Ibid.*

Chapter Ten

1. Spiegel, David, *Op. Cit.*, p. 32.
2. Charmaz, Kathy, *Op. Cit.*, p. 178.
3. Sarton, May, *After the Stroke: A Journal* (New York: Norton, 1988), p. 78.
4. Sontag, Susan, *Illness as Metaphor* (New York: Vintage Books, 1977), p. 3.
5. Charmaz, Kathy, *Op. Cit.*, p. 220.
6. Taylor, Shelley E., *Positive Illusions: Creative Self-Deception and the Healthy Mind* (New York: Basic Books, 1989), p. 162.
7. Schoolman, Jenilu, *Within Measured Boundaries*, Community Breast Health Project website at *http://www-med.stanford.edu/CBHP/Personal_Stories/Jenilu.html*.
8. Charmaz, Kathy, *Op. Cit.*, p. 76.
9. *Ibid.*, p. 101.
10. Audre Lorde, *The Cancer Journals* (San Francisco: Spinsters/Aunt Lute, 1980), pp. 21–22.

Chapter Eleven

1. Lipstein, Owen, "Loss: An interview with Froma Walsh," *Psychology Today*, Vol. 25, No. 4, p. 64, July 1992.
2. Charmaz, Kathy, *Op. Cit.*, pp. 81–82.
3. Yalom, Irvin D., *Existential Psychotherapy* (New York: Basic Books, 1980), pp. 31–32.
4. Colburn, Don, "The Grace of a 'Good Death' Escapes Many," *The Washington Post*, December 5, 1995, p. Z07.
5. Callahan, Daniel, "Pursuing a Peaceful Death," *The Hastings Center Report*, Vol. 23, No. 4, p. 33, July 1993.
6. "A Controlled trial to improve care for seriously ill hospitalized patients: The Study to Understand Prognoses and Preferences for Outcomes and Risks of Treatments (SUPPORT)," *Journal of the American Medical Association, JAMA*, Vol. 274, No. 20, p. 1591, November 22, 1995.
7. "Too Many Americans Die Alone, in Pain, Attached to Machines," The Robert Wood Johnson Foundation, at *http://www.dash.com/netro/nwx/tmr/tmr1295/death1295.html*.
8. Callahan, Daniel, "Once again, reality: now where do we go? Dying Well in the Hospital: The Lessons of SUPPORT," *The Hastings Center Report*, Vol. 25, No. 6, p. S33, November 1995.
9. Nuland, Sherwin B., *How We Die: Reflections on Life's Final Chapter* (New York: Knopf, 1994), p. 257.
10. *Ibid.*, p. 223.
11. *Ibid.*, p. 234.
12. Callahan, Daniel, *The Troubled Dream of Life: In Search of a Peaceful Death* (New York: Simon & Shuster, 1993), p. 51.
13. Skelly, Flora Johnson, "The good things about death," *American Medical News*, Vol. 35, No. 40, p. 41, October 26, 1992.
14. *Ibid.*, p. 41.
15. Nuland, Sherwin B., *Op. Cit.*, p. 258–59.
16. *Ibid.*, p. 228–9.
17. Broyard, Anatole, *Intoxicated by My Illness and Other Writings on Life and Death* (New York: Fawcett, 1992), p. 57.
18. Foley, Kathleen M., "Competent Care for the Dying Instead of Physician-Assisted Suicide," *New England Journal of Medicine*, Vol. 336, No. 1, January 2, 1997.
19. "What is Hospice?" *Boston Globe*, June 20, 1996.
20. *Ibid.*

Chapter Twelve

1. Moyers, Bill, *Healing and the Mind* (New York: Doubleday, 1993), p. 319.
2. Kleinman, *Op. Cit.*
3. Remen, Naomi, as quoted in Moyers, *Op. Cit.*, p. 239.

4. Charmaz, Kathy, *Op. Cit.*, p. 178.
5. Yalom, Irvin, *Op. Cit.*
6. Remen, Naomi, in Moyers, Bill, *Op. Cit.*, p. 351.
7. Lewis, CS, *A Grief Observed* (New York: Bantam, 1961), pp. 12–13.
8. Broyard, Anatole, "Good Books About Being Sick," *The New York Times*, April 1, 1990, 7:1.
9. Lorde, Audre, *The Cancer Journals* (San Francisco: Spinsters/Aunt Lute, 1980), pp. 21–22.
10. Frankl, Viktor, *The Will to Meaning: Foundations and Applications of Logotherapy* (New York: Penguin, 1970), p. 17.
11. Cassell, Eric. J., *The Nature of Suffering and the Goals of Medicine* (Oxford University Press, 1991), p. 44.
12. Charmaz, Kathy, *Op. Cit.*, pp. 258–259.

Glossary

Please note: The use of italics indicates that a term is defined under its own entry in this glossary.

ABMT
    See *autologous bone marrow transplant.*

Acute
    Occurring suddenly or in a short space of time, as opposed to *chronic.*

Adenocarcinoma
    A general term for a cancer formed from glandular tissue, including breast cancer.

Adjuvant
    Refers to surgery, *radiation*, *chemotherapy*, hormonal or other treatment used in, after, and in addition to *primary* cancer treatment. Most often used to refer to chemotherapy.

Alkaline Phosphatase Test
    A *tumor marker* test that assists in diagnosis of *bone* and *liver metastases.*

Alkylating
    Characteristic of one group of *chemotherapy* drugs, referring to a particular way in which these drugs interfere with cell growth and reproduction. Cytoxan is a common alkylating agent.

Alopecia
    The medical name for the hair loss that accompanies cancer treatment, as a *side effect* of *chemotherapy* or *radiation* therapy.

Amenorrhea
    Stopping of menstruation, usually as a result of *chemotherapy.*

Analgesic
    A general term for a drug that relieves pain.

Androgen
> A male hormone, sometimes used in the treatment of metastatic breast cancer.

Anecdotal Evidence
> Reports of individual cases. While often providing interesting leads, case reports do not provide scientific evidence in and of themselves. Such evidence comes from *clinical trials*.

Anemia
> A lowered *red blood cell* count, often the result of *chemotherapy*. Lowered oxygenation in anemia results in symptoms of *fatigue*, shortness of breath, weakness, loss of energy, skin pallor.

Angiogenesis
> A process by which cancerous tumors send out chemical signals to induce the growth of blood vessels to feed the tumor.

Anorexia
> Loss of appetite, caused by treatment or the cancer itself.

Antiangiogenic
> Referring to a new class of substances that inhibit the chemical signals sent by tumors to create their own blood supply.

Antidepressant
> A drug used to relieve feelings of depression, despair and hopelessness.

Antiemetic
> A drug that reduces or eliminates nausea and vomiting. Common examples are: *Compazine, Decadron, Zofran, Kytril, Marinol, Ativan*.

Antiestrogen
> A class of drugs, e.g., tamoxifen, that bind with *estrogen receptors* to prevent tumor growth in cases of hormonally sensitive cancer.

Antigen
> A substance that the *immune system* recognizes as foreign to the body.

Antimetabolite
> Characteristic of one group of *chemotherapy* drugs, referring to the way it disrupts cell reproduction. Examples: 5-FU and methotrexate.

Apoptosis
> Programmed cell death, a process occurring in normal body cells.

Aromatase Inhibitors
> These drugs—for example, anastrozole (Arimidex)—inhibit an enzyme called aromatase, which regulates estrogen production in the adrenal glands.

Ascites
Fluid accumulation in the abdomen, usually a result of cancer present in the liver or other tissue. Fluid in the chest is called *effusion*. See also *pleural effusion*.

Aspiration
Drawing fluid into a hollow needle, usually done for testing.

Autologous Bone Marrow Transplant (ABMT)
A *rescue* procedure, now largely replaced by *peripheral stem cell transplant*, whereby the patient's own *bone marrow* is removed, stored and returned following *high-dose chemotherapy*. This latter term is often used to describe the entire procedure.

Axillary Dissection
A diagnostic procedure involving removal or sampling of the axillary *lymph nodes* in the armpit, done with breast cancer surgery to determine the *stage* of the disease.

Biological Response Modifiers
These act to boost the immune system. Examples are: antibodies, *monoclonal antibodies*, vaccines, *colony stimulating factors*.

Biopsy
Microscopic examination of tumor tissue taken from the body for evidence of the presence of cancer cells, done by a *pathologist*. Apart from identifying the presence and type of cancer, tissue or cells may be processed for a number of different kinds of studies.

Bisphosphonates
A class of drugs that slow bone loss later in life and strengthen bones damaged by *metastases*.

Blood-Brain Barrier
The thin membrane that protects the spinal fluid and brain from toxic substances. It can interfere with the use of some *chemotherapies* in treating tumors in the central nervous system.

BMT
See *bone marrow transplantation*; *high-dose chemotherapy*.

Bone Cancer
True primary bone cancer is a sarcoma, and is relatively rare. This is not the same as *bone metastases*, spread from cancers elsewhere in the body, most commonly from breast, lung, thyroid, prostate and kidney cancers.

Bone Marrow
Located in the center of the bone, this spongy material is really an important organ system of the body, and is where all the *red blood cells* (erythrocytes), most of the *white blood cells* (leukocytes), and all the

platelets (thrombocytes) are made. Primitive stem cells in the bone marrow are the progenitors for all the blood cells in the body.

Bone Marrow Biopsy

A test used to determine the presence of *cancer cells* in the *bone marrow.* Usually done in a doctor's office under a local anesthetic, it involves inserting a hollow needle into one of the large bones, usually the hip. The term *aspiration* is used sometimes when a smaller sample is taken.

Bone Marrow Depression (or Suppression)

A *side effect* of *chemotherapy* treatment, where the *bone marrow* isn't able to make a normal number of *red* and *white blood cells* and *platelets.*

Bone Marrow Harvest and Transplantation

Bone marrow withdrawn, or "harvested," from the patient herself (autologous) under general anesthesia is frozen and later transplanted (re-introduced into the blood stream) to support the patient's own bone marrow that has been severely compromised by *high-dose chemotherapy (HDC).* Peripheral or circulating *stem cells* gathered through a process called "pheresis" are now more commonly used in most *autologous transplants.* See also *autologous bone marrow transplant* and *high-dose chemotherapy.*

Bone Metastasis

Spread of cancer to the bone, a common site of metastatic breast cancer. Most commonly presents with pain, and can be confirmed by *CT Scan, MRI* and *x-ray* studies. Sometimes a *biopsy* is done to confirm the diagnosis. Treatments include *radiation* and chemo-hormonal therapy.

Bone Scan

A harmless radioactive tracer substance is injected prior to this test to give a picture of the entire skeleton, showing areas of increased "uptake" of the radioactive substance, such as *bone metastases* where cells are dividing rapidly. "Hot spots" that show up on a bone scan may also be caused by arthritis, infection or injury.

Brain Metastasis

Spread of cancer to the brain, another site of metastatic breast cancer. Symptoms may include headaches, visual disturbances, vomiting, seizures, loss of balance and other neurological signs. Diagnosed through *CT Scans* and *MRI*, and most often treated with *radiation* therapy.

BRCA1 and BRCA2

Two *genes* that have recently been shown to be associated with a high rate of familial breast cancer.

Breast Calcifications

Small flecks of calcium in the breast, visible on mammograms, that may be signs of cancer in a small number of cases.

CA 15-3

A *tumor marker* that can be monitored in the majority of patients with metastatic breast cancer, indicating the progression, regression or stability of the disease. Like all the tumor markers, it can be assessed from a blood sample.

CA 27-29

A *tumor marker* similar to CA 15-3 above, used to monitor disease progression in metastatic breast cancer. Also known as the Truquant test.

CA 125

A *tumor marker* used to monitor ovarian cancer, highly predictive of *recurrence* for most ovarian cancer patients.

Cachexia

A so-called "wasting syndrome" that often accompanies the very advanced stages of cancer, characterized by weight loss, emaciation, weakness and *fatigue*, and loss of appetite.

Cancer Cell

A cell that divides and reproduces abnormally, with uncontrolled growth, and that may spread to other parts of the body.

Cardiomyopathy

A *chronic* disorder of the heart muscle, which can result in heart failure, embolism, enlargement or arrhythmias.

Cathepsin D

A protein secreted by breast cancer cells, thought to indicate a poorer prognosis.

CEA (carcinoembryonic antigen)

A monoclonal *tumor marker* sometimes used to monitor breast cancer patients. Because it can also indicate other cancers and certain inflammatory conditions, it is not considered specific enough to be the sole indicator.

Cerebrospinal fluid

Fluid that surrounds and bathes the brain and spinal cord and provides a cushion from shocks.

Chemoembolization

Process by which *chemotherapy* drugs are delivered by *infusion* directly to the area where the tumor is, sometimes used in treating *liver metastases*.

Chemoresistance or Chemoinsensitivity

In time, *cancer cells* develop the capacity to withstand and expel *chemotherapy* drugs, and are said to be *chemoresistant* or *chemoinsensitive*.

Chemosensitivity Testing

Experimental *in vitro* (in the laboratory, literally, "in glass") testing of tumor tissue to show its response to various cancer drugs. While it is extremely promising, many physicians feel this testing process is not yet accurate enough for general use.

Chemosensitizers

Drugs or chemicals that enhance *chemotherapy's* effects.

Chemotherapy

A general term used to refer to drugs that act in different ways to kill or inhibit the growth of *cancer cells* by interrupting the cell cycle of reproduction. These drugs are called *systemic treatments*, because they act throughout the body, as opposed to localized treatments, like surgery or *radiation*, that act only on a particular tumor and surrounding tissue. Different types of drugs are active against different phases in cancer cell reproduction, one reason that *combination chemotherapy* is often more effective than single agent chemotherapy. Different types of chemotherapy include: *alkylating* agents, *antimetabolites*, antibiotics, alkaloids, hormones and others. These drugs may be administered orally, by *injection* or *infusion* into a muscle or vein (often through an *indwelling catheter*), or into body cavities or organs, the spinal fluid, or applied topically, as with some treatments for *inflammatory breast cancer*. Chemotherapy may be offered on many different schedules, from daily or by continuous infusion to weekly, biweekly or monthly, according to the method and dosage that scientific studies have shown is most effective. Since it affects all rapidly dividing cells, chemotherapy can have many *side effects*, including *bone marrow depression*, *stomatitis*, *neutropenia*, *thrombocytopenia*, *anemia*, *alopecia*, *anorexia*, *fatigue*, infection, and nausea and vomiting.

Chronic

A repeating or constant condition, lasting a long time.

Clinical Trial

See *Phase I clinical trial*; *Phase II clinical trial*; *Phase III clinical trial*.

Colony-Stimulating Factors (CSF)

Also called "growth factors," these are natural substances that stimulate the *bone marrow's* production of *white* and *red blood cells* and *platelets*. In recent years, the use of these factors has made higher, more effective doses of *chemotherapy* safer, since they foster more rapid recovery of the bone marrow. In common use are *G-CSF* (Neupogen), which stimulates white blood cell production and *erythropoetin* (Epogen), which stimulates red blood cell production. Still in *clinical trials* is thrombopoetin, which stimulates the production of platelets, or clotting factors.

Combination Chemotherapy

Using more than one kind of *chemotherapy* drug is often more effective than a single agent, because each drug acts in a different way on the cancer reproductive process, making it less likely that some cells that are resistant to treatment will survive, or that cells that do survive can repair the damage.

Complete Blood Count (CBC)

A blood test that gives results of *white* and *red cell* counts, *platelets*, hemoglobin and other factors.

Comprehensive Cancer Centers

Medical centers designated by the National Cancer Institute share a number of characteristics—strong clinical and laboratory research programs, including conducting clinical studies and trials, ongoing training of cancer physicians and other clinical staff, and community programs in prevention, information and outreach. The Cancer Information Service of the NCI will supply an up-to-date list of these facilities at (800) 4-CANCER.

Consolidation Strategies

Attempts to further eradicate cancer at previous tumor sites by means of treatment.

Continuous Infusion

A drug or drugs that need to be administered continuously; for example, some kinds of *chemotherapy* or medications to control pain can be given through an *infusion* pump worn by patients 24 hours a day.

CT Scan (also called CAT Scan)

Computerized axial tomography, a diagnostic test, is a computerized *x-ray* that shows cross sections, giving doctors a three-dimensional view of the entire body. It is much more detailed than x-rays, and can visualize minutely detailed structures anywhere in the body. It usually does not require injection of a contrast medium.

Cytology

The study of cells.

Cytotoxic

A substance that causes cells to die.

Differentiation

The degree to which a *cancer cell* resembles a normal cell. In general, poorly differentiated cancer cells are more aggressive.

DNA

The part of every body cell that carries our genetic information.

Dose-Response Ratio

The concept that treatment effectiveness increases with higher doses of *chemotherapy* drugs.

Doubling Time

The time it takes *cancer cells* to reproduce themselves, and tumors to double in size. The range of doubling time for breast cancer cells is from 23 to 209 days.

Drug Resistance

When *cancer cells* are insensitive to cancer drugs, either initially or as a result of prior treatment, they are said to be resistant. "Cross-resistance" occurs when cancers develop resistance to a drug after exposure to a related drug.

Dyspnea

Shortness of breath, or difficulty breathing.

Edema

A swelling because of an accumulation of fluid in body tissues, often a result of some hormonal therapies. See also *lymphedema*.

Effusion

An accumulation of fluid in the body cavities, with metastatic breast cancer most commonly manifested by a *pleural effusion*, where fluid accumulates in the pleural cavity surrounding the lungs. This can be relieved by *thoracentesis* where the fluid is drained through a hollow needle, and *biopsied* for evidence of *malignant* cells.

Erythrocytes

See *red blood cells*.

Erythropoietin

Epogen, Procrit. A *growth factor* that promotes the *red blood cell* count and reduces the need for transfusions.

Estrogen Dependent

A tumor that grows, or grows more rapidly, in the presence of estrogen. Considered a positive indicator, as it permits hormonal treatment for control of the tumor, increasing options for treatment.

Estrogen Receptor Positive (or Negative)

This is often written as ER+ or ER- and is a measure of the degree to which a given tumor is dependent upon estrogen for its growth, measured by an estrogen receptor assay (ERA). The number of hormone receptors on the tumor are measured to determine this. See also *progesterone receptors*.

Extravasation

Leakage of an intravenous drug into the surrounding tissue.

Fatigue

A feeling of extreme tiredness, weariness, or exhaustion, common in metastatic breast cancer patients in connection with treatments or undiagnosed cancer progression. *Anemia* from *metastases* to the *bone marrow* and other causes, tissue repair following *radiation treatment, bone marrow depression* associated with *chemotherapy* treatment, inadequate nutrition, depression and anxiety are some of the important causes.

First-line Treatment

First treatment given following *adjuvant* treatment, when there is a *recurrence*.

Flow Cytometry

A test of *cancer cells* to determine the number that are in the S-Phase or dividing stage, and to look at the *DNA* content, called "ploidy." These factors are correlated to aggressiveness of tumor growth.

G-CSF

Neupogen, or granulocyte *colony-stimulating factor*, that helps the *white blood cells* recover rapidly following *chemotherapy* treatments.

Gene

The fundamental unit of *DNA* that contains inherited characteristics.

Growth Factors

See *colony-stimulating factors*.

Hematologist

A physician specializing in blood diseases. Many medical oncologists are hematologists.

HER-2/neu

Also known as c-erB-2, this *gene* is thought to contribute to some breast cancers. Anti-HER-2/neu humanized *monoclonal antibody* has completed *clinical trials* and is expected to be approved by the FDA.

Herceptin

The anti-HER-2/neu drug developed to treat breast cancer patients who over-express *HER-2/neu*.

Heterogeneity

Refers to the fact that there are many different types of cells with differing properties in any breast cancer.

Hickman Catheter

An external line (tubing) with one end outside of the chest and the other inserted into a large chest vein and threaded to the heart, used for drawing blood and administering medications painlessly. While it can be left in place for many months or years, it must be carefully cared for to prevent infection.

High-Dose Chemotherapy

A form of treatment, still in *clinical trials*, used with high-risk (Stage III) and metastatic breast cancer patients in which the goal is to eradicate all the *cancer cells* in the body by using very high doses of *chemotherapy*, so high that without the use of *growth factors* and transplantation of the patient's own *stem cells*, patients would not survive the treatment. Also referred to by the *rescue* procedures such as *bone marrow transplant (BMT)* or *autologous bone marrow transplant (ABMT)*.

Hospice

First begun in England, these programs, usually home-based, provide services by a team of professionals for the care of terminally ill patients and their families. The goal is to improve quality of life, relieve pain and other troublesome symptoms and make the dying process easier for patient and family.

Hyperalimentation

Also called total perenteral nutrition (TPN), this means giving nutrition intravenously, for patients unable to eat normally.

Hypercalcemia

Bone loss from progressing *bone metastases* can result in higher levels of calcium in the blood, causing this metabolic disorder, characterized by *fatigue*, muscle weakness, nausea, *anorexia*, constipation and, in severe cases, disorientation and coma. New medications such as Aredia are used in its treatment.

Immune System

A multi-faceted, incompletely understood system which functions to protect the body from any foreign invaders, such as bacteria, viruses, toxins and cancers.

Immunosuppressed

A lowered resistance to disease, often because of *chemotherapy* treatments.

Immunotherapy

Experimental treatments that attempt to use the body's own defenses to control the cancer. Also known as immunomodulation.

Induction Chemotherapy

Treatment given prior to *high-dose chemotherapy*. The purpose is twofold: to assess the patient's response to treatment before administering very high doses, and to decrease the tumor burden, the amount of cancer in the body, prior to high-dose chemotherapy, thus giving the best chance for *remission*.

Indwelling Catheter
A tube which is threaded through a large chest vein to the heart so that blood can be drawn and drugs, including those for *chemotherapy* and medications for other purposes, can be given without needing to repeatedly find a vein. Indwelling catheters can be either the external type, such as the *Hickman catheter*, or subcutaneous (under the skin). This latter type is generally called a *port*.

Infiltrating Ductal Carcinoma
The most common form of invasive breast cancer.

Infiltrating Lobular Carcinoma
Less common, this breast cancer originates in the lobules, rather than the ducts of the breast.

Inflammatory Breast Cancer
An aggressive form of breast cancer, occurring in about one percent of all diagnoses, that rapidly spreads into the *lymphatic* channels in the breast, causing the tissue to appear reddened and swollen, resembling a rash or infection.

Informed Consent
The legal right of a patient to be informed by medical personnel about a treatment or a procedure before giving consent to undergo it. With experimental treatments and most surgical procedures, this is put into writing.

Infusion
Administering drugs into a vein or artery slowly, over a period of time, sometimes using a pump. Note: Both infusion and *injection* can be intra-arterial, into an artery; intramuscular, into a muscle; intraperitoneal, into the abdominal cavity; intrapleural, into the space around the lungs; intrathecal, into the spinal fluid; or intravenous, into a vein.

Injection
Administering drugs into a vein or artery all at once. See the note under *infusion*.

In vitro
Literally, "in glass." Taking place outside the body, in a laboratory.

In vivo
Taking place in the body, or in another living organism.

Lesion
A general term indicating a change in the structure of any body tissue, often used as a synonym for cancer.

Leukopenia
Decrease in the *white blood cell* count.

Liver Metastases

Breast cancer can metastasize to the liver, which often presents as being enlarged or tender, and can be diagnosed by a *liver scan*, ultrasound, *CT scan* and *alkaline phosphatase tests*.

Liver Scan

A radioactive tracer is injected into the bloodstream that enhances the *x-ray* picture of the liver.

Lung Metastases

Because all the blood is filtered through the lungs, breast cancer also spreads to the lung and *pleura* surrounding the lung. Shortness of breath and a persistent cough are among the symptoms. Scans and *x-ray* are commonly used for diagnosis, although sometimes a lung *biopsy* may be advised for definitive diagnosis.

Lymph Nodes

Small, bean-shaped organs that filter bacteria and *cancer cells* circulating in the *lymphatic system*. When the axillary lymph nodes are positive in breast cancer, this is an indicator that the disease has already begun to spread beyond the breast.

Lymphatic System

The collection of ducts, *lymph nodes*, and other organs that drain the tissue fluid called lymph into the bloodstream.

Lymphedema

Women who have had the axillary lymph nodes sampled or removed at the time of lumpectomy or mastectomy, or who have had the axillary area radiated, may at any time later develop this condition, caused by damage to the *lymphatic system's* capacity to move lymphatic fluid. The hand, arm and tissues of the upper chest can become swollen and painful. While it can be controlled with the use of compression sleeves and a massage technique called manual lymphatic drainage, it cannot be cured. Lymphedema can also occur in the feet and legs as a result of node removal in the groin or pelvic area.

Malaise

A state of extreme tiredness and loss of well-being.

Malignant

Another term for cancer, less commonly used.

Metastasis

The spread of a cancer from the part of the body where it originally appeared (the *primary* site) to another part (the metastatic site, or secondary tumor).

Molecular Biology
A relatively new field of scientific investigation where the basic structure of the *cancer cell* is being studied.

Monoclonal Antibody
An antibody drawn to *cancer cells* specifically, used to target treatments. An example is the *HER-2/neu* monoclonal antibody, currently in *clinical trials*.

MRI (Magnetic Resonance Imaging)
A computerized body-imaging process, using radio waves and powerful magnets to provide three-dimensional images of the body. It is higher definition than a *CT scan* and considered safer, because it does not use *radiation* or contrast dyes.

Mucositis
See *stomatitis*.

Nadir
The lowest point in *white blood cell*, *red blood cell* and *platelet* counts following treatment, often occurring ten days to two weeks following *chemotherapy* or *radiation*. Patients are often cautioned to be extra careful with exposure to infection and avoiding anything that could cause bleeding during this time. Sometimes, *growth factors* are given to encourage the *bone marrow* to regenerate cells more rapidly.

Necrosis or Necrotic
Referring to tissue that has died.

Neupogen
See *G-CSF*.

Neutropenia
A low *white blood cell* count of neutrophils, the cells most crucial in the body's fight against infection, usually caused by *chemotherapy* drugs. This is a potentially serious complication, and patients should avoid exposure to situations that may put them at risk.

Oncogene
One of a number of *genes* believed to be responsible for the uncontrolled cell growth of cancers.

Oncologist
A doctor who specializes in the diagnosis and treatment of cancer. Medical oncologists treat patients with *chemotherapy* and hormones and usually coordinate patient care. *Radiation oncologists* specialize in the use of *radiation* and nuclear medicine treatments. Surgical oncologists are most likely to be involved in *primary* cancer treatment of localized disease.

Oophorectomy

Surgical removal of the ovaries; it used to be a common treatment for metastatic breast cancer prior to the newer estrogen and progesterone antagonists.

Orchiectomy

Surgical removal of the testicles in male breast cancer patients, no longer much used with the hormonal treatments available.

Osteoblastic

A type of *bone metastasis* in which there is abnormal bone growth. Both *osteolytic* and osteoblastic lesions can occur in the same person.

Osteolytic

A type of bone metastasis in which the bone is eaten away, producing a characteristic "moth-eaten" appearance. Untreated, there is a likelihood of fractures over time. See also *osteoblastic*.

Ovarian Ablation

Surgery, *radiation* or drug treatment to stop ovarian production as a treatment for breast cancer. Not as frequently done, with the newer hormonal drugs.

p53

A "gatekeeper" *gene* for many cancers. When this gene is mutated, cells tend to grow without normal controls.

Paget's Disease

About three percent of breast cancer patients have this form of the disease, involving the nipple.

Palliative

That which relieves pain and other symptoms of disease, or controls the disease without likelihood of cure. In palliative care, the patient's quality of life is paramount.

Pathologist

A doctor who specializes in the interpretation of cellular changes in disease.

Peripheral Stem Cell Support or Transplant

Reinfusion of a patient's own *stem cells*, following *high-dose chemotherapy*.

Phase I Clinical Trial

Following *in vitro* and animal testing, this is the first level of the clinical trials procedure by which new drugs or combinations of drugs are tested and approved in human beings. A small number of patients are given a new treatment. The focus is on determining safety, dosage and short-term effectiveness.

Phase II Clinical Trial

The second level of clinical trials testing in human beings. A larger number of participants are enrolled than *Phase I*. Phase II trials also focus on effectiveness and on chronic *side effects* over a longer period.

Phase III Clinical Trial

The final level of clinical trials testing. Here, there is a comparison of experimental treatments with an established testing treatment for safety, effectiveness, dosage and *side effects*. Usually such trials are multi-centric and involve large number of patients. Optimally, they are "blinded" so that neither researchers nor patients know which treatment they are receiving. This is not always possible.

Photo-dynamic Therapy (PDT)

A new therapy whereby a light source activates targeted delivery of a *chemotherapy* drug. Used with skin *metastases*.

Physician's Data Query (PDQ)

A database maintained by the National Cancer Institute providing the latest treatment information. See Appendix B, *Resources*, for more information.

Placebo

A harmless or inert substance used in place of an active drug to offer comfort or to compare for effectiveness. It is an established clinical fact that placebos show some success, probably as a result of patient expectations. This mechanism is as yet poorly understood. Because of this placebo effect, the best *clinical trials* are "blinded," meaning that neither patients nor researchers know which treatment is being administered until the conclusion of the study. Clinical trials where a new treatment is being tested against established treatments do not use placebos.

Platelet

Disc-shaped blood cell which aids in blood clotting.

Pleura

The membranous lining around the lungs.

Pleural Effusion

Fluid that has accumulated around the lungs in the pleural cavity, often the result of metastatic spread of cancer to the lungs. See also *effusion*.

Polychemotherapy

See *combination chemotherapy*.

Port (Infuse-a-Port, Mediport or Port-a-cath)

A device implanted beneath the skin with a catheter threaded through a large vein to the heart, it permits medications to be given and blood to be drawn without having to find a vein. The entrance to the port is covered with a rubber septum, into which a needle can be inserted through the chest. While ports don't carry the same risk for infection as external catheters, they must be flushed periodically to avoid the formation of blood clots.

Primary Breast Cancer

In breast cancer, the primary cancer occurs in the breast, the site from which *metastatic* or secondary cancer can spread.

Procrit

See *erythropoietin*.

Progesterone Receptor Positive (or Negative)

This is often written as PR+ or PR- and is a measure of the degree to which a given tumor is dependent upon progesterone for its growth. The number of hormone receptors on the tumor are measured to determine this. See also *estrogen receptors*.

Prognosis

The expected or probable outcome of a disease, usually based on statistical analysis of large groups of patients.

Protocol

The treatment outline or plan. In research, a study designed to answer a treatment hypothesis under controlled conditions.

Quadrant

To indicate the position in which a clinical observation, such as a tumor, may be found, doctors divide the part of the body, for example, the breast or abdomen, into four quarters. For example, breast cancer is most commonly found in the upper, outer quadrant of the breast. To visualize this, think of lines that cross at the nipple, defining the four areas: inner, outer, upper and lower.

Radiation Oncologist

A physician who specializes in the treatment of cancer with high energy x-rays. A radiologist, by contast, is expert in the diagnosis of diseases through the use of x-rays.

Radiation Simulation

Before *radiation treatment* starts, the location on the body, dosage and precise positioning of the body are "rehearsed."

Radiation Treatment

In metastatic breast cancer patients, radiation treatment is most often used to control *bone metastases*, but can be used to treat other isolated areas of tumor as well. *Side effects* include *fatigue* and loss of appetite, and inflammation of the surrounding tissue.

Randomized

In research studies and *clinical trials*, this means that patients are chosen at random by a computer to receive an experimental treatment or to be in a control group that receives conventional treatment against which the experimental treatment is being tested.

RAS Inhibitors

Substances that inhibit the activity of the RAS *oncogene*, which promotes cancer growth.

Recurrence

The reappearance of the disease. In breast cancer, recurrence following *primary breast cancer* can be local (in the same place), *regional* (in surrounding tissue) or *metastatic* (in some other part of the body).

Red Blood Cells (erythrocytes)

These blood cells circulate oxygen breathed in through the lungs throughout the body.

Regional Recurrence

The cancer recurs in nearby tissue, for example, in *lymph nodes* or on the chest wall.

Regression

A decrease in the disease or its symptoms.

Reinfusion

Another term for the reintroduction of preserved *stem cells* or *bone marrow* following *high-dose chemotherapy*.

Relapse

The *recurrence* of the cancer after a disease-free period.

Remission

This term is used to describe a decrease or disappearance of the cancer, for any period of time. In *clinical trials*, a partial remission (PR) means a decrease in observed illness by at least 50 percent, and a complete remission (CR) means no measurable evidence of cancer is present in the body.

Rescue (as in Stem Cell Rescue)

The *infusion* of a substance to restore or preserve a patient's *bone marrow* following *chemotherapy*. Most commonly used with *stem cells*, bone marrow, and leukovorin, a derivative of Vitamin A that protects the body from the effects of large doses of methotrexate, an anticancer drug.

Retinoids

Substances that induce cell *differentiation* in cancer ·treatment. Also known as retinoic acid.

Risk/Benefit Ratio

Initially examined in the process of setting up *clinical trials*, this term is now widely used as a way of conceptualizing the pros and cons of a particular procedure or treatment.

Second-Line Treatment

Second treatment given after *first-line treatment* has failed. This may be followed by third-line, fourth-line, and so forth. Treatment efficacy tends to decrease with each exposure, as the cancer mutates to become *chemoresistant*.

Second Opinion

An expert consultation to confirm treatment or suggest alternatives at times when treatment decisions may be indicated. Most good doctors encourage their patients to seek second opinions. Many physicians work on a team basis, where they regularly consult with other physicians as a routine part of their practice. Metastatic breast cancer patients frequently seek second opinions from nationally recognized specialists at major cancer centers and/or from *pathologists*.

SEER (Surveillance, Epidemiology and End Results)

This is the National Cancer Institute's primary method for tracking, gathering and reporting cancer incidence and mortality. Statistics are published periodically on incidence and mortality for all cancers.

Side Effect

A secondary and undesired result of treatment that can be painful, unpleasant or potentially harmful.

Staging

When first diagnosed, all breast cancers are classified according to their stage, to determine the most effective treatments. Stage I means that the cancer is no bigger than 2 centimeters and has not spread beyond the breast. Stage II means a 2 to 5 centimeter cancer with or without spread to *lymph nodes* under the arm, or a smaller tumor with spread to axillary lymph nodes. Stage IIIA means either a 2 to 5 centimeter tumor where the cancer has grown beyond the axillary lymph nodes to surrounding structures, or a larger than 5 centimeter tumor with spread to the axillary nodes. Stage IIIB means that the cancer has spread to regional tissue such as the skin, chest wall, muscles or the lymph nodes along the clavicle. Stage IV connotes spread to distant sites, such as bone, lung, liver, brain and other sites. Stage IV breast cancer represents around 10 percent of diagnosed cases.

Stem Cells

Cells from which all blood cells develop.

Stereotactic Radiosurgery
Focused, multiple low-intensity beams of radiation programmed to converge on a tumor site in the brain that may be inaccessible to surgery. Also referred to as "gamma knife" surgery.

Stomatitis
Mouth sores from *chemotherapy* treatments, also called mucositis.

Supraclavicular Lymph Nodes
Located above the collarbone, they are a frequent site for the spread of *regional* disease.

Systemic Treatment
A treatment like *chemotherapy* or hormonal therapy that affects the whole body or system, as opposed to localized treatment, such as surgery or *radiation*.

Terminal
Now used infrequently to describe far-advanced metastatic disease where there is a very limited time before death anticipated.

Thoracentesis
A pleural tap, where fluid is removed from the chest cavity with a long, hollow needle. This is done either for diagnostic purposes or to relieve shortness of breath and pain caused by fluid accumulation. Often the fluid returns, however, which can be resolved by a process known as "schlerosing" the lining of the lung.

Thrombocytopenia
A potentially serious complication of *chemotherapy* and *radiation*, as well as in certain types of cancer, involving a drop in the level of *platelets*, the blood cells responsible for clotting. People with this condition must avoid any situation that could result in bleeding, internal or external.

Tumor Board
A hospital-based panel of medical experts that makes treatment recommendations in difficult cases.

Tumor Marker
One of several substances in the body that usually increases with tumor growth and decreases with tumor regression. Examples for breast cancer are *CEA* and *CA 27-29* or *CA 15-3*.

Tumor-suppresser Gene
One of a number of *genes* responsible for controlling cell growth in the body. If damaged or mutated, this can lead to cancer.

Viscera
Term meaning the internal organs of the abdominal cavity.

White Blood Cells

Cells that help the body fight infection and disease.

X-rays

Short-length high-energy electromagnetic waves used both diagnostically and for treatment of disease. In lower doses, they permit the visualization of parts of the body to monitor disease, and in higher doses they are used for treatment, most commonly in metastatic breast cancer to control and stabilize *bone metastases*. See *radiation treatment*.

Index

employment. *See* work
ethics
    cultural attitudes affect, 74-75
    disclosure of diagnosis, 73-77
    disclosure of prognosis, 77-83
    informed consent, aggressive
        treatment, 89

F

faith and spirit
    as comfort, *xxv-xxvi*, 358-359,
        386-389
    control and surrender, 362-363
    future always uncertain, 16-19
    life never the same, 19-23
    living in the moment, 365-369
    meaning, finding, 386-389
    surrender and letting go, 364-365
    trust, 27-32
family and friends
    as "second-order patients," 257-
        259
    caregivers, care for, 257-260
    children
        for extended support, 258-
          259
        help for during illness, 258-
          259
        resources for, 424-425
    communication, problems in,
        236-243, 297-300
    death and dying
        communication about death
          and dying, 297-300
        dishonesty about, 298-299
        end-of-life dilemmas and
          directives, 305-311
        hospice care, 323-327
        statements to/from loved one,
          326
        stories of final days and
          dying, 327-355
    deepening of love, 246-249
    fear and emotional distancing, 21

    fears of high-risk patient, not
        acknowledging, 20-21
    help, asking for, 225-231, 269,
        271
    needs and priorities, conflicting,
        252-257
    partners, stories of relationships,
        249-252
    stress, cycles of illness and
        remission, 233-236
    support from, 267-272
    withdrawal, denial, 260-266
    See also partners
fears. *See* emotions, coping with
Feldman, Laurie
    help, asking for, 225
    side effects of treatment, 204
financial assistance
    drug purchases, 450-451
    resources, 417-420
Fisher, Jacque
    hospitalization, 214
    side effects of treatment, 204
    treatment decisions, 146
Foley, Dr. Kathleen
    respect patients' decisions to end
        treatment, 317
Folkman, Dr. Judah
    anti-angiogenesis factor research,
        127, 128
Frank, Arthur
    limits of modern medicine, 6-7,
        171
    physician communication, 94
Frankl, Dr. Viktor
    humor, value of, 379
    meaning is essential for life, 357
friends. *See* family and friends

G

Gelbwasser, Bonnie
    families, how cancer affects, 253,
        259
    hospitalization, 213-214

Hagler, PJ (*continued*)
    testing, pain of, 196
    withdrawal of friends and family,
        262, 299-300
Harpham, Dr. Wendy S.
    cancer-related fatigue, 200
HDC. *See* high-dose chemotherapy
healing, not cure, 189
help, asking for, 225-231, 269, 271
heroes, as ordinary people, *xxiii*, 389-
        392
Hiebert, Pam
    ceremony at time of shaving head,
        68-69
    complementary treatment
        choices, 166-167
    couples, conflicting needs of,
        254-255
    diagnosis with Stage IV cancer,
        38-39
    emotional response to recurrence,
        55-56
    emotional ups and downs, 179
    faith, finding new sense of, 388-
        389
    family members, changes in roles,
        230
    fears, facing and releasing from,
        286
    living moment to moment, 369
    meaning and support at
        diagnosis, 67-68
    pain treatment, 222-224
    poems
        "I do not want this dance,"
            72
        "Discovery is a journey...,"
            189
        "What if they find
            something...," 38-39
        "Who am I to have...," 281
    profile, 401
    prognosis, disclosure by
        physician, 78-79
    research to contain fears, 85-86
    retelling cancer experience, 280

support group, description of,
    186
work, performance and meaning,
    291-292
See also Rainwater, Sylvan
high-dose chemotherapy, 129-138
    aggressive vs. conservative
        philosophies, 111-113,
        130, 131, 135
    clinical trials, 132-138
    decisions by patients, 138-141
    remission following, 132-138
    resources for, 433
    safety of, 132-133
    side effects, 131, 135
    See also chemotherapy
Hirshaut, Dr. Yashar
    high-dose chemotherapy,
        assessing benefit, 134-
        135
    second opinions, importance of,
        89
holistic treatments. *See*
        complementary therapies
hope
    claims for miracles, unscrupulous,
        159-161
    complementary therapies, 151,
        158-163
        choices, 158-163
        healthy lifestyle approaches,
            160-161
        unscrupulous claims, 159-
            161
    continuing treatment, 300-305
    expectations of cure
        from modern medicine, 152
        miracle claims, 159-161
    healing and cure, 189
    keeping hope alive, 379-380
    new and experimental treatments,
        113-129
    transformation of, to new goals,
        381-384
    words that heal, words that harm,
        153-154

Kleinman, Dr. Arthur
  emotions from deep losses of
      illness, 359
knowledge. *See* research; treatment
      decisions
Kolenburg, Joleene
  communication with husband,
      237-238
  diagnosis of lung metastases, 49-
      50
  families, effect of cancer on, 259-
      260, 269-270
  help, asking for, 226
  profile, 402
  reactions to illness, 262-263
  retiring from paid work, 290
  side effects of treatment, 209-210
  treatment decisions, 148-149

L

Lane, David
  molecular oncology, hope for
      cure, 120
Langer, Amy
  chronic disease, metastatic breast
      cancer as, 9
laughter, 377-379
Leach, Chris
  Pat's final days, 345-349
  profile, 402-403
  See also Leach, Pat
Leach, Pat
  emotional response to recurrence,
      58, 170
  emotional ups and downs, 178-
      179
  hope, maintaining, 362-363
  hormonal changes from
      chemotherapy, 244
  hospitalization, 211
  profile, 402-403
  recurrence, 22, 58
  second opinion, importance of,
      90

testing, anxiety of, 195
testing, pain of, 196
See also Leach, Chris
Lebow, Penny
  recurrence, 46-47
  support at diagnosis, 67
Lederberg, Dr. Marguerite
  families as "second order
      patients," 258-259
legal issues
  end-of-life dilemmas and
      directives, 305-311
  resources for, 417-420
  work and retirement, 287-293
Lerner, Michael
  evaluating complementary
      therapies, 161-162
  healing vs. curing, 189
  high-dose chemotherapy,
      treatment decision, 140-
      141
Lewis, CS
  illness can be managed, moment
      to moment, 368
Listserv, Breast Cancer, *xv-xvii*, 425-
      427
liver metastases, 50-52
living in the moment, 365-369
  sense of time in illness, 278-279
loneliness and isolation, 260-266,
      275, 297-300
Lorde, Audre
  courage to tell experiences, 294
  "Transformation of Silence into
      Language and Action,"
      294
  truth-telling, 377
Love, Dr. Susan
  course of individual's illness
      impossible to predict, 27
  lung metastases, 47
  secondary response to stopping
      hormonal drugs, 109
  symptoms of recurrence, 23, 45
lung metastases, 47-50

poems (*continued*)

"My Heart Knows," 181-182

"My Hospital Bag," 214-215

"Now Maybe," 274-275

"On the trail…," 31

"This Is a Day," 197-198

valentine poem, 379

"What if they find something…,"
38-39

"Who am I to have…," 281

politics of breast cancer. *See* advocacy
for breast cancer patients

prescription drugs. *See* drugs

priorities

family, conflicting with, 252-257

setting, 373-379

profiles of people interviewed, 393-
410

prognosis

course of illness impossible to
predict, 27

disclosure of by physicians, 73-
77, 153-158

end-of-life dilemmas and
directives, 305-311

factors, 39-40

improved odds over statistics
cited, 82-83

increasing longevity, group
support, 27-31

statistics, 77-83

withholding can isolate patient,
297-300

See also hope; medical treatments;
research; uncertainty

Q

Quirarte, Barbara

hospice services, what offer, 325-
326

R

Ragland, Barbara

priorities, 374, 376

profile, 404-405

recurrence, 23-24, 42

remission, long-term, 283

support at diagnosis, 66-67

survival, 283

volunteering, 376

work, benefits and planning
retirement, 292-293

Rainwater, Sylvan

couples, conflicting needs of,
253-254

living moment to moment, 370-
371

physical pain of partner, 224

poem, "Now Maybe," 273-275

testing, anxiety, 192-194

work during chemotherapy,
Pam's, 292

See also Hiebert, Pam

Rait, Douglas

families as "second order
patients," 257-259

recurrences

diagnosis, responses to, 54, 55-72

bad news, 55-57

coping and resilience, 70-72

grief, 57-63

where to start?, 63-71

emotional response, 57-63

fear of, 16-19

fears of friends, family, 20-21

vigilance vs. denial, 23

monitoring for physical
symptoms, 23-27

signs and symptoms, 23-27

work (*continued*)
    resources for legal issues, 417-420
    retirement from paid work, leaves
        of absence, 287-293
Wortman, Camille
    fear or misunderstanding
        common responses to
        cancer patients, 21

X, Y

Yalom, Dr. Irvin
    denial of death robs us, 300
    physicians and dying patients,
        314
    the present is the only reality, 366
Yandell, Sandra
    disease progression, 321-322
    finding a balance in cancer, 361
    humor, finding, 378
    perspective, change of, 322
    physical appearances and new
        love, 245
    profile, 409-410
    reflections on survival, 391-392
    risking a new beginning,
        marriage, 370

Z

Zakarian, Beverly
    caution on for-profit treatment
        searches, 100-101
    clinical trials, look for your best
        interests, 116
Zujewski, Nelson, Abrams, Drs.
    HDC, review of literature, 137-
        138

About the Author

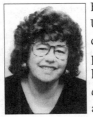Before completing her MFA in the Writing Division at Columbia University, Musa Mayer worked for many years as a Master's level counselor in the Ohio Community Mental Health system, with a particular focus on groups and women's issues. Her two prior published books were both memoirs. The first, *Night Studio: A Memoir of Philip Guston* (Knopf, 1988; Penguin, 1990; DaCapo, 1997), was about growing up as the daughter of a well-known painter in the New York art world of the 1950's. The second, *Examining Myself: One Woman's Story of Breast Cancer Treatment and Recovery* (Faber & Faber, 1993), was Musa's own journey with breast cancer that led her to participate in the Breast Cancer Listserv on the Internet, where she developed the idea for a book about metastatic breast cancer and met most of the people she interviewed.

Her experiences as teacher, counselor and writer of memoirs have given her an abiding faith in the transformative and healing power of telling life stories. Musa also regularly teaches memoir writing, and leads writing workshops and retreats for people with life-threatening illnesses.

Favorite activities include gardening, golf, theater and travel. She remains very involved with her father's work, traveling widely for exhibitions of his paintings and drawings. She lives in New York City with her husband, Tom, a neuropsychologist who works with people with head injuries. Her two sons, David and Jonathan, live nearby.

Photo by Tom Mayer

Colophon

Patient-Centered Guides are about the experience of illness. They contain personal stories as well as a mixture of practical and medical information.

The cover of *Advanced Breast Cancer: A Guide to Living with Metastatic Disease* was designed by Edie Freedman using Photoshop 5.0 and QuarkXPress 3.32. Cover photos are from Rubberball and Photodisc. The fonts used on the cover are Onyx BT and Berkeley.

The interior layout for the book was designed by Nancy Priest and Edie Freedman. The interior fonts are Berkeley and Franklin Gothic. The text was prepared by Edie Freedman, Mike Sierra, and Nancy Wolfe Kotary, using QuarkXPress and FrameMaker 5.5.

The revised sections of this second edition were copyedited by Lunaea Hougland and proofread by Claire Cloutier LeBlanc and Ellie Maden. Interior composition was done by Claire Cloutier LeBlanc and Trisha Manoni. Clairemarie Fisher O'Leary and Sheryl Avruch provided quality assurance. The index was written by Linda Lamb.

Patient-Centered Guides™

Questions Answered
Experiences Shared

We are committed to empowering individuals to evolve into informed consumers armed with the latest information and heartfelt support for their journey.

When your life is turned upside down, your need for information is great. You have to make critical medical decisions, often with what seems little to go on. Plus you have to break the news to family, quiet your own fears, cope with symptoms or treatment side effects, figure out how you're going to pay for things, and sometimes still get to work or get dinner on the table.

Patient-Centered Guides provide authoritative information for intelligent information seekers who want to become advocates of their own health. They cover the whole impact of illness on your life. In each book, there's a mix of:

- **Medical background for treatment decisions**
  We can give you information that can help you to intelligently work with your doctor to come to a decision. We start from the viewpoint that modern medicine has much to offer and also discuss complementary treatments. Where there are treatment controversies we present differing points of view.

- **Practical information**
  Once you've decided what to do about your illness, you still have to deal with treatments and changes to your life. We cover day-to-day practicalities, such as those you'd hear from a good nurse or a knowledgeable support group.

- **Emotional support**
  It's normal to have strong reactions to a condition that threatens your life or changes how you live. It's normal that the whole family is affected. We cover issues like the shock of diagnosis, living with uncertainty, and communicating with loved ones.

Each book also contains stories from both patients and doctors — medical "frequent flyers" who share, in their own words, the lessons and strategies they have learned when maneuvering through the often complicated maze of medical information that's available.

We provide information online, including updated listings of the resources that appear in this book. This is freely available for you to print out and copy to share with others, as long as you retain the copyright notice on the print-outs.

http://www.patientcenters.com

Other Books in the Series

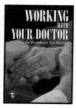

Working with Your Doctor
Getting the Healthcare You Deserve
By Nancy Keene
ISBN 1-56592-273-5, Paperback, 6" x 9", 382 pages, $15.95

"Working with Your Doctor *fills a genuine need for patients and their family members caught up in this new and intimidating age of impersonal, economically-driven health care delivery.*"

—James Dougherty, MD
Emeritus Professor of Surgery,
Albany Medical College

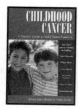

Childhood Cancer
A Parent's Guide to Solid Tumor Cancers
By Nancy Keene
ISBN 1-56592-531-9, Paperback, 6"x 9", 544 pages, $24.95

"*I recommend [this book] most highly for those in need of high-level, helpful knowledge that will empower and help parents and caregivers to cope.*"

—Mark Greenberg, MD
Professor of Pediatrics,
University of Toronto

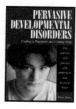

Pervasive Developmental Disorders
Finding a Diagnosis and Getting Help
By Mitzi Waltz
ISBN 1-56592-530-0, Paperback, 6" x 9", 592 pages, $24.95

"*Mitzi Waltz's book provides clear, informative, and comprehensive information on every relevant aspect of PDD. Her in-depth discussion will help parents and professionals develop a clear understanding of the issues and, consequently, they will be able to make informed decisions about various interventions. A job well done!*"

—Dr. Stephen M. Edelson
Director,
Center for the Study of Autism,
Salem, Oregon

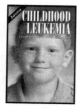

Childhood Leukemia
A Guide for Families, Friends, and Caregiver, 2nd Edition
By Nancy Keene
ISBN 1-56592-632-3, Paperback, 6" x 9", $24.95, 564 pages

"*What's so compelling about* Childhood Leukemia *is the amount of useful medical information and practical advice it contains. Keene avoids jargon and lays out what's needed to deal with the medical system.*"

—The Washington Post

Patient-Centered Guides
Published by O'Reilly & Associates, Inc.
Our products are available at a bookstore near you.
For information: **800-998-9938** • **707-829-0515** • info@oreilly.com
101 Morris Street • Sebastopol • CA • 95472-9902

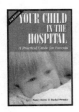

Your Child in the Hospital
A Practical Guide for Parents, Second Edition
By Nancy Keene and Rachel Prentice
ISBN 1-56592-573-4, Paperback, 5" x 8", 176 pages, $11.95

"When your child is ill or injured, the hospital setting can be overwhelming. Here is a terrific 'road map' to help keep families 'on track.'"

—James B. Fahner, MD
Division Chief,
Pediatric Hematology/Oncology,
DeVos Children's Hospital,
Grand Rapids, Michigan

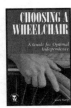

Choosing a Wheelchair
A Guide for Optimal Independence
By Gary Karp
ISBN 1-56592-411-8, Paperback, 5" x 8", 192 pages, $9.95

"I love the idea of putting knowledge often possessed only by professionals into the hands of new consumers. Gary Karp has done it. This book will empower people with disabilities to make informed equipment choices."

—Barry Corbet
Editor,
New Mobility Magazine

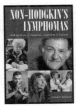

Non-Hodgkin's Lymphomas
Making Sense of Diagnosis, Treatment & Options
By Lorraine Johnston
ISBN 1-56592-444-4, Paperback, 6" x 9", 584 pages, $24.95

"When I gave this book to one of our patients, there was an instant, electric connection. A sense of enlightenment came over her while she absorbed the information. It was thrilling to see her so sparked with new energy and focus."

—Susan Weisberg, LCSW
Clinical Social Worker,
Stanford University Medical Center

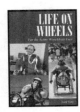

Life on Wheels
For the Active Wheelchair User
By Gary Karp
ISBN 1-56592-253-0, Paperback, 6" x 9", 576 pages, $24.95

"Gary Karp's Life On Wheels is a super book. If you use a wheelchair, you cannot do without it. It is THE wheelchair-user reference book."

—Hugh Gregory Gallagher
author of FDR's *Splendid Deception*

Patient-Centered Guides
Published by O'Reilly & Associates, Inc.
Our products are available at a bookstore near you.
For information: **800-998-9938 • 707-829-0515 • info@oreilly.com**
101 Morris Street • Sebastopol • CA • 95472-9902

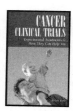

Cancer Clinical Trials
Experimental Treatments and How They Can Help You
By Robert Finn
ISBN 1-56592-566-1, Paperback, 5" x 8", 216 pages, $14.95

"I highly recommend this book as a first step in what will be for many a difficult, but crucially important, part of their struggle to beat their cancer."

—From the foreword by Robert Bazell
Chief Science Correspondent for NBC News
and author of *Her-2: The Making of Herceptin, a Revolutionary Treatment for Breast Cancer*

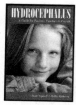

Hydrocephalus
A Guide for Patients, Families & Friends
By Chuck Toporek and Kellie Robinson
ISBN 1-56592-410-X, Paperback, 6" x 9", 384 pages, $19.95

"Toporek, a medical editor, and wife Robinson, a writer and hydrocephalus patient, fill a void of information on hydrocephalus (water on the brain) for the lay reader. Highly recommended for public and academic libraries."

—Library Journal

"In this book, the authors have provided a wonderful entry into the world of hydrocephalus to begin to remedy the neglect of this important condition. We are immensely grateful to them for their groundbreaking effort."

—Peter M. Black, MD, PhD
Franc D. Ingraham Professor of Neurosurgery,
Harvard Medical School
Neurosurgeon-in-Chief,
Brigham and Women's Hospital,
Children's Hospital,
Boston, Massachusetts

Patient-Centered Guides
Published by O'Reilly & Associates, Inc.
Our products are available at a bookstore near you.
For information: **800-998-9938** • **707-829-0515** • **info@oreilly.com**
101 Morris Street • Sebastopol • CA • 95472-9902